Minor Surgery
a text and atlas

'The extraction of the stone'. Painting by Jan de Bray (17th century). Museum Boymans – van Beuningen, Rotterdam. (Photograph: Wellcome Institute Library, London.)

Minor Surgery
a text and atlas

Fourth edition

John Stuart Brown MBE
OStJ, MB, BS(Hons), MRCS, LRCP, FRCGP, DCH, D(Obst)RCOG,
AKC

*General Medical Practitioner, Thornhills Medical Group,
Larkfield, Aylesford, Kent*

A member of the Hodder Headline Group
LONDON
Co-published in the United States of America by
Oxford University Press, Inc., New York

First published in Great Britain in 1986
Second edition 1992
Third edition 1997
Fourth edition 2000 published by Arnold,
a member of the Hodder Headline Group
333 Euston Road, London NW1 3BH

http://www.arnoldpublishers.com

Distributed in the United States of America by
Oxford University Press Inc.,
198 Madison Avenue, New York, NY 10016
Oxford is a registered trademark of Oxford University Press

Whilst the advice and information in this book are believed to be true and
accurate at the date of going to press, neither the authors nor the publisher
can accept any legal responsibility or liability for any errors or omissions
that may be made. In particular (but without limiting the generality of the
preceding disclaimer) every effort has been made to check drug dosages;
however it is still possible that errors have been missed. Furthermore,
dosages schedules are constantly being revised and new side-effects
recognized. For these reasons the reader is strongly urged to consult the
drug companies' printed instructions before administering any of the
drugs recommended in this book.

British Library Cataloguing in Publication Data
A catalogue record for this book is available from the British Library

Library of Congress Cataloging-in-Publication Data
A catalog record for this book is available from the Library of Congress

ISBN 0 340 76113 X

1   2   3   4   5   6   7   8   9   10

Commissioning Editor: Nick Dunton
Production Editor: Lauren McAllister
Production Controller: Iain McWilliams
Project Manager: Gray Publishing
Cover Design: Terry Griffiths

Typeset in 10/12 pt Dutch766 and produced by Gray Publishing, Tunbridge Wells, Kent
Printed and bound in India by Ajanta Offset, New Delhi

To Anne

Contents

Contributors   xvii
Acknowledgements   xviii
Preface to the fourth edition   xx
Preface to the first edition   xxi
Foreword by Barry Jackson   xxii

PART ONE: BASIC TECHNIQUES   **1**

1 Introduction   **3**
  1.1   Scope and limitations of minor surgery   6
  1.2   Advantages and disadvantages   7
  1.3   Organization within the practice   8

2 Instruments   **10**
  2.1   Choice of instruments   10
  2.2   Instrument and equipment manufacturers
         (Appendix A)   16
  2.3   Sources of supply   16
  2.4   Advantages of instrument packs   17
  2.5   Care of instruments and equipment   20
  2.6   Care of stainless steel   20
  2.7   Electrical safety   21
  2.8   Rechargeable battery packs   21

3 The Minor Operating Theatre   **22**
  3.1   Fixtures and fittings   22
  3.2   The operating-theatre table   25
  3.3   Illumination   26
  3.4   The electrocautery   28
  3.5   The 'Hyfrecator' or unipolar diathermy   31
  3.6   The radiosurgery unit   32
  3.7   Resuscitation facilities   32
  3.8   Sterilizers   34
  3.9   The cryoprobe   35
  3.10   Use of Entonox   35
  3.11   Disinfectant dispensers   35
  3.12   Syringes and needles   36
  3.13   Tourniquets   36
  3.14   'Sharps' containers   36
  3.15   Clinical waste disposal   36
  3.16   Hot-air hand driers   36
  3.17   Alternative layouts for minor operating theatres   37

3.18	First-aid box	37
3.19	Comparison of different instruments	38
3.20	Monitoring of vital signs during operations	39
3.21	Tape or CD player to provide music	40

4   The Role of the Practice Nurse/Operating Theatre Assistant   **41**
4.1	Management of the treatment room/minor operating theatre	41
4.2	Sterilizing instruments	42
4.3	Supplies	42
4.4	Time management	42
4.5	Documentation	43
4.6	Nurse–patient relationship	43
4.7	Assisting at operations	43

5   Infection Control   **46**
5.1	Common pathogens	46
5.2	Hepatitis viruses	47
5.3	HIV infection	47
5.4	Infection control guidelines	48
5.5	Procedures in the case of accidental contamination	49
5.6	Infection book	49

6   Sterilizing and Disinfecting Instruments   **50**
6.1	Antiseptic solutions	50
6.2	Boiling	50
6.3	Hot-air ovens	51
6.4	Autoclaves	52
6.5	Guidelines for selecting sterilizers	52
6.6	Use of CSSD facilities	53
6.7	Improvised methods of sterilization	53

7   Assessment, Preoperative Preparation and Skin Preparation   **55**

8   Anaesthesia   **57**
8.1	Freezing	57
8.2	Topical or surface anaesthesia	57
8.3	Topical anaesthetic creams	58
8.4	Infiltration anaesthesia	58
8.5	Mechanism of action of local anaesthetics	60
8.6	Which local anaesthetic?	60
8.7	Maximum dose of local anaesthetics	60
8.8	Toxicity of local anaesthetics	61
8.9	Nerve blocks	61
8.10	Technique of posterior tibial nerve block	62
8.11	Ulnar nerve block	62
8.12	Radial nerve block	63
8.13	Median nerve block	64
8.14	Digital nerve blocks	65
8.15	Local infiltration and bloodless field	65
8.16	Analgesia	66

8.17	Entonox inhalation	67
8.18	General anaesthesia	68
8.19	Local anaesthetic technique in general practice	68
9	**Surgical Techniques**	**69**
9.1	Haemostasis	70
9.2	Tissue healing	71
9.3	Surgical technique using pigs' trotters	71
9.4	Surgical technique using skin simulators	71
10	**Incisions**	**76**
10.1	Technique of skin incision	78
10.2	Deeper dissection	79
10.3	Excision	79
10.4	Technique for removal of a 'dog-ear'	80
11	**Skin Closure**	**81**
11.1	Sutures	82
11.2	Suture materials	84
11.3	Skin closure strips	86
11.4	Skin closure clips	86
11.5	Drains	87
11.6	Stitchcraft and knots	87
11.7	The use of tissue adhesive	92
12	**Suturing Lacerations**	**95**
12.1	Instruments required	96
12.2	Technique for suturing lacerations	96
12.3	Technique for closure with 'glue'	97
12.4	Choice of skin closure	100
13	**Dressings**	**101**
13.1	Reasons for using dressings	101
13.2	Types of dressing	102
14	**Suture Removal**	**105**
14.1	Technique of suture and clip removal	105
15	**Chemical Cauterization**	**107**
15.1	Silver nitrate	107
15.2	Phenol (carbolic acid)	109
15.3	Monochloroacetic acid	110
16	**Electrocautery**	**111**
16.1	Uses of electrocautery	116
16.2	Comparison between instruments	119
16.3	Hazards with inflammable antiseptics	120
17	**The Unipolar Diathermy**	**121**
17.1	Advantages of high-frequency currents	123
17.2	Disadvantage of high-frequency currents	124
17.3	Some applications of high-frequency treatment	124
18	**Cryotherapy**	**126**
18.1	Mechanism of action	126
18.2	Indications for cryosurgery	127

18.3	Cryosurgical equipment	128
18.4	Contraindications and dangers of cryosurgery	137
18.5	Cryobiopsy	138
18.6	Success rates for curing lesions	139

19 Histology — **142**
19.1	Histological appearances of common lesions	142
19.2	The histology book	149

20 Statistical Analysis — **150**
20.1	Record-keeping	150
20.2	Organizing a minor operating list	151
20.3	Informing the patient	151
20.4	Complications	156
20.5	Bravery certificates	156

21 Audit — **158**

PART TWO: ROUTINE MINOR SURGERY — **161**

22 Injections and Aspirations — **163**
22.1	Choice of steroid	163
22.2	Landmarks	164
22.3	Indications for use	164
22.4	Contraindications for the use of steroids	164
22.5	Tennis elbow (lateral epicondylitis)	164
22.6	Golfer's elbow (medial epicondylitis)	167
22.7	Olecranon bursitis	167
22.8	Intra-articular injections	167
22.9	The painful shoulder	168
22.10	Injection of the carpal tunnel	170
22.11	Injection of trigger finger	173
22.12	Injection for DeQuervain's disease	175
22.13	Radiocarpal joint	175
22.14	First carpometacarpal joint (thumb base)	175
22.15	Metacarpophalangeal joints	176
22.16	Interphalangeal joints	177
22.17	Injection of tendon sheaths in the hand	177
22.18	Injection of small ganglia	178
22.19	Injections around the hip joint	178
22.20	Meralgia paraesthetica	179
22.21	Aspiration and injection of the knee	179
22.22	Semimembranosus bursitis (popliteal or baker's cyst)	181
22.23	Prepatallar bursitis	181
22.24	The foot	181
22.25	Miscellaneous joint injections	183
22.26	Miscellaneous soft-tissue injections	183
22.27	Abdominal ascites	183
22.28	Aspiration of pleural effusions	188
22.29	Needle biopsy	189
22.30	Aspiration of cysts and bursae	190

23 Incision of Abscesses — **193**

24 Dermatological Minor Surgery **195**
24.1 Normal skin 195
24.2 Lesions suitable for treatment 196
24.3 Lesions to avoid 197
24.4 Lesions that do not require treatment 198
24.5 Lesions where there is doubt about the diagnosis 198

25 Skin Lesions **199**
25.1 General technique for excision 200
25.2 Curette and cautery 203
25.3 Intradermal naevi and pigmented naevi 203
25.4 Histiocytoma (dermatofibroma) 204
25.5 Cylindroma (turban tumour) 204
25.6 Solar keratosis 204
25.7 Seborrhoeic warts 204
25.8 Keratoacanthoma 205
25.9 Granuloma pyogenicum (eruptive angioma) 206
25.10 Spider naevi 207
25.11 Haemangioma 209
25.12 Molluscum contagiosum 209
25.13 Removal of tattoos 209
25.14 Juvenile melanoma 209
25.15 Malignant melanoma 209
25.16 Basal cell carcinoma (rodent ulcer) 211
25.17 Squamous cell epithelioma 212
25.18 Carcinoma *in situ* (Bowen's disease) 212
25.19 Keloids 213
25.20 Skin biopsy 213

26 Skin Tags and Papillomata **215**

27 Warts and Verrucae **219**
27.1 Medical treatments 219
27.2 Surgical treatments 219

28 Sebaceous Cysts **227**
28.1 Technique for removal of sebaceous cysts
on the scalp 228
28.2 Alternative method for removal of
sebaceous cysts 230
28.3 Histology 230

29 Excision of Lipoma **232**

30 Minor Operations on the Toes **234**
30.1 Treatment of ingrowing toe-nails 234
30.2 Onychogryphosis 246
30.3 Subungual exostosis 247
30.4 Soft corn 248
30.5 Fungal infection of the toe-nails 248

31 Biopsy Techniques **249**
31.1 Shave biopsy 250
31.2 Punch biopsy 251

31.3 Incisional biopsy, including curettage 254
31.4 Excisional biopsy 256
31.5 Needle biopsy 257
31.6 Cytological examination of fluids 257

32 Epistaxis **258**
32.1 Silver nitrate cauterization 258
32.2 Electrocauterization of Little's area 259
32.3 Diathermy of Little's area 259
32.4 Cryosurgery to Little's area 259
32.5 Photocoagulation of Little's area 259
32.6 Radiosurgical coagulation 259
32.7 The acute bleed 260

33 Use of the Proctoscope **261**
33.1 Disposable proctoscopes 261
33.2 Non-disposable proctoscopes 261

34 Sigmoidoscopy **263**
34.1 Indications for use 263
34.2 Preparation of the patient 265
34.3 Technique of sigmoidoscopy 266

35 Thrombosed External Haemorrhoids **267**

36 Treatment of Internal Haemorrhoids **269**
36.1 Types of haemorrhoid 269
36.2 Treatment of internal haemorrhoids by injection of sclerosing fluid 270
36.3 Cryosurgical treatment of internal haemorrhoids 270
36.4 Infrared photocoagulation of internal haemorrhoids 271
36.5 Neoprene band ligation of internal haemorrhoids 273
36.6 Manual dilatation of the anus 274

37 Varicose Veins **275**
37.1 Anatomy 275
37.2 Selection of patients 277
37.3 Sclerotherapy 278
37.4 Stab avulsion for varicose veins 281

38 Minor Surgical Procedures in Gynaecology **283**
38.1 Cervical cytology 283
38.2 Endometrial cell samplers 283
38.3 Brush cytology 284
38.4 Cauterization of cervical erosions 284
38.5 Cryosurgery for cervical erosions 284
38.6 Electrocautery of cervical erosions 285
38.7 Diathermy of cervical erosions 285
38.8 Vaginal vault granulations following hysterectomy 285
38.9 Genital warts 286
38.10 Repair of episiotomy 286

38.11	Bartholin's cysts and abscesses	286
38.12	Urethral caruncle	287
38.13	Insertion of intrauterine contraceptive devices	288
38.14	Removal of the 'lost' coil	290
38.15	Hormone implants	290
38.16	Removal of endocervical polypi	294

39 Vasectomy — **295**

39.1	Preoperative counselling	295
39.2	Technique	297
39.3	Postoperative care	302

40 Lymph-Gland Biopsy — **303**

40.1	Selection of patients	303
40.2	Technique for excision of gland	304

41 Treatment of Ganglia — **305**

41.1	Indications for treatment	305
41.2	Choice of treatments for ganglia	306
41.3	Technique for aspiration and sclerosant injection	308
41.4	The mucous cyst (ganglion) on the finger	309

42 Radiosurgery — **311**

42.1	Background	311
42.2	Different waveforms	313
42.3	Learning the technique of radiosurgery	318
42.4	Warnings	320
42.5	Avoidance of complications	321
42.6	Cleaning electrodes	321
42.7	General guidelines for radiosurgery	323
42.8	Care of electrodes after use	323
42.9	Preparation of the patient	323
42.10	Anaesthesia	324
42.11	Applications of radiosurgery	324
42.12	Radiosurgery in conjunction with cryosurgery	330
42.13	Intradermal naevi	331
42.14	Ingrowing toe-nails	332
42.15	Recurrent 'spicules' of nail	334
42.16	Telangiectasia and thread veins	334
42.17	Epilation	335
42.18	Rhinophyma	336
42.19	Xanthelasmata	336
42.20	Seborrhoeic keratoses	336
42.21	Cervical dysplasia	336
42.22	Miscellaneous other uses for radiosurgery	337

43 Miscellaneous Minor Surgical Procedures — **338**

43.1	Subungual haematoma	338
43.2	Removal of subungual splinters	339
43.3	Small scalp lesions	340
43.4	Xanthelasmata	340

43.5	Removal of foreign bodies in ears and noses	340
43.6	Stone in the salivary duct	341
43.7	Ear-lobe cysts	341
43.8	Haemangioma of the lip	341
43.9	Skin grafting	342
43.10	Nasal polypi	342
43.11	Congenital extra digits	342
43.12	Accessory auricles	343
43.13	Supernumerary nipples	344
43.14	Removal of pacemaker	344
43.15	Foreign-body removal utilizing a bloodless field	345
43.16	Circumcision	345
43.17	Removal of fish-hooks	346
43.18	Pinch-grafts to varicose ulcers	346
43.19	Spider naevi	349
43.20	Biopsy of the temporal artery	350
43.21	Division of tongue-tie	351
43.22	Chondrodermatitis helicis chronicus	352

44 Resuscitation   **353**

44.1	The vasovagal attack	354
44.2	Profound vasovagal attack leading to convulsion	354
44.3	Major epileptic convulsion	354
44.4	Myocardial infarction	354
44.5	Allergic reactions to drugs administered	355
44.6	Anaphylactic reaction	355
44.7	Pulmonary embolism	355
44.8	Concealed haemorrhage	355
44.9	Cerebrovascular attack	355
44.10	The acute psychiatric crisis	356
44.11	Cardiac arrest	356

PART THREE: ADVANCED MINOR SURGERY   **361**

45 Decompression of the Carpal Tunnel   **363**

45.1	Instruments	364
45.2	Technique for producing anaesthetic bloodless field	364
45.3	The operation	365

46 Release of Trigger Finger   **369**

46.1	Instruments	369
46.2	Technique for producing anaesthetic bloodless field	370
46.3	The operation	371

47 Stab-Avulsion Varicose Veins   **372**

47.1	Instruments	372
47.2	Operative technique	373

48 Excision of Ganglia   **378**

48.1	Instruments	379

48.2	Technique for producing anaesthetic bloodless field	379
48.3	The operation	380
48.4	Excision of rheumatoid synovioma	382

49 Caudal Epidural and Intravenous Regional Anaesthesia **383**
| 49.1 | Epidural anaesthesia | 383 |
| 49.2 | Intravenous regional anaesthesia (Bier's block) | 385 |

PART FOUR: SPECIALIST MINOR SURGERY **389**

50 Plastic and Reconstructive Surgery
R.W. Smith and I.H. Whitworth **391**
50.1	Choice of incision	391
50.2	Suturing techniques	393
50.3	Postoperative care	394
50.4	Scarring	395

51 Minor Operations in Ophthalmology
C. Jones **397**
| 51.1 | Examination techniques | 397 |
| 51.2 | Surgical procedures | 399 |

52 Dental Problems in General Practice
A.B. Miller **404**
52.1	Introduction	404
52.2	Medical history	404
52.3	Extraoral signs	404
52.4	Differential diagnosis of swellings of the face	405
52.5	Differential diagnosis of facial pain	405
52.6	Dental history and intraoral examination	405
52.7	Symptoms, possible diagnosis and treatment	406
52.8	Dental caries	406
52.9	Trauma	407
52.10	Treatment of dental abscesses	407
52.11	Dental extractions	407
52.12	Complications of extractions	416
52.13	Some dos and don'ts	416
52.14	Bleeding and suturing	417
52.15	Prophylactic antibiotic cover against bacterial endocarditis	417
52.16	Antibiotic regime for infections	417
52.17	Recommended instruments	418

PART FIVE: ADMINISTRATION **421**

53 Providing Information to the Patient **423**

54 Medicolegal Aspects of Minor Surgery
Based on the booklet by P. Dando, S. Green & J. Price MDU **443**
| 54.1 | Surgical skill | 443 |

54.2	Preoperative assessment of the patient	443
54.3	Consent	444
54.4	Histology	444
54.5	Danger areas	445
54.6	Infection	445
54.7	Anaesthetics	446
54.8	Product liability	446
54.9	Mishaps	446
54.10	Risk management analysis	447
54.11	Minimizing the risk of a claim	447

55 The General Practitioner and the National Health Service — **449**

55.1	Remuneration	449
55.2	1990 contract	451
55.3	Minor surgery procedures	452
55.4	Offering a minor surgery service to colleagues	452
55.5	Obtaining help from health authorities	453
55.6	Collaboration with consultant colleagues	453
55.7	The private patient	453

Appendix A Surgical Instrument and Equipment Suppliers — **454**

	UK	454
	North America and Canada	455

Appendix B Corresponding Trade Names for Drugs Named in the Book — **457**

References — **458**

Selected Further Reading — **460**

Index — **462**

Contributors

Miss Carole A. Jones FRCS, FRCOphth
Consultant Ophthalmic Surgeon, Kent County Opthalmic & Aural
Hospital, Church Street, Maidstone, Kent ME14 1DT

Mr Alwyn B. Miller BDS
Dental Surgeon, West Malling Dental Practice, 23/27 Swan Street,
West Malling, Kent ME19 6JU

Roger W. Smith MCh, FRCS
Consultant Plastic and Reconstructive Surgeon, McIndoe Surgical
Centre, Holtye Road, East Grinstead, West Sussex RH19 3EB

Mr Ian H. Whitworth BSc, MS(Plast), FRCS
Senior Registrar, McIndoe Surgical Centre, Holtye Road, East
Grinstead, West Sussex RH19 3EB

Dr Patrick Dando, Stephen Green and Julie Price
The Medical Defence Union Ltd.

Acknowledgements

The first edition of this book was based on a series of articles on minor surgery in the *Pulse* reference section, 1984, and my grateful thanks are due to the staff of *Pulse* who gave me so much help and advice and, in particular, to Cynthia Clarke for her medical illustrations, Philip Fraser Betts and Paul Thorpe for many of the photographs.

To Mrs Vaux and Mrs Harrison, state-registered chiropodists in Maidstone, my grateful thanks for their tuition on the method of treating ingrowing toe-nails.

My thanks are also due to Mr W. Keith Yeates for allowing me to use his slides illustrating vasectomy in the first and second editions and to his widow Mrs J. Yeates for her permission to use the slides in this section; also to Dr Philip Hopkins for his advice on liquid nitrogen cryosurgery.

The new chapter on the histological appearance of various skin lesions was made possible with the help I received from Dr R. J. Cairns who allowed me to use his slides of skin lesions, and Dr Trevor Telfer who personally made the photomicrographs of all the histological specimens and gave me invaluable advice. To both of them, I extend my sincere thanks.

Chapter 54 on medicolegal aspects of minor surgery is based on the booklet 'Problems in general practice – minor surgery' by Patrick Dando, Stephen Green and Julie Price of the Medical Defence Union Ltd and I am extremely grateful to them for their help. Copyright in the material is retained by the Medical Defence Union Ltd.

Mr Maurice Frohm showed me the technique for stab avulsions for varicose veins and I am grateful to him for his advice.

I am very grateful to my partners, and to all the nurses who have worked with us at Larkfield and given so much help and advice, also to all our receptionists and staff for their help.

I am especially grateful to Mrs Sylvia Smith, practice manager of the Thornhills Medical Group for over 25 years, for her invaluable help in typing, reading and correcting the manuscripts for the first and second editions, a task which she did meticulously.

Finally, a special word of thanks to my wife, Anne, who has given me so much help throughout the preparation of all four editions, and without whose assistance it would not have been possible.

The new section on Specialist Minor Surgery contains chapters by Mr Roger Smith, Consultant plastic surgeon, Mr Ian Whitworth,

Senior registrar, Miss Carole Jones, Consultant ophthalmologist, and Mr Alwyn Miller, General dental surgeon – I am particularly grateful to them for their help in producing these.

I would like to thank Mrs Gillian Cowell, Mrs Jennifer Tourney, and Mrs Angela Howitt the practice nurses at Thornhills Medical Group for their help in writing the Chapter on the role of the Practice Nurse/Operating Theatre Assistant.

J.S.B.

Preface to the fourth edition

Further changes and additional procedures have been included in the fourth edition of *Minor Surgery – A Text and Atlas* to reflect improved techniques, and also to help those doctors who wish to increase the scope of their minor surgery.

A new chapter on the role of the Practice Nurse/Operating Theatre assistant is included – this acknowledges the vital role these colleagues play in the day-to-day running of a Minor Surgical service.

There is also an additional chapter on Biopsy Techniques, which are becoming increasingly important with the increasing incidence of skin malignancies where a prompt accurate histological diagnosis of a skin lesion may accelerate treatment and improve overall prognosis.

There is a new departure from previous editions in a section entitled *Specialist Minor Surgery,* where specialists in their field have been invited to contribute a chapter giving additional information which, it is hoped, will improve still further the doctor's results in minor surgery. This section also includes a chapter on dental minor surgery, which is important if a doctor is in an isolated situation where there are no dental facilities.

Preface to the first edition

This book provides an illustrated step-by-step guide to minor surgery. It covers all minor surgical conditions and treatments encountered by the author over 25 years in general practice.

The selection of suitable instruments and equipment is described, followed by methods of instrument sterilization, skin preparation, choice of incisions and a comprehensive description of methods of anaesthesia, including intravenous regional anaesthesia, nerve blocks and infiltration anaesthesia.

Wound closure and the use of different suture materials are described, together with a section on the timing of suture removal to obtain the neatest scars. Follow-up and statistical analysis of the types of operation feasible in general practice are covered.

Individual minor surgical procedures are then described with illustrations. The practitioner is taken through each operation, commencing with simple injection techniques, through excision of cysts, biopsies, ingrowing toe-nails and varicose veins to more complex minor operations including decompression of the carpal tunnel, release of trigger finger and excision of ganglion.

Finally, simple diagnostic procedures such as proctoscopy, sigmoidoscopy and biopsy are described.

This volume provides a valuable reference book for all general medical practitioners, both in practice and in training.

Although all the operations described can be performed under general or local anaesthesia, the author has described local anaesthetic techniques almost exclusively.

Foreword

I first opened the pages of this book during a damp winter's weekend and found myself immersed for many more hours than I had expected, such was the clarity of the text and the excellence of the illustrations. No wonder *Minor Surgery* is now in its fourth edition since it was first published in 1986!

Surgery carried out by general practitioners and junior hospital doctors is called minor surgery, but for patients it is often believed to be far from minor. Indeed, it has been said that for a patient there is no such thing as a minor operation. This important consideration shows throughout the book, especially in the section on providing information to the patient, and in the chapters on the need for the correct equipment and environment, thus ensuring safe practice.

The heart of the volume, of course, lies in the illustrated descriptions of operations – these are a triumph. The writing is lucid and the many coloured photographs are of the highest quality. Practitioners everywhere, be they general practitioners in well-equipped surgeries, surgical trainees in hospitals, or doctors in isolated rural communities, will find this text and atlas of the greatest value in preparing for and undertaking the operations described within. I just wish it had been available when I set out on my surgical career.

Barry Jackson MS, PRCS, FRCP, President
The Royal College of Surgeons of England

Basic techniques

Introduction

> If thou examinest a man having a gaping wound in his head, penetrating to the bone, thou shouldst lay thy hand upon it and thou shouldst palpate his wound. If thou findest his skull uninjured thou shouldst say regarding him 'an ailment which I will treat'
>
> *Edwin Smith, Surgical Papyrus, 3000–2500 BC*

All doctors have seen many minor operations performed, and as medical students, resident housesurgeons and trainee general practitioners (GPs) have performed many of them personally. Before the advent of the National Health Service (NHS) in the UK, most family doctors undertook their own minor surgery: incising boils and abscesses, excising cysts and suturing lacerations. Some had contracts with the local hospitals and performed all their own minor surgery, together with many major surgical procedure. Patients expected their family doctors to operate, and family doctors themselves expected to undertake most minor surgical procedures – including delivering babies at home, and even 'tonsillectomies on the kitchen table'!

In recent years, there has been a gradual move away from GP minor surgery. Family doctors in hospitals have been replaced by specialist consultant colleagues and fewer GPs were now undertaking their own minor surgery, preferring instead to refer the majority of their patients with such conditions to hospital. Inevitably, as this trend increased, hospital surgical waiting lists increased. Interestingly, with the latest developments in the NHS in the UK and the formation of primary care groups with the provision of services outside traditional hospitals, there is now an increasing interest in minor surgery within general practice again.

In many instances, because the patient realizes that his or her condition is not serious and knows that there are long delays, he or she may not even consult the family doctor, preferring to keep the 'cyst' or 'mole' or 'veins'. In recent years, however, there has been a renewed interest by general medical practitioners in minor surgery; with training now taking up to 10 years, and many doctors moving into purpose-built premises complete with treatment rooms, and working with attached community nurses or practice nurses, many now feel that they would like to undertake their own minor operations again. This has been welcomed by the patients, who now find they can receive treatment for their minor lesions promptly, in familiar surroundings, and done by a doctor whom they know well, with follow-up by the nurses whom they know already.

Figure 1.1 The treatment room, Thornhills Medical Group, Larkfield, Kent. (1) Operating theatre table, (2) dressing trolley, (3) dressing trolley, (4) instrument cupboard, (5) handwash basin, (6) work surface, (7) storage cupboards, (8) paper towel dispenser, (9) lights and (10) wastebin.

Because of the great variety of minor surgical procedures, there is a good chance that doctors will never have seen some of them performed, and if they wish to learn the techniques they may have to refer to 12 or more specialized textbooks of surgery. For example, a GP would need to consult a surgical instrument catalogue for the choice of instruments, equipment firms for sterilizers, tables and lights, textbooks on general surgery for the excision of sebaceous cysts, and reference books on ophthalmic surgery for the treatment of meibomian cysts.

Removal of intradermal naevi might be found in a textbook of dermatology or general surgery, whereas intra-articular steroid injections might be found in books on rheumatology, general medicine or orthopaedics, proctoscopy, sigmoidoscopy and the injection of haemorrhoids could be covered in three separate textbooks, while the treatment of ingrowing toe-nails might be included in books on general surgery, orthopaedics, dermatology and chiropody. Skin tumours and their management would be found in specialist books on oncology,

Figure 1.2 The treatment room, Thornhills Medical Group, Larkfield, Kent.

dermatology, general surgery, plastic surgery and even lasers in medicine, while injection of the carpal tunnel would be included in books on rheumatology, neurology, physical medicine or general surgery. Practitioners wishing to learn the technique of cryotherapy might have difficulty in knowing which specialized textbook to consult, as they would if they wished to sterilize instruments or equipment. Thus, although each procedure may correctly be classified as minor surgery, nevertheless the term embraces many different specialities, and hence the reason for this book: it is an attempt to bring together under one cover all the minor operations and practical surgical procedures that GPs might wish to perform themselves.

With a few exceptions, all the minor operations described can be performed single-handed by the practitioner or with the assistance of an 'unscrubbed' nurse.

The techniques described and the instruments used are those which the author has found most suitable over 40 years performing more than 20 000 minor operations personally. The choice of firms supplying instruments and equipment is always difficult as there are many excellent firms in both the UK and the USA; thus, only a representative sample has been included in the book, mainly of suppliers that the author has used himself.

1.1 SCOPE AND LIMITATIONS OF MINOR SURGERY

All the minor operations described in this book are well within the capability of any general medical practitioner, housesurgeon, casualty officer or trainee GP as well as the specialist. Some require purchase of a special item of equipment such as an electrocautery, while others require a special instrument, for example chalazion ring forceps for meibomian cysts. Above all, practitioners must satisfy themselves that they can safely carry out any particular surgical procedure before attempting it. Thus it may be helpful, as well as referring to texts and photographs to watch a procedure being performed by a colleague and obtain expert tuition before embarking on it themselves.

As experience grows, so the number and variety of minor operations attempted will increase, and the final decision of what to attempt, and not to attempt will rest entirely with the doctor. A single-handed practitioner will be inadvised to attempt any operation involving intravenous regional anaesthesia, where an assistant is mandatory, and although the majority of operations described can safely be performed single handed, nevertheless, if an assistant such as a nurse or colleague can be available, it helps both the patient and operator considerably. For this reason, if the doctor contemplates undertaking minor surgery to any extent, it is a good idea at the outset to reserve a time for an operating session or 'list'; this may be daily, weekly or once a month depending on numbers and circumstances. General anaesthesia has not been included in this book as it was assumed that most GPs would not have adequate recovery beds and facilities in the average surgery. However, all of the procedures described can easily be performed very safely and comfortably using local anaesthetic techniques.

Where the patient can have a short rest afterwards and transport can be arranged, there are very few minor operations which cannot readily be performed in the GP's consulting or treatment room. Where the patient is too ill (e.g. malignant ascites) or too handicapped (e.g.

Figure 1.3 In the past it was not considered necessary to wear gloves for some procedures, but it is now recommended that gloves be worn for all minor operations.

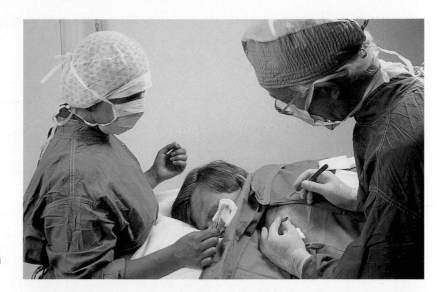

Figure 1.4 For others, such as excision of lipoma, opening joints or vasectomy, sterile gloves and gowns may be used, together with masks.

Figure 1.5 Sterile drapes, either paper or linen, will ensure less risk of infection.

confined entirely to bed) it may be preferable to bring the equipment and instruments to the patient's home rather than bringing the patient to the doctor's premises, and in this respect, minor surgery lends itself admirably.

1.2 ADVANTAGES AND DISADVANTAGES

There are considerable advantages where the patient's doctor undertakes minor surgery (Table 1.1). First, the patient and doctor are already well known to each other, and this immediately allays much anxiety, particularly with very young patients. Secondly, there is saving of time for both the patient and the hospital; the patient can generally choose a convenient time and the hospital, by not seeing the patient, can offer the time saved to another patient. Thirdly, there are

Table 1.1 Advantages of GP minor surgery

1. Staff already known to patient
2. Saving of time for patient and hospital
3. Financial savings to local hospital
4. Continuity of care
5. Less infection
6. Greater job satisfaction
7. Greater efficiency
8. Offering a better service
9. Rapid biopsy and histology results
10. Greater patient satisfaction

Table 1.2 Disadvantages of GP minor surgery

1. Lack of suitable training
2. Lack of suitable equipment and premises
3. The risk of missing serious pathology
4. Allocating sufficient time
5. Worry should complications occur (with medicolegal implication)
6. Financial disincentives

considerable financial savings, particularly to the hospital budget. It has been shown that one GP performing only a few minor operations per week can save the local hospital a significant amount of money [1, 2] and that, on average, it is 15 times cheaper to perform the same operation in general practice than in a hospital. Fourthly, there is a continuity of care; the doctor performing the operation is the same doctor who initially saw the patient, the nurse assisting at the operation is likewise already known to the patient and is the same nurse who will remove any sutures and undertake any further follow-up, and, when the patient is ready to return to school or work, it is the very same doctor who will check that all is well and discharge the patient.

Cross-infection outside hospital is much less of a problem than inside hospital, commonly less than 1 or 2%. Other advantages could include greater job satisfaction, greater efficiency, offering a better service, rapid biopsy and histology results, and greater patient satisfaction.

Offset against these many advantages are a few disadvantages (Table 1.2). Some of the most commonly voiced worries are lack of suitable training, lack of suitable equipment and premises, the risk of missing serious pathology, worry about medicolegal implications should complications occur, and finding sufficient time. However, the advantages greatly outweigh any disadvantages, and rarely does one find a doctor who has started to undertake surgery thinking of abandoning it.

1.3 ORGANIZATION WITHIN THE PRACTICE

Some procedures such as injection of tennis elbow, golfer's elbow and carpal tunnel take so little time that it is usually preferable to perform these at the time of the initial consultation. Similarly, if the electrocautery and an ampoule of local anaesthetic are available easily, small skin tags, papillomata and warts and naevi may all be dealt with in less than 5 min.

Where a number of operations is to be performed, or where a procedure is likely to take longer than the initial consultation appointment time, it is easier and preferable to set aside a certain time each week, and to make a minor operations list at which the practice nurse and/or an assistant can help. With a little experience the doctor will soon know how long each procedure takes and will able to offer appropriate appointments accordingly.

Accurate records of all operations performed should be kept, together with any drugs used, and types of sutures and dressings; a register of operations enables the doctor to analyse his or her work and produce an annual breakdown of the type of work being carried out (Chapter 20).

Many elementary procedures are described in this book and lists of instruments are often repeated throughout the book. This is a deliberate policy to avoid the reader having to refer back to several previous sections.

CHAPTER 2

Instruments

> When thou meetest a tumour that has attacked a vessel... say 'I will treat the disease with the knife, poultice it with fat, and burn it with fire so that it bleeds not too much'.
>
> *Ebers Papyrus, 1500 BC.*

2.1 CHOICE OF INSTRUMENTS

Every doctor has a favourite selection of instruments, and what suits one surgeon does not always suit another. One practitioner may prefer small fine-toothed delicate instruments, whereas another is happier with larger instruments. However, certain basic sets of instruments seem to be generally popular, and the following are included as being the most commonly used by the author (Fig. 2.1):

- 1 size 3 scalpel handle
- scalpel blades 15, 10, 11

Figure 2.1 A basic instrument pack. (1) Scalpel handle, size 3; (2) scapel blades, sizes 10, 11 and 15; (3) 5 in. (12.7 cm) toothed dissecting forceps; (4) 5 in. (12.7 cm) standard stitch scissors, pointed; (5) 5 in. (12.7 cm) straight artery forceps (Halstead's); (6) 5¼ in. (13.3 cm) Kilner needle holder.

- 5 in. (12.7 cm) toothed dissecting forceps (Treves)
- 5 in. (12.7 cm) standard (sharp/sharp) stitch scissors
- 5 in. straight artery forceps (Halstead) (12.7cm)
- $5^{1}/_{4}$ in. (13.3 cm) Kilner needle holder.

These five instruments plus scalpel blades form the nucleus of most minor operating sets; they can be used for simple suturing of lacerations and excision of most dermal lesions. Where the practitioner intends to build up various instrument packs to be sterilized by the central sterile supplies department (CSSD) several such basic packs should be made up.

Next to the scalpel, the needle holder will be the most frequently used instrument during a doctor's working life in minor surgery; it is, therefore, worth spending relatively more on this instrument in order to have the best quality available. In particular, it is essential to check the jaws to ensure that they not only hold the finest needle accurately, but importantly hold the finest suture without slipping or traumatizing. Nothing is more frustrating than trying to tie a knot in 6/0 monofilament nylon only to find the suture material slipping through the jaws of the needle holder.

The Gillies combined needle holder and scissors is a very popular instrument, although it sometimes takes practice to learn the technique of using it. Where the surgeon is working with limited assistance, the Gillies can be used as a needle holder, to tie the knot and to cut the suture, all without having to change instruments.

The next most useful instruments are the sharp-spoon Volkmann curette and electrocautery, which between them enable the practitioner to remove most warts, verrucae, papillomata, granulomata, keratoses and similar intradermal lesions. The curette is generally easy to choose, depending on the doctor's preference, but selection of an electro-cautery can be difficult as there are many excellent models on the market (Chapters 3 and 16).

Where smaller instruments are required for fine surgery, Adson's $4^{3}/_{4}$ in. (12 cm) toothed dissecting forceps are ideal, together with a pair of Iris scissors, fine $4^{1}/_{2}$ in. (11.4 cm) straight or curved. Similarly, the fine (12.7 cm) Halstead mosquito forceps, curved or straight, are most useful instruments.

Sebaceous cysts and lipomata can be dissected using a pair of curved 7 in (17.8 cm) McIndoe scissors, which may also double up for cutting the threads of intrauterine contraceptive devices after they have been inserted (Fig. 2.2).

At some stage, the practitioner will need some small retractors: these may be either self-retaining such as the Kocher's thyroid retractor, West Weitlander $5^{1}/_{2}$ in. (14 cm), or the baby Kilner/Dickson Wright spring self-retaining retractor, or single/double retractors which will need to be held by an assistant. Of these, the Gillies skin-hooks $6^{1}/_{2}$ in. (16.5 cm) are popular, as are the double-ended Kilner Senn Miller 6 in. (15.2 cm) (so-called cat's paw retractors).

To complete the list of small general instruments is the McDonald double-ended $7^{1}/_{2}$ in. (19 cm) dissector, which is extremely versatile and useful for many minor procedures.

All doctors regularly see patients suffering from meibomian cysts (chalazion); normally such patients would need to be referred to a

Figure 2.2 Some of the most commonly used instruments in addition to the basic set. (1) Allis tissue forceps 3 × 4 teeth 6 in. (15.2 cm); (2) self-retaining retractor (Krocher's thyroid or equivalent); (3) McDonald's double-ended dissector 7½ in. (19 cm); (4) Retractor: double-ended Kilner Senn Miller 6 in. (15.2 cm) (so-called cat's paw retractor); (5) Adson's toothed dissecting forceps 4¾ in. (12 cm); (6) 5 in. (12.7 cm) curved fine artery forceps (Halstead's mosquito); (7) Iris scissors, straight, 4½ in. (11.4 cm); (8) Curved 7 in. (17.8 cm) McIndoe's scissors; (9) Electrocautery burner and handle (Mark Hovell's); (10) Volkmann double-ended sharp spoon curette.

ophthalmic surgeon, but the treatment of incision and curettage is so simple and quick that it can be one of the most rewarding conditions to treat, provided the practitioner has the necessary instruments. These comprise a pair of chalazion ring forceps, a small chalazion curette, no. 3 scalpel handle with the pointed no. 11 blade, together with a syringe and needle for administering local anaesthetic (Fig. 2.3).

Another valuable instrument, although not used as frequently as the above, is the abdominal trocar and cannula for draining abdominal ascites. More recently, with the introduction of plastic intravenous cannulae, a less traumatic aspiration may be obtained by the using one of these instead. In general practice the most common cause of ascites is inoperable malignant disease, and great relief, albeit temporary, can be offered by the judicious tapping of ascitic fluid when symptoms of pressure become distressing (Fig. 2.4).

Figure 2.3 Instruments required for incision and curette of meibomian cyst (chalazion).

Figure 2.4 Trocar and cannula used for draining abdominal ascites.

As the treatment of haemorrhoids is included in the textbook, a choice of proctoscope, sigmoidoscope and haemorrhoid injection syringe should be considered. There are many different sigmoidoscopes and proctoscopes on the market with a variety of methods of illumination and magnification, some disposable, some non-disposable, and costs vary considerably. Where a practitioner is considering purchasing such instruments, it is often helpful to ask the advice of the local general surgeon and ask for a demonstration.

The Lloyd-Davies stainless-steel sigmoidoscope has been in use for many years and is a popular, virtually indestructible instrument. Illumination can be by fibre-optic cable, filament bulb, or tungsten or quartz halogen lamp: they are rigid, reasonably priced and interchangeable (Fig. 2.5). More recently, flexible, fibre-optic sigmoidoscopes have been marketed, but the cost is still high, and probably outside the price range of the average practitioner. However, the illumination and view are excellent and more of the sigmoid colon can be visualized than with the rigid instrument.

Naunton Morgan's proctoscope is ideal for the general practitioner. As with the sigmoidoscope, illumination may be from either a fibre-optic cable or a filament bulb. It is an excellent instrument to use if the practitoner contemplates injecting haemorrhoids. For this latter procedure, Gabriel's haemorrhoid syringe is used. It has the advantage of good fine control, although many simpler disposable haemorrhoid syringes have now been introduced with Luer-lock fittings to prevent the needle being expelled under pressure (Fig. 2.6).

As all of the operations described in this book are performed under local anaesthesia, it is important that this be made as discomfort free as possible. To this end, the finest possible needle should be used for

(a)

(b)

Figure 2.5 (a) The Lloyd-Davies stainless-steel rigid sigmoidoscope. (b) Flexible fibre-optic sigmoidoscope with light source (Welch Allyn UK Ltd).

Figure 2.6 St Mark's Hospital pattern proctoscope with Gabriel's haemorrhoid injection syringe and needles. Illumination by tungsten filament 3.5 V bulb, or fibre-optic cable and light.

infiltration anaesthesia, and there is no better needle to use than the 30 swg (0.3 mm) needle mounted on a dental syringe loaded with a cartridge of local anaesthetic. If the injection is given slowly and gently, it can be virtually pain-free – a point greatly appreciated by the younger patient (Fig. 2.7).

Where larger volumes of local anaesthetic need to be injected, the initial 'bleb' or 'weal' can still be raised with the dental syringe and needle. Larger needles merely traumatize the tissues, cause unnecessary pain, delay healing and increase the risks of infection.

Finally, before leaving this section on the choice of instruments, mention must be made of two invaluable instruments in the surgical treatment of ingrowing toe-nails, these are the nail chisel and the Thwaites nail nipper (Figs 2.8 and 2.9). With these two instruments plus a pair of straight artery forceps the practitioner can offer a treatment for ingrowing toe-nails which carries a 99% cure rate (Chapter 30).

Figure 2.7 Dental syringe with cartridges of local anaesthetic and 30 swg needles, ideal both for children and for digital nerve blocks (Nova Instruments).

Figure 2.8 Thwaites nail nipper (English pattern, Nova Instruments).

Figure 2.9 Nail chisel (Nova Instruments).

2.2 INSTRUMENT AND EQUIPMENT MANUFACTURERS (Appendix A)

The list given at the end of this book is far from comprehensive; it includes all of the firms which the author has used during the past 39 years, however each practitioner will have his or her own favourite suppliers, and it is certainly worth 'shopping around' for the 'best buy'. All items of equipment and surgical instruments described in this book can be obtained from firms included in this list.

2.3 SOURCES OF SUPPLY

To build and equip a minor operating theatre using all new materials and instruments could be prohibitively expensive for most general practitioners (GPs), particularly as they are unlikely to be able to recoup much of the expenditure either from grants, item-of-service payments or patients' fees.

However, by making careful enquiries and contacting various agencies, a very acceptable treatment room can be equipped for a fraction of what it would cost new. Major items such as operating theatre tables, trolleys, sterilizers and lights may often be obtained from the local hospital supplies officer who knows of obsolete items of equipment no longer required by the hospital. They may often be purchased for a nominal sum, and although classified as 'obsolete' as far as the hospital is concerned, may prove to be exactly what is needed in a small minor operating room.

Often equipment has been purchased for use in hospital, only to be superseded by an improved model after several years; the original is then relegated to the stores, yet is still perfectly serviceable. Similarly, it is worth contacting large surgical equipment manufacturers to see whether they have any reconditioned, obsolete or demonstration models available at a reduced price. Medical representatives from these firms are always most helpful if they can see what is needed, and it is always worth contacting them, usually through the operating room supervisor or theatre sister at the nearest hospital.

Charitable organizations will often be prepared to raise money and purchase a piece of equipment, particularly if they can see the benefits which will accrue locally if an improved surgical service is offered.

Finally, when all else fails, it is still possible to advertise for equipment and instruments in the various journals and weekly magazines, and be successful.

2.4 ADVANTAGES OF INSTRUMENT PACKS

Where a doctor is performing a regular number of minor operations and particularly if the CSSD facilities can be used, there is much to commend compiling a number of 'instrument packs', e.g. suture pack, ingrowing toe-nail pack, meibomian cyst pack and abdominal paracentesis pack. In this way, just the instruments which are required are sterilized and used in a more efficient way. Individual packs may be sterilized and kept for future use as well as being available for use either at the surgery or in the patient's home. It is also easier to check the contents of each pack at the end of each operation to ensure that no instruments have been lost. Unfortunately, the smaller autoclaves are not suitable for instrument packs as they do not have a vacuum cycle and will therefore not dry the instruments, so the practitioner will normally have to rely on a hospital autoclave, or failing this a hot-air oven.

The following instrument packs will be found to be most useful for the GP undertaking minor surgery.

2.4.1 Basic suture pack (Fig. 2.10)

- 1 scalpel handle size 3
- Kilner needle holder 5$\frac{1}{4}$ in. (13.3 cm)
- stitch scissors, pointed, 5 in. (12.7 cm)
- 1 toothed dissecting forceps 5 in. (12.7 cm)
- 1 straight artery forceps 5 in. (12.7 cm)
- 1 scalpel blade size 10
- 1 sterile Prolene suture. Ref. Ethicon WB020T (1.5 metric) with curved cutting needle 26 mm (or equivalent)

2.4.2 Meibomian cyst pack (Fig. 2.11)

- 1 pair chalazion ring forceps
- 1 scalpel handle size 3
- 1 pair iris scissors, curved 4$\frac{1}{4}$ in. (11.4 cm)
- 1 chalazion curette
- 1 scalpel blade size 11
- 1 sterile eye pad and bandage sterile gauze swabs

2.4.3 Abdominal paracentesis pack

- 1 scalpel handle size 3
- 1 scalpel blade size 15
- 1 trocar and cannula or intravenous cannula
- connecting tubing and screw clip
- sterile gauze swabs.

Figure 2.10 Basic instrument set, ready for autoclaving (Rocket of London Ltd).

Figure 2.11 Meibomian cyst pack, ready for autoclaving (Rocket of London Ltd).

2.4.4 Ingrowing toe-nail pack

- 1 scalpel handle size 3
- 1 scalpel blade size 15
- 1 pair artery forceps, straight 5 in. (12.7 cm)
- 1 pair stitch scissors, sharp/sharp 5 in. (12.7 cm) or Thwaites nail nipper (English pattern) $5^1/_8$ in. (13 cm) (Nova Instruments)
- 1 nail chisel (Nova Instruments)
- 1 Volkmann sharp-spoon curette
- 2 wooden applicators with cotton-wool sterile gauze swabs.

2.4.5 Minor operations pack (Fig. 2.12)

- 1 pair Rampley sponge forceps $9^1/_2$ in.(24.1 cm)
- Mayo towel clips
- 3 Dunhill artery forceps 5 in. (12.7 cm)
- 3 Halstead mosquito forceps straight 5 in.(12.7 cm)
- 3 Halstead mosquito forceps curved 5 in.(12.7 cm)
- 2 Allis tissue forceps 6 in. (15.2 cm)
- 1 McDonald's dissector
- 1 McIndoe dissecting forceps 6 in. (15.2 cm)
- 1 Gillies dissecting forceps 6 in. (15.2 cm)
- 1 McIndoe's scissors, curved 7 in. (17.8 cm)
- 1 Mayo scissors straight $5^1/_2$ in. (14 cm)
- 2 Gillies skin hooks
- 2 Kilner, double-ended retractors
- 1 Volkmann scoop
- 1 Kilner needle holder

Figure 2.12   A comprehensive minor operation set of instruments in tray, ready for autoclaving (Rocket of London Ltd).

Figure 2.13 General minor surgical set in stainless-steel case which may be autoclaved for immediate use (Chas Thackray Ltd).

- 1 scalpel handle size 3
- scalpel blades 10 and 15
- sterile drapes, gauze swabs
- 1 sterile Prolene suture. Ref. Ethicon W 8020T (1.5 metric) with curved cutting needle 26 mm (or equivalent)

Certain manufacturers make comprehensive instrument packs in stainless-steel containers ready for immediate autoclaving (Fig. 2.13).

2.5 CARE OF INSTRUMENTS AND EQUIPMENT

Like all mechanical and electronic equipment, surgical instruments require regular care and maintenance to retain their efficiency and prolong their useful life. Dirty, rusty forceps are not only a potential source of infection, but look unsightly, are difficult to use and ultimately break prematurely.

2.6 CARE OF STAINLESS STEEL

Stainless steel is the material of choice for most surgical instruments; it combines a high resistance to corrosion and rust with an attractive finish. Even under ideal conditions the finest stainless-steel instruments can become pitted and stained, so great care is needed with washing and cleaning, polishing and lubrication. Rough handling or the use of abrasives can permanently mark stainless steel, so initially all instruments after use should be cleaned with a hard brush under running cool water. Very hot water will cause coagulation of blood and exudate and make subsequent cleaning harder. If an ultrasonic cleaning bath using instrument detergents is available, this will be ideal and restore a high polish to most instruments (see Fig. 4.1). After washing, instruments should be carefully dried to avoid water remaining in any joint and causing corrosion. Lubrication using a water-soluble lubricant is strongly recommended and will greatly prolong the useful life of any instrument.

Saline solutions are a major cause of pitting, and instruments should never be soaked in them, nor should a saline solution be allowed to dry on an instrument.

Whenever cleaning or washing instruments, one should keep all ratchets unlocked and box joints open, and similarly avoid using wire wool or abrasives, iodine, bromine, aluminium chloride or barium chloride. The same advice applies to surgical blades and needles, both of which may rust and corrode more easily than stainless-steel instruments. Serrated surfaces on artery forceps and needle holders can be effectively cleaned with a small brass wire brush obtainable from shoe shops.

Plastic instruments or plastic parts of instruments are particularly vulnerable to corrosive agents, heat, rough handling and abrasive cleaners. They should be treated with great respect; in general, washing with warm soapy water with a soft cloth is sufficient. Sterilization may be by either soaking in antiseptic solutions or autoclaving at a lower temperature [115°C under 9 lb/in^2 (62 kN/m^2) for 30 min] than is used for steel instruments. Cleaning and polishing should only be undertaken using recommended cleaners and polishers, as even ordinary domestic polishes can abrade Perspex and similar plastics. Most plastics are best stored in a dry state rather than under prolonged soaking in antiseptic solutions.

2.7 ELECTRICAL SAFETY

It cannot be stressed enough that there should be the utmost regard for electrical safety at all times. Many modern instruments and pieces of equipment operate from mains voltage, 110 or 240 V a.c. All such instruments have to pass stringent safety tests during and after manufacture and can be assumed to be electrically safe on delivery. However, with use, cables become frayed, earth connections work loose or break, internal components move with vibration, or accidental damage or unauthorized alteration to the circuitry or safety fuses occurs, resulting in potentially lethal voltages and currents reaching the patient. Obvious simple checks of plugs, fuses and cables should be made regularly, and routine maintenance performed by a qualified person at standard intervals as recommended by the manufacturer. Water and electricity do not mix, so it is imperative that all mains electrically operated instruments be kept dry. Low-voltage battery equipment is generally safe and may even be designed to work in damp or humid conditions. Earth connections and safety fuses should be regularly checked, making sure that the correct loading fuses are being used. Any frayed cables should be immediately replaced and any loose components such as switches and sockets dealt with. All equipment working from mains voltage should have a circuit breaker in the supply lines.

Cardiac defibrillators deliver a high voltage of several thousand volts, together with a relatively high current, making a lethal combination to the operator if any serious electrical fault should occur. It is thus even more imperative that servicing and maintenance of these instruments be entrusted to a qualified electrical engineer.

Electronic components comprising microchips and integrated circuits are generally very rugged and will withstand rough handling; they also operate at low voltages so are relatively safe, but they respond badly to high temperatures. Overheating should therefore be avoided and any ventilation apertures left uncovered; given these safeguards, they should give good service.

2.8 RECHARGEABLE BATTERY PACKS

Increasingly, rechargeable nickel–cadmium batteries are being used for items of medical equipment. These are relatively expensive and have a limited life, although are electrically safe. Rechargeable batteries are capable of delivering a very high current on discharge, so should not be shorted, as this might result in fire. Another feature is that their life is extended by regular discharging and recharging. Thus, any piece of equipment containing rechargeable batteries should be regularly switched on, fully discharged and then fully recharged. As they can fail without warning, back-up batteries for essential pieces of equipment are a good idea.

The minor operating theatre

> There are two kinds of light, the common and the artificial – the common is not at our disposal – the artificial is at our disposal.
>
> *Hippocrates, 460–377 BC*

The physical dimensions of the treatment room will ultimately determine what equipment can be accommodated, thus the smallest room compatible with reasonable operating conditions would have a floor area of 13 m^2 (140 square feet) and in most cases, the larger the room, the better the facilities. It should be emphasized that a separate operating room is not an essential prerequisite; indeed, many minor surgical procedures described in this book may be performed in the doctor's consulting room using the examination couch as an operating table, and an anglepoise lamp fitted with a reflecting spotlight as the source of illumination. Where presterilized instrument packs are used, the standard of asepsis can be extremely high.

However, there is no doubt that where a purpose-built treatment room is available, a much more satisfactory service can be offered to the patient; not only can all the instrument packs be assembled in readiness, but sterilizers, resuscitation equipment, trolleys, illumination and recovery facilities can also be prepared.

In general practice this room has the advantage that it can double as a nurse's treatment room, chiropody clinic, examination or recovery room, and immunization or family-planning clinic, so the maximum use can always be made of the facilities.

3.1 FIXTURES AND FITTINGS

Fitted cupboards and a good working surface are essential. Wall-mounted cupboards can be used if space is at a premium; these are used to store instrument packs, dressings, bandages, suture materials, equipment such as sphygmomanometers and electrocauteries, as well as resuscitation equipment.

A glass-fronted instrument cupboard, although not essential, makes selection of instruments and drugs very much easier, and this too can be permanently fixed to the wall. One X-ray viewing box is a relatively inexpensive item and if not used for viewing X-ray films, can still be used for viewing colour transparencies. Sufficient hooks for coats should be provided and a separate clothes locker would be even better.

A good-quality, stainless-steel hand wash-basin is essential, with hot and cold running water, preferably with an elbow-operated mixer tap,

Figure 3.1 Elbow-operated mixer-taps help to avoid cross-infection.

Figure 3.2 A large waste-bin with disposable bin-liners is very useful (Kimberley-Clark).

Figure 3.3 A separate container is necessary for all needles, broken glass and 'sharps'.

and an antiseptic/soap dispenser fitted above. Waste disposal is usually by means of bins with plastic liners (Figs 3.1–3.3).

Disposable paper hand towels and paper sheets are becoming more popular. Several of the large paper manufacturers produce wall-mounted dispensers and holders for the rolls of paper; likewise, disposal bags and stands are made by the same firms. The large disposable sheets are excellent for placing on the operating theatre table underneath the patient, for protecting pillows and for covering trolley shelves (Figs 3.4–3.7). Sufficient electric power sockets should be fitted and a minimum of eight outlets provided.

Figure 3.4 (a–e) A selection of paper hand-towels: economical and hygienic (Kimberley-Clark).

Figure 3.5 The wider paper towelling is useful for couches and covering the operating theatre table (Kimberley-Clark).

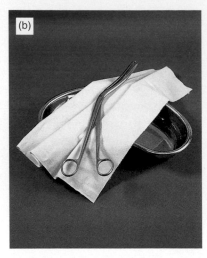

Figure 3.6 (a) Paper dressing-towels may also be included in CSSD instrument packs (Kimberley-Clark). (b) Paper towels used to dry instruments and dishes.

Background illumination may be provided by fluorescent strip lighting which will complement natural light from windows. An extractor fan is not a luxury: there are many procedures such as opening perineal abscesses, sigmoidoscopy and the use of electrocautery where a rapid change of air is desirable; because of this it is better to choose an extractor fan one or two sizes larger than recommended by the manufacturers. Finally, included amongst the fixtures and fittings is a small dangerous-drugs cupboard or drawer; this is recommended as some surgical procedures may require a premedication injection of such drugs as midazolam (Hypnovel) and fentanyl (Sublimaze).

Figure 3.7 Paper towelling being used to cover examination couch and operating area (Kimberley-Clark).

3.2 THE OPERATING-THEATRE TABLE

The most important item in any minor operating room is the table (Fig. 3.8) or couch for the patient. New operating theatre tables are expensive for the average practitioner, but by contacting local hospitals and clinics, a second-hand table may be found which will be more than adequate for minor surgery. The ability to raise and lower the patient and, in particular, to be able to put the patient in the head-down position and elevate the lower limbs, is a decided advantage over the fixed examination-couch type tables, and where possible it is worth waiting until a second-hand theatre table becomes available. In addition, it is wise to position the operating theatre table so that there is free space on all sides for an assistant, trolleys, and additional lights or equipment.

Having acquired the table, certain simple accessories such as an arm rest or lithotomy stirrups can be obtained and greatly increase the scope of the operations to be performed. Where space is restricted, a small Mayo-type tray which fixes to the side of the operating theatre table is a useful addition which can be recommended. One or two instrument trolleys should be purchased, preferably glass topped or stainless steel. Instruments for any operation may then be prepared in advance and the trolley brought to the patient for the operation. Again, new trolleys need not be felt to be essential as many very good second-hand ones can be found in most hospitals, perhaps needing slight repairs such as welding or repainting.

One operator's stool, adjustable in height, is needed; most minor operations can be readily performed with the patient lying down and the operator standing, but where any intricate surgery is being done, a comfortable stool for the surgeon makes the task easier.

As many minor operations are performed on the lower limbs, a chiropodist's chair for the patient would be a great help; as they are fairly bulky, however, a large treatment room would be necessary.

Figure 3.8 Operating theatre table.

3.3 ILLUMINATION

As previously mentioned, it is worth spending money on a good-quality operating spotlight. For superficial minor surgical procedures, it is not necessary to install the large shadowless main operating theatre lights, but one or two good-quality, low-voltage spotlights are essential, preferably mounted permanently to the wall or ceiling (Figs 3.9 and 3.10). Most are now fitted with a plastic heat filter, tinted to give a more natural wavelength of light, and many also have adjustable focus. Low-voltage (24 V) bulbs are preferred, especially the quartz halogen lamps, but each will need a special step-down transformer or rechargeable battery which needs to be fitted separately (Fig. 3.11).

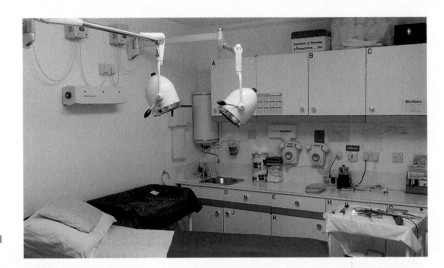

Figure 3.9 Wall-mounted spotlights are ideal for most minor surgical procedures.

Figure 3.10 Anglepoise-type spotlights are adequate where space is restricted, and give very good illumination (Ledu Lamps).

Figure 3.11   (a) A useful spotlight using low-voltage reflector bulb; may be wall or ceiling mounted or on castors. (b) Wall-mounted 'shadow-less triple spot-light' LS-200 (Welch Allyn). (c) The LS-200 floor-mounted spot-light (Welch Allyn).

In recent years, circular fluorescent lights surrounding a central 5 in. (12.7 cm) convex lens have been introduced, and these give excellent illumination coupled with magnification, particularly valuable for eye surgery and intricate hand surgery. Several firms make such lights, and each will provide lenses of different (or even combined) magnifications depending on the needs of the operator (Fig. 3.12). These lights have the added advantages that no heat is generated, the light wavelength approximates to natural daylight, and they are light and manoeuvrable. Their only disadvantage is that they have to be interspersed between the patient and operator; and, where short focal length lenses are used, there is a risk of the operator's hands and instruments accidentally touching the undersurface of the unit.

Small head-mounted spotlights are favoured by some surgeons; the source of illumination may be a tungsten filament bulb or quartz halogen bulb mounted behind a convex lens, or a fibre-optic transmission system from a light source adjacent to the operator. Although giving good illumination, particularly inside cavities, they have the disadvantage that the operator is connected to the batteries, transformer or light source and is not able to move about freely.

Figure 3.12 (a) Fluorescent circular magnifying light; extremely valuable for fine work e.g. eyes and removing splinters. (b) Welch Allyn surgical headlight with fibre-optic light source. (c) Welch Allyn 'Lumiview' combination head-light, magnifier and stereoscopic imaging system.

3.4 THE ELECTROCAUTERY

One of the most useful instruments for minor surgical procedures is the electrocautery. It consists essentially of a platinum wire which can be heated to red heat by means of an electric current (Figs 3.13–3.16).

Application of the red-hot wire to tissues will either cut them or seal any bleeding points by coagulation. It is thus ideal for removing small skin tags and papillomata, and for controlling the bleeding following curetting warts, granulomas and similar lesions.

The earliest electrocauteries used a standard battery and a rheostat to control the temperature of the tip; subsequently with the change in domestic electricity supplies from direct current (d.c.) to alternating current (a.c.) it was possible to use step-down transformers and rheostats as the source of current, with the great advantage that it avoided 'flat' batteries, provided the patient was within reach of a mains voltage socket.

Figure 3.13 Electrocautery transformer and selection of burners (Rimmer Bros Ltd).

Figure 3.14 Alternative electrocautery transformer with pistol-grip handle (Down Bros).

LENGTH		MODEL C28 BURNERS
47 mm	120 mm	(HIGH ENERGY 125 SERIES)
ORDER CODES		
B281		PUNCTURE POINT
	B287	
B282		RING CUTTER
	B286	
B283		STRAIGHT CUTTER
	B284	
B288		COAGULATION BALL
	B285	
56 mm ONLY		COLD POINT
B289		

Figure 3.15 A selection of the five most useful burners. For most minor surgery work the short 47 mm length is the easiest to handle. The longer (120 mm) burners are useful for gynaecological procedures.

More recently, with the introduction of nickel–cadmium rechargeable batteries with their ability to withstand high current drain without damage, several firms now produce portable rechargeable electrocauteries, with a variety of different burners (Fig. 3.17a, b).

One great advantage of the rechargeable cautery is the absence of long, trailing wires, and the fact that it can easily be carried between consulting rooms, or even to the patient's home for immediate use. The batteries may be kept on continuous low-current charge, and when fully charged will give 100 or more burns before requiring recharging.

Figure 3.16 The C28 rechargeable electrocautery; quick and simple to use (Warecrest Ltd).

Figure 3.17 (a) The C28 cordless cautery in use (Warecrest Ltd). (b) Two of the most useful instruments for skin surgery: electrocautery and curette.

A variety of different-shaped platinum burners is produced for different applications, some with a short and others with a long extension. In general, the short burners give better control, and the most useful shapes are (Fig. 3.15):

- ball-ended burner: ideal for sealing some bleeding vessels and for destroying small, superficial lesions
- cutting electrodes (ring and straight): suitable for dividing tissues. No force is needed – the heat of the tip does the cutting
- small puncture electrode: suitable for releasing subungual haematomata, spider naevi, and dividing small papillomata
- 'cold point' tip, consisting of a central firm needle-type electrode surrounded by a coil of platinum wire. Heat is transferred by

conduction to the tip which, as its name implies, does not reach such as a high temperature as the platinum wire itself. The cold point burner is ideal for treating spider naevi and for releasing subungual haematomata.

All of these burners will last for many years with careful use; they do not corrode, and may be immediately sterilized merely by switching on the current and heating the tip to red heat for a few seconds.

3.5 THE 'HYFRECATOR' OR UNIPOLAR DIATHERMY

Most surgeons will be familiar with the standard bipolar diathermy apparatus in use in most large operating theatres. In this, a very high-frequency current is passed through the patient's body and generates heat. By making one electrode relatively large and strapping it firmly to one limb, and by making the other electrode a pointed movable tip, sufficient heat is generated at the tip to coagulate or cut tissues. For major surgery such coagulating/cutting is standard practice, but the equipment is expensive, has to pass stringent tests for electrical safety, and is not really necessary or ideal for minor surgery.

One answer has been to use the unipolar diathermy or the Hyfrecator (Fig. 3.18). This is a small, portable instrument which, by means of an adjustable spark gap or solid-state circuitry and trans-former, produces a very high voltage and low current, sufficient to cause a spark to pass from the electrode tip to the patient without needing a second large pad electrode to complete the circuit. Three types of electrode are commonly used: The first is a fine wire electrode which may be inserted into the lesion to be destroyed. Passing a current through the tissues generates heat, which in turn coagulates the blood and cells; this 'desiccation' is particularly suitable for vascular haemangiomata. The second type of electrode is larger than the needle electrode, and is held a short distance away from the tissues; when the current is switched on, a stream of hot sparks passes between the patient and the electrode, and this is sufficient to destroy small areas of tissue. This technique is referred to as fulguration. Thirdly, the Hyfrecator can be used for coagulation by using a double electrode which is connected to a lower voltage winding on the high-frequency transformer. By placing this double electrode on the surface to be treated and passing a slightly heavier current between the poles of the electrode, the underlying tissues are coagulated and destroyed.

The advantage of using the Hyfrecator is the absence of bleeding; its effect is very similar to that of the electrocautery, and the heat generated automatically sterilizes the treated area; a sterile dry dressing or no dressing at all is, therefore, all that is needed to promote healing. The disadvantage is that histological examination of the treated lesion is not usually possible owing to the distortion of the cells from the heat; thus, a preliminary biopsy needs to be done where the diagnosis is in doubt.

Figure 3.18 The Birtcher Hyfrecator Model 733 on stand 708-1 (Birtcher Corporation, USA: Schuco International, London).

Figure 3.19 The Ellman Surgitron FFPF radiosurgical instrument with footswitch assembly. Surgitron hand-piece, coated passive antenna and electrodes (Ellman International, Hewlett, USA).

3.6 THE RADIOSURGERY UNIT

Radiosurgery units (Fig. 3.19) use high-frequency electric currents (3.8 MHz) to cut and coagulate tissues. There is much less tissue damage than with conventional electrocauteries and diathermy, and excellent cosmetic results can be obtained (Chapter 42). Cutting is by means of a fine-gauge needle or tungsten wire loop, and haemostasis by a ball-ended electrode. The instruments are small, portable and inexpensive. Where radiosurgery is used regularly, a Vapor-Vac smoke extraction unit is advisable as plumes of smoke are generated. Unlike in the electrocautery, the electrode remains cold throughout the surgical procedure. No pressure is needed and the surgeon needs to learn a completely new technique to use this equipment.

3.7 RESUSCITATION FACILITIES

Every doctor's surgery should possess some form of simple resuscitation equipment. Because patients suffering from a variety of diseases are constantly passing through the premises, sooner or later one will collapse with a myocardial infarction, major epileptic convulsion, cardiac arrest, simple haemorrhage or just a vasovagal faint. Where any form of treatment is being offered, be it one hypodermic injection or a minor surgical procedure, the practitioner must be prepared for the patient who will faint, or suffer an unexpected allergic reaction to the treatment. Should a patient collapse on the premises the first prerequisite is a room or area sufficiently large to be able to allow the patient to lie on the floor with sufficient space around him or her for equipment, doctors and assistants. The second requirement is the management of the unconscious patient: to maintain an airway and circulation, prevent the inhalation of secretions or vomit, establish a diagnosis and render treatment.

Fortunately, the majority of 'attacks' will be vasovagal, all of which will be expected to recover rapidly once the patient is lying with or without elevation of the legs to assist venous return to the heart.

A clear resuscitation sheet, based on first-aid manuals [3] and supplemented with additional information for cardiac arrest and anaphylactic reactions, should be displayed on a wall in the treatment room for all staff to see.

Resuscitation equipment should comprise syringes and needles, a selection of drugs to be administered including diazepam, benzodiazepine antagonists (Anexate, flumazenil), morphine, adrenaline, lignocaine, atropine, verapamil, plasma expanders and hydrocortisone, together with intravenous cannulae, intravenous giving sets, bandages and adhesive plasters. Simple disposable airways are valuable, and an Ambu-type positive pressure resuscitator is worth having. Where funds permit, and particularly where regular surgery sessions are undertaken, additional resuscitation equipment such as electric suction, electrocardiographic (ECG) machines, oxygen giving sets and cardiac defibrillators are a good idea, even though the need for any of them hardly ever arises. In general practice it would be difficult to justify the purchase of such items as cardiac defibrillators, but this type of equipment is often donated by charitable organizations or groups of patients, and the possession of more sophisticated types of resuscitation equipment adds greatly to the practitioner's (and patient's) peace of mind (Figs 3.20–3.22).

Figure 3.20 (a) Resuscitation equipment should always be available. This figure shows a combined cardiac monitor and cardiac defibrillator (Physio Lifepak 5). (b) Contents of a simple resuscitation box. Main drugs, syringes, etc., are kept separately.

Figure 3.21 Portable resuscitation kits have the added advantage that they can be taken to the patient's home in addition to use at the surgery.

Figure 3.22 Adequate suction equipment is valuable (Chas F. Thackray).

3.8 STERILIZERS

Some means of sterilizing or disinfecting instruments and equipment should be included in the minor operating theatre. In recent years there has been a trend towards Central Sterile Supplies Department (CSSD) packs, where the instruments are cleaned, prepared and packed at a central sterilizing department, autoclaved in sealed paper envelopes and delivered to the treatment room or surgery. Where such an arrangement can be made by the practitioner, this is ideal; every instrument is guaranteed to be sterile, together with all dressings, drapes, towels and gowns which are included in the pack. Where CSSD facilities do not exist, alternative methods can be employed.

Traditionally, the method of disinfecting instruments was by boiling in water for 5 min; however, bacterial spores and viruses may not be destroyed and thus the term sterilization should not strictly be employed. Most hot-water disinfectors have a variable heat control indicator light and thermostat together with trays to hold instruments. Alternatively, a dry-heat oven may be employed, heating the instruments to 160°C (320°F) for 1 h; this is better than boiling, but has the disadvantage that plastics, paper drapes and dressings tend to be damaged. Where heat cannot be used for certain instruments such as fibre-optic cables and endoscopes, soaking in a solution of glutaraldehyde is acceptable.

Perhaps the most efficient method of sterilizing instruments in a small treatment room is by using a small portable autoclave (Fig. 3.23). These use the same principle as the larger hospital equipment, i.e. steam under pressure resulting in temperatures of 136°C (277°F) under a pressure of 30 lb/in^2 (207 kN/m^2) for 2.5 min. This destroys all known organisms and can be used for most instruments. However, it has the disadvantage that instruments cannot be packed with dressings and drapes inside a sealed paper envelope as the smaller machines do not have a vacuum cycle to extract all of the air.

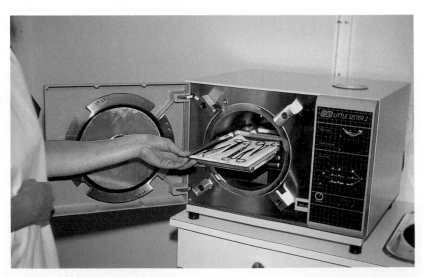

Figure 3.23 Instruments being loaded into 'Little Sister Mk II' autoclave.

Figure 3.24 Liquid nitrogen cryosurgical equipment; may be used as either cryoprobe or cryospray.

3.9 THE CRYOPROBE

In recent years there has been a renewed interest in cryotherapy, where superficial lesions are destroyed by freezing. The common cryogens are carbon dioxide, nitrous oxide and liquid nitrogen. The carbon dioxide and nitrous oxide equipment may be kept on the premises for immediate use. Liquid nitrogen on the other hand gives better results for many skin lesions, but some means of storage in a vacuum flask has to be arranged and where this is not available, small quantities of liquid nitrogen need to be collected in advance. This has the slight disadvantage that patients need to be booked in advance for a session (Fig. 3.24).

3.10 USE OF ENTONOX

An Entonox giving set is a very useful additional piece or equipment for any minor operating theatre. Originally designed for the relief of pain during labour, the equipment may be used for both adults and children in uncomfortable or painful procedures. Consciousness is not lost, the gas is self–administered and recovery is rapid (Fig. 3.25).

3.11 DISINFECTANT DISPENSERS

Surgical scrub solutions are recommended for routine washing and hand-scrubbing before each operation, the two most commonly used agents being Hibiscrub (chlorhexidine gluconate 4% in detergent base) and Betadine surgical scrub (povidone–iodine 7.5% in detergent base). Each is supplied in a standard container which may be affixed to a wall-mounted dispenser, usually provided free of charge by the manufacturers.

Figure 3.25 Entonox (50:50 nitrous oxide:oxygen) is valuable for pain relief for procedures such as incision of abscesses, injections and painful dressings.

3.12 SYRINGES AND NEEDLES

Standard 1, 2, 5, 10 and 20 ml syringes with Luer fittings are needed for local anaesthetics, intravenous drugs and sclerotherapy of varicose veins. Three standard-size Luer fitting needles are recommended: 25 swg × 5/8 in. (0.5 × 16 mm), 23 swg × 1 in. (0.6 × 25 mm) and 21 swg × 1½ in. (0.8 mm × 40 mm). In addition, a standard dental syringe and 30 swg × ¾ in. (0.3 × 19 mm) needle will be found to be invaluable for giving local anaesthetics in fingers and toes, and particularly for children. Dental cartridges of local anaesthetic can be quickly inserted in the syringe, and as nearly a painless injection as is possible can be made.

3.13 TOURNIQUETS

Where a bloodless operating field is required, such as for ingrowing toe-nails, excision of ganglia, removal of foreign bodies, or exploration a tourniquet is required. For fingers and toes, this need only be a length of rubber tubing, rubber strip, a wide rubber band, or even a surgical rubber glove with the tip cut off and rolled down the digit. However, for a whole limb, a proper orthopaedic tourniquet should be used (Fig. 3.26).

Figure 3.26 Orthopaedic pneumatic tourniquet; this is better than a blood-pressure sphygmomanometer if regional intravenous anaesthesia is undertaken.

3.14 'SHARPS' CONTAINERS

Needles, broken glass ampoules and other 'sharps' need to be disposed of safely. They should be placed in a cardboard or plastic receptacle such as a 'burn-bin', which is subsequently incinerated (Fig. 3.3).

3.15 CLINICAL WASTE DISPOSAL

Blood-stained and contaminated dressings and paper drapes can be collected in plastic bin-liners for eventual disposal by incineration (Fig. 3.2). Most local authorities provide special clinical waste-disposal sacks and arrange for regular collection.

3.16 HOT-AIR HAND DRIERS

Unless the doctor uses separate sterile paper towels with each instrument pack, there is a possible risk of cross-infection and contamination from hand towels. A simple method for drying hands after washing is to use an electric wall-mounted hot-air hand drier. Slight disadvantages are the noise and the small risk of airborne droplet infection.

Labels within figure:
Mobile equipment
Weighing machine
TREATMENT
ADMINISTRATION & COUNSELLING
Clinical basin
Couch
UTILITY
Preparation
Worktop
Refrigerator

Figure 3.27 Where space permits improved minor surgery facilities may be offered by dividing the space into three separate areas as shown.

3.17 ALTERNATIVE LAYOUTS FOR MINOR OPERATING THEATRES

Where new premises are being designed, and where there are sufficient funds and space available, much improved minor operating facilities may be considered. There is much to commend dividing the total floor area into three separate areas, namely: 1. administration and counselling; utility and preparation; and treatment. This division provides extra comfort for the patient, relatives and nurses, allows all the paperwork to be done away from the treatment area, allows more than one patient to be treated simultaneously, allows instruments and trolleys for the next case to be prepared outside the main treatment room area, and reduces the risks of cross-infection (Fig. 3.27).

3.18 FIRST-AID BOX

It is often forgotten that, under the Health and Safety (First Aid) Regulations 1981, even doctors' surgeries need to have first-aid provisions. There should be a nominal appointed person to take charge of any accident, to ensure that it is reported and recorded, and a simple first-aid box installed in the building. It is not a good idea to rely on treatment room first-aid supplies.

The first-aid box should contain:

- a guidance card on resuscitation
- individually wrapped sterile adhesive dressings
- triangular bandages
- medium-sized sterile wound dressings
- large sterile wound dressing
- safety pins
- sterile eye-pads and bandages

First-aid boxes should not contain medications of any kind.

3.19 COMPARISON OF DIFFERENT INSTRUMENTS

There are now several instruments on the market which offer to treat skin lesions successfully – cryosurgery, electrocautery, hyfrecation and radiosurgery (plus laser for those who can afford it) – and it can be quite difficult for a practitioner to decide which instrument will be the best for his or her situation (Tables 3.1 and 3.2).

3.19.1 Cryosurgery

Liquid nitrogen will treat most superficial skin lesions including viral warts. Results are good, cryobiopsies can be obtained for histology, there is minimal scarring and most treatments are given without prior anaesthesia, although it can be quite painful and unacceptable to young children. More than one treatment may need to be given and supplies of liquid nitrogen need to be available easily. Maintenance costs are minimal and running costs are just the cost of the liquid nitrogen. The equipment is very portable and may be taken to the patient's home.

Table 3.1 Comparison of cryotherapy, electrocautery, diathermy and radio-surgery and the different characteristics of each.

Table 3.1 Comparison of cryotherapy, electrocautery, diathermy and radiosurgery and the different characteristics of each

Characteristic	Cryosurgery	Cautery	Hyfrecator	Radiosurgery	Scalpel
Cutting	No	Yes	No	Yes	Yes
Control of bleeding	No	Yes	Yes	Yes	No
Ability to obtain biopsies	Yes	Yes	No	Yes	Yes
Self-sterilizing	No	Yes	No	Yes	No
Production of sterilized cut	No	Yes	No	Yes	No
Healing time	Same	Same	Same	Same	Same
Production of scar tissue	No	Yes	Little	No	Yes
Ability to plane soft tissue	No	No	No	Yes	Yes
Initial costs	+++	++	+++	++++	+
Running costs	+	+	+	++	+
Need for local anaesthesia	No	Yes	Yes	Yes	Yes

Table 3.2 Comparison of cryotherapy, electrocautery, diathermy and radiosurgery in the treatment of different skin lesions

Uses	Cryosurgery	Cautery	Hyfrecator	Radiosurgery	Scalpel
Intradermal naevi	Yes	Yes	Yes	Yes	Yes
Spider veins	No	Yes	Yes	Yes	No
Viral warts	Yes	Yes	Yes	Yes	Rarely
Ingrowing toe-nails	Some	No	Some	Yes	Yes
Keratoses	Yes	Yes	Yes	Yes	Yes
Basal cell carcinoma	Yes	Yes	Yes	Yes	Yes
Skin tags	Some	Yes	Some	Yes	Yes
Keratoo-acanthoma	Yes	Yes	Yes	Yes	Yes
Molluscum contagiosum	Yes	Yes	Yes	Yes	No
Pyogenic granuloma	Some	Yes	Yes	Yes	No
Seborrhoeic warts	Yes	Yes	Yes	Yes	Yes
Cervical erosions	Yes	Yes	Yes	Yes	No

3.19.2 Electrocautery

The small, hand-held, cordless rechargeable cautery is an ideal instrument to start minor surgery. It can both cut and coagulate, is immediately available and can be used for the removal of most skin lesions, either alone or with a curette or scalpel. Local anaesthesia is necessary for many lesions. Maintenance costs are minimal and, with care, the burners last for years. Running costs are also minimal, only the cost of electricity to recharge the batteries – and one single rechargeable cell needs replacing after several years of use. Electrocautery produces thermal damage to delicate tissues with some degree of scarring. Histological specimens may be obtained in most cases. The equipment is very portable and may be taken to the patient's home. Burners are self-sterilizing. One disadvantage is the smell of burning and the use of an extractor fan is advisable.

3.19.3 Hyfrecator

This is very useful instrument which is ideal for treating all superficial skin lesions, including keratoses, angioma, warts, molluscum, Bowen's and basal cell carcinomata. Local anaesthesia is necessary for all but the smallest lesions. Thermal damage occurs with consequent mild scarring. The electrodes are not self-sterilizing. It is excellent for vascular lesions and for haemostasis and epilation. The disadvantages include difficulty in obtaining specimens for histology and the smell of burning, so a good extractor fan or vacuum extractor unit is advisable. Maintenance and running costs are minimal, consisting only of the occasional replacement of flexible leads. The equipment is portable and may be taken to the patient's home.

3.19.4 Radiosurgery

This combines both cutting and coagulation. There is minimal thermal damage to tissues and excellent cosmetic results are achieved with virtually no scarring. Lesions may be 'planed' down to skin level. There is minimal postoperative pain with rapid healing. Local anaesthesia is needed for most lesions. Specimens may be obtained for histology. Electrodes are self-sterilizing. Maintenance costs are minimal, mainly the cost of replacing wire electrodes and flexible cables. Running costs are also minimal, only the cost of electricity used. The smell of burning is more pronounced than with electrocautery or diathermy so a good extractor fan and vacuum extractor unit are necessary. The equipment is semiportable and may be taken to the patient's home.

3.20 MONITORING OF VITAL SIGNS DURING OPERATIONS

For the majority of minor operations, done on fit healthy young adults under local anaesthesia, there is no need to monitor vital signs, but

Figure 3.28 Welch Allyn vital signs monitor.

Figure 3.29 Welch Allyn 'Atlas monitor'.

where intravenous sedation is used, or the patient is elderly, frail or on complex medication, has cardiac or respiratory problems or is particularly anxious, regular monitoring of pulse, blood pressure, oxygen saturation and possibly ECG is an added safeguard and is recommended (Figs 3.28 and 3.29). This is also useful if a particular operation is likely to take longer than average. It is essential that the doctor and all nursing staff are familiar with the instruments and aware of their limitations, and can take appropriate action if problems arise. As with all medical equipment, but even more so with these types of monitor, they should be regularly checked, calibrated and serviced by qualified personnel.

3.21 TAPE OR CD PLAYER TO PROVIDE MUSIC

For many patients, there is no such thing as a minor operation. For them, it is a major event and can create considerable anxiety. The playing of relaxing music quietly in the background can be of immense benefit for both patient and staff. This can be in the form of a standard tape player or CD player. Some doctors provide a personal stereo and ask the patients to bring along one of their favourite tapes.

The role of the practice nurse/ operating theatre assistant

For all but the most minor procedures, an assistant is advisable, and in many cases essential for the smooth running of the procedure, and for the safety and comfort of the patient. In most situations this person will be the practice nurse or operating theatre assistant. Their role is vital and becoming increasingly skilled. The majority will have a nursing training with additional skills in minor surgery and the care of instruments together with sterilizing procedures. There is also an added advantage if the same operating team of doctor and nurse works regularly together so that the individual preferences and surgical techniques of the doctors are known in advance.

4.1 MANAGEMENT OF THE TREATMENT ROOM/ MINOR OPERATING THEATRE

The nurse should be responsible for supervising and ensuring adequate cleaning of all floors, walls, working surfaces and operating theatre lights, and reporting any defects or faults. He or she should also choose suitable dressing trolleys (a minimum of two is essential) and ensure that they run smoothly and have easily cleaned surfaces (stainless steel or plate glass). There should be a suitable operating-theatre table or couch which is fully adjustable and which has the ability to raise or lower, as well as tilt head downwards in the case of a patient who feels faint. This needs to be movable and ideally positioned with a clear margin on all sides. If patients are going to be left on this couch after their operation, some form of restraint such as side-rails should be provided to prevent the patient falling off the couch and injuring themselves.

Figure 4.1 An ultrasonic cleaning bath. This is an excellent method of keeping surgical instruments clean prior to sterilizing.

4.2 STERILIZING INSTRUMENTS

As mentioned in Chapters 2, 3, 5 and 6 it is essential to guarantee sterile instruments; this may be achieved by a portable autoclave or by using sterilizing facilities at a local hospital. Where an autoclave is used, a regular contract for servicing must be taken out to meet Health and Safety regulations. It is also a good idea to have some means of checking temperature and sterilizing conditions within the autoclave such a test-paper which will change colour when the correct temperature has been reached. Autoclaves are not washing machines, so only clean instruments should be put in for sterilizing (Fig. 4.1), and it is also necessary to regularly clean the inside of the sterilizing chamber regularly, as well as the distilled water containers.

4.3 SUPPLIES

4.3.1 Sterile supplies manager

One of the most useful contacts for the practice nurse will be the local or district hospital sterile supplies department manager. This person will have access to surgical instrument suppliers, and in many cases will be able to obtain new instruments at a better discount than the doctor can obtain. They will also be able to make arrangements for the sterilizing of any instrument packs, and for a reliable, efficient delivery and collection service. By using the sterile supplies department, supplies of sterile linen drapes, dressings, gloves and sutures can be obtained at a very reasonable cost.

4.3.2 Stock control

The practice nurse or operating theatre assistant is probably in the best position to check supplies of sutures, dressings, anaesthetics, dressing packs and instrument packs, and to reorder when supplies are running low.

4.4 TIME MANAGEMENT

4.4.1 Planned sessions

Planned operating sessions are preferable to random fitting-in during normal surgery times. They are a better use of time and more efficient, and less time is wasted trying to synchronize both doctor and nurse appointments. A planned session also enables the nurse/assistant to prepare the room in advance for each procedure and to check essential equipment. It also reduces the risk of possible cross-infection if the previous patient has had an infected lesion which needed dressing.

4.4.2 Protected time

Some 'protected time' is essential for cleaning and restocking the treatment room. It also allows for the unexpected emergency and encourages safe practice.

4.5 DOCUMENTATION

4.5.1 Recording

It is good practice to send every specimen for routine histological examination, and to this end the name, address and date of birth of every patient, together with the nature of the specimen, should be entered in a record book such as a histology register. Ideally, this should be done at the time of the operation, or immediately afterwards. As the histology results are returned, these must be entered in this book, and any omissions noted and acted upon promptly.

4.5.2 Postoperative information leaflets

These should be readily available and may be given to each patient at the end of their operation. The nurse/assistant should check regularly that there are sufficient supplies and that each is still up-to-date with current practice.

4.6 NURSE–PATIENT RELATIONSHIP

4.6.1 Reassurance

There is no such thing as a 'minor operation' as far as the patient is concerned. Most are extremely anxious and will welcome reassurance from the practice nurse/operating theatre room assistant. The patient will greatly appreciate such courtesies as introducing members of the team when the patient arrives, explaining what is going to happen, how long the procedure is expected to take, what time they will be ready to go home, the form of anaesthetic and/or sedation to be used, any unfamiliar equipment such as a radio-surgery unit, fibre-optic instruments, or any electronic monitoring procedures, asking whether they have any questions or concerns, and general reassurance. Where there is a language barrier, the use of a translator will also be appreciated.

4.6.2 Recovery and after-care

The nurse should be responsible for giving the patient all information leaflets postoperatively, and for making any follow-up appointments for suture removal or dressings. The patient should also know that they are free to contact the nurses at any time during the postoperative period if they have any concerns, and may have any dressings checked during that time if necessary.

4.7 ASSISTING AT OPERATIONS

4.7.1 Positioning the patient on the operating table or couch

Both the patient and surgeon must be comfortable during any operation. For the majority of surgical procedures, it is better to have the patient lying down rather than sitting upright to reduce the possibility of fainting. Lesions on the face, the front of body and the limbs can be treated with the patient lying comfortably on their back, with the head supported by a pillow. However, lesions on the back of the head, back, buttocks, thighs and the back of the lower limbs mean that the patient may have to lie face downwards. In this situation it is worth spending a little time making the patient completely comfortable in this position, as well as giving best exposure of the lesion to be treated, without causing undue tension on the skin in any direction. The practice nurse can ensure that the patient is in the best position, and can also check at regular intervals that no discomfort is present. Additional pillows or supports are helpful when it is necessary to have the patient in the semiprone position, or on their side. At this stage it may be necessary to shave any hair in the operation site, or clip a few strands of hair from the scalp to expose an underlying sebaceous cyst, and then to apply any skin antiseptic if this is routinely used.

4.7.2 Preparing anaesthetics

Almost all minor operations will be done using local anaesthetics, and each surgeon will have preferred anaesthetic agents and means of administration. The practice nurse/assistant will be aware of this, and will be able to prepare any ampoules, syringes and needles, intravenous cannulae and dressings. For simple infiltration anaesthesia to the skin, many doctors are happy for their assistant to perform this while they are scrubbing up, which will save time. In any event, where local anaesthetics are used, particularly those with added adrenaline, it is vital that both doctor and nurse check that the correct solution is being administered, and that the maximum dose for that particular anaesthetic agent is not exceeded.

4.7.3 Preparing instruments and instrument packs

One of the essential roles of any practice nurse/assistant is preparing all necessary instruments and instrument packs which are likely to be used for the operation. The choice of sutures should be discussed in advance, together with dressings, dressing towels and drapes, and any postoperative dressings and bandages. Where extra-fine sutures are to be used (e.g. 6/0 or finer) it may be necessary to select a needle holder which will grip the suture material without slipping. Likewise, if above-average bleeding is anticipated, additional gauze swabs should be available. Any monitoring equipment such as a pulse oximeter, blood pressure monitor or electrocardiograph should be connected at this stage and the reasons explained to the patient.

4.7.4 Scrubbed or unscrubbed

For most minor operations it is not necessary that the assistant be scrubbed and wearing sterile gloves, but for procedures where an additional pair of hands is necessary, the nurse/assistant should scrub up and don sterile gloves exactly as the surgeon. In this situation, it might even be helpful to have a third 'unscrubbed' person within earshot in case an additional instrument, suture or anaesthetic is needed.

4.7.5 The role of the assistant during an operation

As well as reassuring the patient at all times, the nurse/assistant will be required to assist at many operations. This may involve holding simple skin retractors, applying pressure to any bleeding vessels, cutting sutures, inserting sutures if appropriate, cleaning the skin at the end of the operation, or applying skin-closure strips, aerosol skin cover, and/or dressings and bandages.

4.7.6 Role of the assistant at the completion of an operation

Following any surgical procedure, the nurse/assistant should clear away any instruments and dressings, dispose of any sharps and then escort the patient from the operating couch to an adjacent recovery area. Where any premedication drugs have been used, it is vital that the patient be kept under close observation until these have worn off and the patient is fully in control of their movements and balance.

4.7.7 Record-keeping

All specimens which have been taken must be carefully labelled with the patient's name and address, and the site of the specimen. Histology forms should be completed at this stage giving as much information as possible to the pathologist, and an entry made in the 'histology book' with similar details. Usually the surgeon will be responsible for writing details of the operation in the patient's notes, but a good practice nurse/assistant will check that this has been done.

4.7.8 At the end of the 'list'

At the end of the operating list, the practice nurse/assistant should be responsible for sorting instruments, cleaning if appropriate, packing in readiness for sending for sterilizing, and completing all paperwork, cleaning and sterilizing any surfaces which may have been contaminated, and leaving any specific advice or requests for the cleaners.

Any doctor who has been faced with a minor operation without the help of an assistant will realize what an essential role the practice nurse/assistant plays in the smooth running of this service for their patients.

Infection control

> I tried the application of carbolic acid to the wound to prevent decomposition of the blood.
>
> *Lord Joseph Lister, 1827–1912, letter dated 27 May 1866 to his father*

Infection in general practitioner (GP) minor surgery is very rare; nevertheless, unless consistently high standards of preoperative, operative and postoperative care are adopted, the incidence of infection and cross-infection will rise, producing anything from minor irritation to a major disaster.

Most cases of infection can be avoided by careful surgical technique, and meticulous attention to sterilization of instruments and dressings.

However, as well as the problems of common bacterial pathogens, doctors are now having to address the problems of methicillin-resistant *Staphylococcus aureus* (MRSA), viral agents such as hepatitis B, hepatitis C, herpes and immunodeficiency virus (HIV) infection, which may have very much more serious consequences.

Infection is also not always a one-way problem of patients infecting doctors or other patients; in a few instances an infected surgeon can infect the patient or other colleagues. It is therefore important for all involved with minor surgery to be aware of the possible causative agents of infection and to know how to avoid or treat them [4].

5.1 COMMON PATHOGENS

Bacterial pathogens include staphylococci and streptococci and are responsible for the majority of cases of cellulitis and abscesses seen on the skin. Most respond to appropriate antibiotics such as flucloxacillin. Abscesses in the perineal area are frequently infected with anaerobic and mixed organisms; in these situations metronidazole or similar antibiotics may be necessary.

Where infection is suspected, a bacterial swab should be taken: this will often be helpful in ascertaining whether the infective agent was present before or after the surgical treatment, and will also guide the doctor to the most appropriate treatment.

Fungal infection of toe-nails and finger-nails may be easily recognized by sending nail clippings or even the complete nail for mycology. Such action may avoid the need for surgery and establish a definitive diagnosis.

Candida infections are generally not seen in minor surgery, and if so are readily treated with any of the antimycotic agents.

5.2 HEPATITIS VIRUSES

5.2.1 Hepatitis B (serum hepatitis)

This is one of the most infective viruses, causing serious illness. It may be transmitted from patient to patient by as little as 0.0001 ml of infected blood. The virus remains active for up to 6 months in dried blood, consequently, instruments which have been poorly cleaned or disinfected may be responsible for infecting other patients, whilst poor surgical technique may result in the doctor becoming infected from the patient, or vice versa.

It has been estimated that there are possibly 200 million carriers of hepatitis in the world, representing up to 20% of the population in African, Pacific and other tropical countries, and 0.5% of the population in northern Europe. Thus, statistically the doctor has a 1 in 200 chance of treating a hepatitis B carrier.

Worse still, if the doctor becomes accidentally infected with the hepatitis B virus, not only may the disease develop but the doctor may become a hepatitis B carrier and be a serious risk to patients.

For this reason, every doctor and nurse undertaking minor surgery should have a full course of hepatitis B vaccine and a follow-up blood test to confirm immunity. It is probably good practice to be retested after 5 years to confirm continued protection.

5.2.2 Hepatitis C

Hepatitis C has recently been isolated as another blood-borne virus, capable of causing liver cirrhosis and liver failure. At the present time there is no vaccine available to protect against this organism.

5.3 HIV INFECTION

The acquired immune deficiency syndrome (AIDS) was first described in 1981 and the human immunodeficiency virus (HIV) was first identified in 1983. Also in 1983 the receptor cell for the virus was identified as the CD4 or T-helper cell. Antibody tests were subsequently developed which revealed the HIV status of the individual. In 1986 a second strain, HIV-2, was isolated.

Like hepatitis B, the virus is present in blood and body fluids, but unlike hepatitis B is relatively easily destroyed outside the body and is not as infectious as the hepatitis B virus. Infection of the surgeon can occur from contamination from infected blood or body fluids, either through an open wound, from aerosol sprays, or from a puncture wound or needle-stick injury.

Following infection there is an asymptomatic period during which antibody to the virus is not yet present in the blood, and thus HIV tests will be negative. After approximately 6 months the infected individual may seroconvert and the HIV antibody may be detected. A high proportion will then progress to develop AIDS.

A common presenting feature in AIDS sufferers is Kaposi's sarcoma, with an incidence of between 25% and 50%. Biopsy of such lesions may be the first contact the doctor has with this disease as far as minor surgery is concerned. Kaposi's sarcomas present as pink to purple blotches like a bruise or blood blister. They may be flat or raised. They are skin cancers arising from the endothelial cells such as those lining blood vessels. Histologically, malignant transformation causes the endothelial cells to become stippled with spindle-shaped tumour cells; lymphatic obstruction may occur, but they do not metastasize, and remain multifocal, both on the skin and in the alimentary tract.

Despite the worry of surgeons about risks of infection, these remain small. Surgeons have been shown to contaminate themselves with blood in 8.7% of cases and sustain penetrating injuries in 1.7% cases, yet statistically the risk of seroconversion for a surgeon is one infection every 8 years in a high-risk area with a caseload of 15 000 patients per year, and as small as one infection every 80 years in a low-risk area. Thus, the risk to the GP minor surgeon is exceptionally low.

5.4 INFECTION CONTROL GUIDELINES

Where the doctor suspects or knows that the patient may be HIV positive, additional infection control protocols are carried out. This may not be entirely logical, and it is better to assume that every patient is potentially infectious, and to use the same standards of care and sterility throughout. In this way the unsuspected HIV-positive patient will not put either the doctor, the staff or other patients at risk. As a general guide, therefore, the following procedures would seem to be reasonable.

- For all patients the doctor should wear latex/vinyl gloves and a plastic apron for all procedures in which exposure to blood and/or body fluids is anticipated.
- All sharps must be discarded into a good-quality plastic sharps container. Needles must never be resheathed after use. Syringes should not be broken, but syringe and needle discarded in one piece. Where the needle needs to be removed, a pair of forceps or needle-holding device should be used. The sharps container must be incinerated.
- Specimens from patients infected with HIV or hepatitis should be placed in a sealed plastic bag and marked with warning tape.
- Contaminated dressings and waste material should be placed in a yellow plastic bag for incineration via the local Environmental Health Department.
- Any linen contaminated with blood or body fluids should be handled with gloves, and washed in a washing machine at the highest temperature setting.
- To deal with any spillage of blood or body fluids, one should wear an apron, and gently pour undiluted Milton or similar

hypochlorite bleach over the spillage, cover with paper towels, leave for 30 min and wipe up with disposable towels. Alternatively, granular sodium dichlorisocyanate (Na DCC), e.g. Presept granules, may be sprinkled over the spillage and wiped up with paper towels or a disposable cloth.

- Any cuts or abrasions should be covered with a waterproof dressing.

5.5 PROCEDURES IN THE CASE OF ACCIDENTAL CONTAMINATION

Should the operator or assistant be accidentally contaminated, e.g. needlestick injury, the site of entry should be immediately encouraged to bleed, should be thoroughly washed with warm, soapy water, and a sterile dressing applied. An entry should be made in the accident or infection book, with the date, circumstances, names of those present, name of the patient, nature of accident and eventual outcome.

5.6 INFECTION BOOK

A separate infection book is a good idea: all cases of infection should be recorded, particularly the postoperative infection rate. Only by recording every case of infection can an accurate audit be made, and if the rate is unacceptable, steps taken to improve it.

CHAPTER

Sterilizing and disinfecting instruments

> In the course of the year 1864 I was much struck with an account of the remarkable effects produced by Carbolic Acid upon the sewage of the town of Carlisle, destroying the entozoa which usually infest cattle fed upon such pastures.
>
> *Lord Joseph Lister, 1827–1912*

Sterilization is the destruction of all living organisms. Contrary to popular belief an item may only be sterile or non-sterile – it cannot be nearly sterile. Disinfection, by contrast, is the reduction of a population of pathogenic micro-organisms without achieving sterility. Not all bacterial spores are destroyed. There are five methods of sterilizing or disinfecting instruments in general practice:

- antiseptic solutions
- boiling
- hot-air ovens
- autoclave
- use of central sterile supplies department (CSSD) facilities.

6.1 ANTISEPTIC SOLUTIONS

Traditionally, 70% alcohol was the solution most widely used, subsequently with the addition of 0.5% chlorhexidine. This is widely used for emergency disinfection of surgical instruments requiring only 2 min immersion. Where instruments are left for longer periods or stored continuously, the addition of one tablet of sodium nitrite BPC 1 g will prevent rusting. As the tablet dissolves over several days, another is added.

The aldehydes are powerful disinfectors and sterilizers. A solution containing 2% glutaraldehyde will disinfect instruments if they are soaked for 10 min, and sterilize if left soaking for 10 h. The disadvantages are that the solution needs to be fresh and it can cause staining if left on the skin.

6.2 BOILING

This is still the most widely used method of disinfecting instruments in the world; it is simple, quick and reasonably effective, but will not

Figure 6.1 Electric boiling water disinfector with thermostat and removable tray.

destroy certain bacterial spores and certain viruses. Normally, instruments are cleaned and then boiled for 5 min (100°C or 212°F). It is not suitable for dressings, drapes or paper (Fig. 6.1).

6.3 HOT-AIR OVENS

These are thermostatically controlled ovens with an electric heating element, similar to a domestic electric oven. Instruments to be sterilized are heated to 160° C (320° F) for 1 h. Sterilization is achieved, but it is not suitable for rubber, plastic or, to a lesser extent, paper items (Fig. 6.2).

Figure 6.2 Hot-air oven.

Figure 6.3 (a) Portable autoclave 'Little Sister 3'. (b) Portable autoclave 'Instaclave' (Prospect Medical).

6.4 AUTOCLAVES

Now considered to be the most efficient method of sterilizing instruments, packs and dressings, and suitable for most materials, an autoclave is basically a pressure cooker, and there is no reason why a domestic pressure cooker should not be used to sterilize instruments. The small autoclaves produced for the doctor's surgery offer a choice of temperatures, pressures and sterilizing times: typically, a quick cycle would heat the water to 134°C (273°F) for 3.5 min under a pressure of 30 1b/in^2 (207 kN/m^2) whereas a slower cycle, more suitable for plastics, would heat the water to 115°C (239°F) under a pressure of 10 1b/in^2 (69 kN/m^2). In practice, instruments are placed in the trays, and the autoclave is turned on and left for the desired time. At the end of the cycle, the instruments are ready for use. The main disadvantage of the smaller autoclave is that instrument packs cannot be sterilized as there is no vacuum cycle to extract air and dry the packs. However, most materials including rubber, plastics and metal can be readily sterilized, the only exception being sealed containers (Fig. 6.3a, b).

6.5 GUIDELINES FOR SELECTING STERILIZERS

The British Medical Association Board of Science and Education has reviewed the guidance issued by the Department of Health on sterilization and disinfection procedures in general practice [5]. To achieve sterilization using saturated steam (i.e. autoclaving) they recommended 2.2 bar pressure at 121°C for 15 min or 134°C for 3 min. Similarly, using dry heat, they recommended 160°C for 60 min holding time, or 180°C for 30 min.

It is important to re-emphasize that small portable autoclaves used in the general practitioner's (GP's) surgery will only process unwrapped instruments for immediate use, and are not suitable for sterilizing instruments wrapped in any packaging, or for dressings and towels. It is also important to note that sealed containers containing fluids should never be put in a portable autoclave because of the risk of explosion.

Features to look for in the selection of an autoclave in general practice are:

- a preset automatic cycle
- safety interlocks which prevent opening during a sterilizing cycle
- thermocouple entry for testing
- visible instrumentation, giving temperature and pressure readings
- some means of monitoring the sterilising cycle
- cycle/stage fault indicators
- a cycle counter
- empty-chamber performance
- full-load performance
- water reservoir temperature
- safety cut outs
- the ability to sterilize despite cycle interruption
- surface temperature
- electrical safety
- low price.

All sterilizers should be commissioned before use, and regular maintenance carried out by a qualified engineer, recording the dates and results of tests in a hardback book.

It would be a good idea for a doctor to seek written assurance from the supplier that their autoclave meets the recommendations and complies with the British Standards.

6.6 USE OF CSSD FACILITIES

Most hospitals in Europe and North America now use large autoclaves for all routine instrument sterilization. As well as superheated water under pressure, the large machines have two vacuum cycles, a prevacuum pulsing stage which removes air from the load, ensuring efficient steam penetration, and a postvacuum pulse stage which ensures a dry sterile load at the end of the cycle. Thus, dressings, drapes, gowns, sheets and instrument packs can be sterilized and dried at the same time. In practice, instruments are prepacked in plastic or foil trays, together with any selected dressings and drapes, these are then enclosed in a paper envelope which is closed with a heat-sensitive autoclave adhesive tape, and the whole is enclosed in an outer paper envelope, similarly closed with the autoclave marking tape. This tape changes colour if the desired sterilizing conditions have been reached and affords a visible proof of sterilization. This type of autoclave offers the best method of sterilization, and it is well worth the practitioner making arrangements, if at all possible, with a CSSD. Not only will the GP's instruments and drapes be sterilized, but each will be cleaned and repacked in a sterile envelope ready for future use. Such packs may be stored at the surgery and either used on the premises or taken to the patient's home if needed for such conditions as draining malignant abdominal ascites or a minor operation on a housebound patient.

6.7 IMPROVISED METHODS OF STERILIZATION

There will be occasions when the doctor will not have access to CSSD facilities, hot-air ovens or autoclaves, as a result either of

Figure 6.4   'Prestige' autoclaves.

location or failure of existing equipment. Under these circumstances it is possible to improvise techniques for sterilizing instruments as follows.

6.7.1 Hot-air oven

Instruments placed in a metal biscuit tin in a domestic oven and heated to 160°C for 1 h or 180°C for 0.5 h will be adequately sterilized in the majority of cases.

6.7.2 Domestic pressure cooker

Satisfactory sterilization of instruments may be obtained using a domestic pressure cooker, which works on the same principle as an autoclave, i.e. superheated water under pressure. Indeed, one manufacturer of a domestic pressure cooker has produced an autoclave by simple modification (Fig. 6.4).

In general, 15 min at the highest pressure is adequate. For added reassurance, testing strips may be included with the instruments to indicate that sterilizing conditions have been met.

CHAPTER 7

Assessment, preoperative preparation and skin preparation

One of the great advantages of general practitioner minor surgery is that the patient is frequently very well known to the doctor. The latter will therefore be fully aware of the patient's medical condition and what medication, if any, he or she is taking.

It is important to ascertain any relevant past problems with either local anaesthetics, dressings, plaster or skin antiseptics, particularly any known sensitivities.

Of particular relevance is the patient's current medication, especially anticoagulant therapy, and drugs which could react with local anaesthetics such as the tricyclic antidepressants. Also of great importance is any condition which may jeopardize healing, such as a poor peripheral circulation, diabetes, scleroderma, polyarteritis, reduced immunity or a tendency to produce keloid reactions.

At the initial assessment and consultation, a full explanation must be given to the patient of what to expect. It is still surprising to find patients who believe that an operation will leave no scar! The type of scar, its length and situation needs to be discussed, along with any possible complications which could arise. It is wise to record in the medical notes that this information has been given to the patient.

For many procedures skin preparation is probably not necessary; the removal of small skin tags with the electrocautery is certainly better done without applying any antiseptic solution to the skin; indeed, if the electrocautery or diathermy is used shortly after applying an inflammable antiseptic such as alcohol or ether, serious burns could ensue. In any case, the temperature of the electrocautery wire is sufficiently high to sterilize the tissue during use. Similarly, operations on or near the eye are best performed without any prior disinfection of the skin or conjunctive, and rarely does one see any infection.

For the majority of other minor operations some form of skin antiseptic is used; many commercially prepared solutions are available, containing either chlorhexidine 0.5% in isopropyl alcohol (Hibisol; ICI) or povidone–iodine 10% alcoholic solution (Betadine alcoholic solution: Napp). Coloured solutions have the added advantage that the operator can readily see where the antiseptic has been applied. As there are so many preparations are available, the final choice depends on the preference of the individual doctor. Each antiseptic solution may be either painted on the skin using an absorbent swab or sprayed over the area from a pressurized applicator, or the affected part, if small enough, such as a finger or toe, may be immersed in the solution.

Removal of hair by shaving is now rarely necessary and the majority of minor surgical procedures can be performed easily without hair removal. Where sebaceous cysts occur on the head and there is much hair, cutting away the minimum amount with stitch scissors or iris scissors is all that is necessary.

Although normal surgical practice is to apply skin antiseptics only before any operation, occasionally it helps to apply a second application after the skin has been closed, before a final sterile dry dressing is applied, to reduce any bacterial colonies secreted through the pores of the skin or which have contaminated the skin, either air-borne or from the operator or assistant during the operation.

8

Anaesthesia

The powder benumbs the nerves of the tongue depriving it of feeling and taste.

Albert Niemann, first description of cocaine, 1860

Modern anaesthetics have revolutionized surgical practice, and it should now be easily possible to perform any minor operation completely painlessly. It is worth taking time to anaesthetize the area fully and to have the confidence that it has been successful: to repeatedly ask a patient 'Can you feel this?' does nothing for their confidence; they will let the operator know if they can feel any pain!

Many different techniques are available, the most widely used being infiltration; some operations such as those on the eye may require two different methods such as surface anaesthesia of the conjunctive and infiltration of the skin.

8.1 FREEZING

Most doctors have witnessed small abscesses being opened by freezing of the overlying skin with an ethyl chloride spray. Those doctors who have had such a procedure done to them will also say how ineffective it is, and how uncomfortable it is as the tissues thaw out. One suspects that most freezing was performed for the benefit of the operator and had a placebo effect at best for the patient. Ethyl chloride spray freezing was reserved mainly for incision of abscesses; if such abscesses were deeply situated it certainly would not offer much pain relief other than that achieved from the release of pus, and if very superficial probably was unnecessary as the overlying skin was now insensitive to pain. Thus, as a method of anaesthesia it tends to have been superseded by other more effective agents (Fig. 8.1).

8.2 TOPICAL OR SURFACE ANAESTHESIA

Mucous membranes fortunately absorb local anaesthetics very rapidly, efficiently, and painlessly. Thus, the cornea and conjunctive can be readily anaesthetized with local anaesthetic drops, of which there are several varieties. Lignocaine (Xylocaine, UK; Octocaine, USA) is manufactured as a 4% eye-drops solution. Individual applications of oxybuprocaine hydrochloride 0.4% (Minims Benoxinate SNP 0.4%, UK) or amethocaine hydrochloride 0.5% (Minims Amethocaine SNP

Figure 8.1 Ethyl chloride spray; suitable for incision of certain abscesses, but not very effective for the majority of procedures requiring anaesthesia.

0.5%, UK) are manufactured for once-only application. Onset of anaesthesia is rapid and lasts for up to 1 h. The number of instillations is more important than the amount administered for each instillation to achieve anaesthesia.

Similarly, the lining of the nose, buccal mucosa, larynx and pharynx, oesophagus, trachea, tympanic membrane and urethra may all be anaesthetized using topical anaesthetic preparations.

Lignocaine aerosol spray (Xylocaine spray, UK; Octocaine spray, USA) is particularly useful for the nasal cavity, pharynx, and larynx, while lignocaine sterile gel (Xylocaine gel 2%, UK; Octocaine gel 2%, USA) is extremely good for anaesthetizing the urethra.

As with all local anaesthetics, the maximum safe dose which can be given to any particular patient should be known and not exceeded; as doses for different anaesthetic agents differ, the doctor is advised to refer to the manufacturer's data sheet. The patient should be asked whether he or she is on any medication.

8.3 TOPICAL ANAESTHETIC CREAMS

In recent years, topical creams containing local anaesthetics have been introduced with the object of achieving anaesthesia of the skin. Absorption is poor under normal conditions, but by applying an occlusive dressing over the cream, and allowing 1 or 2 h for the cream to be absorbed, satisfactory anaesthesia may be obtained for many superficial procedures.

'Emla' cream containing 25 mg lignocaine and 25 mg prilocaine per gram is manufactured in 5 g tubes, as is 'Ametop' (4% Amethocaine gel), and is effective for anaesthesia of the skin prior to needle puncture or split-skin grafting. For needle puncture, 2 g is applied as a thick layer under occlusion for at least 60 min. For split-skin grafting or pinch grafting 2 g per 10 cm^2 is applied as a thick layer under occlusion for at least 120 min.

Other uses include superficial anaesthesia prior to cauterizing molluscum contagiosum. However, the cream should not be applied to open wounds or mucous membranes or to patients with atopic dermatitis. Where time permits, its most useful application is in children before needle puncture, enabling infiltration anaesthesia to be accomplished painlessly.

8.4 INFILTRATION ANAESTHESIA

Most local anaesthetic agents can be given by injection and this method of infiltration is now widely used for producing anaesthesia, particularly for minor surgery. Certain points need to be borne in mind.

■ The finer the needle, the less the discomfort. If only small volumes of local anaesthetic are needed, a sterile 1 ml diabetic syringe and attached 30 swg needle are ideal (Fig. 8.2a). A small bleb of local anaesthetic is raised in the skin initially before advancing the needle to deeper tissues.

Figure 8.2 (a) For small volumes of local anaesthetic or steroids, sterile single-use diabetic syringes and needles are ideal. (b) Posterior tibila nerve block; excellent for producing anaesthesia of the sole of the foot.

- Injection should be done slowly as the needle advances, as sudden injections of large volumes, even of local anaesthetic, cause pain.
- If possible, the solution to be injected should be at body temperature or at room temperature, as injection of ice-cold solutions taken from a refrigerator causes discomfort.
- An adequate time must be allowed for anaesthesia to develop; so often one sees a rapid injection of local anaesthetic followed immediately by a surgical procedure which can be felt by the patient, only to see full anaesthesia reached after the procedure is completed.
- Single-dose snap-open glass ampoules are preferable to multidose vials; this reduces the risk of cross-infection and reactions to the preservative.
- Only prepacked sterilized disposable syringes and needles should be used.
- Sterilized packs must not be opened until the moment of use.
- Hands should be washed clean with Hibiscrub or similar agent and thoroughly dried; wet hands increase the risk of infection.
- The doctor must not touch the needle at all, and in particular, must not guide the needle with his or her finger.
- Patients should be advised that neither they nor the doctor should talk or cough while the needle is exposed to the air and during the injection; droplet infection can occur otherwise, and for this reason it is still good practice to wear a mask, particularly if aspirating or injecting a joint.
- Where intra-articular injections are to be given, it is still a good idea to swab the skin with an antiseptic such as povidone–iodine in spirit or a similar preparation. For other superficial injections it is probably not necessary to use any skin antiseptic.
- The manufacturer's recommended dose of local anaesthetic must not be exceeded.
- Local anaesthetics with added adrenaline should be avoided, and **never** used for fingers, toes, tip of the nose, ear or penis, in case prolonged vasoconstriction results in ischaemia and gangrene.
- In a vascular area, the doctor should occasionally withdraw the plunger of the syringe to check that the needle is not inside a vein. Probably some 'reactions' and 'allergic responses' to local anaesthetics have been due to inadvertent intravenous injection of the anaesthetic with or without added adrenaline.

- Adrenaline can interreact with certain drugs such as anti-depressants: ask patients if they are taking any medication.
- Caution should be observed in patients with epilepsy.
- Weaker solutions of local anaesthetics cause less discomfort during administration.
- In the presence of infection, e.g. infected ingrowing toe-nail, greater volumes of local anaesthetic are needed owing to increased vascularity.

8.5 MECHANISM OF ACTION OF LOCAL ANAESTHETICS

Chemically, the three most widely used local anaesthetics, lignocaine, bupivacaine and prilocaine, are classified as amides. They are metabolized in the liver. The clearance rate is fastest with prilocaine, followed by lignocaine and slowest with bupivacaine. Prilocaine and bupivacaine are vasodilators, whilst lignocaine appears to have no effect on blood vessels.

It is interesting to speculate how local anaesthetic agents work: their speed of action suggests that they may prevent depolarization and thus non-conduction. Sensory fibres are blocked more rapidly than motor fibres, and their action is slower in inflamed tissues and mucous membranes.

8.6 WHICH LOCAL ANAESTHETIC?

Several well-known local anaesthetic agents are manufactured, and each gives very adequate anaesthesia. Different surveys have shown slight variations in toxicity between different local anaesthetics, but the three most widely used agents are currently lignocaine (Xylocaine, UK; Octocaine, USA) bupivacaine (Marcain, UK; Marcain, USA) and prilocaine (Citanest, UK; Xylonest, USA). Where small volumes are being used, there is little to choose between the three local anaesthetics; where intravenous injections are used, prilocaine appears to be the drug of choice at present.

Each of the above anaesthetics is also manufactured with added adrenaline as an option; this has the effect of causing localized vasoconstriction and thus prolonging the action of the anaesthetic drug. However, as previously emphasized, any of the preparations with adrenaline should be treated with great respect and should never be used for digital anaesthesia, as the constriction of digital arteries could result in gangrene of fingers or toes. This also applies to the tip of the nose, tip of the ear, or penis. For this reason, as an added safeguard, all local anaesthetics containing adrenaline should be kept separately from the plain injections, and should be clearly marked.

8.7 MAXIMUM DOSE OF LOCAL ANAESTHETICS

As a guide, the maximum safe dose of each of the three local anaesthetics is shown below for an average adult of 70 kg:

- lignocaine 200 mg
- bupivacaine 140 mg
- prilocaine 400 mg.

This represents, respectively, 20 ml of 1% lignocaine (or 40 ml of 0.5% lignocaine), 28 ml of 0.5% bupivacaine (or 56 ml of 0.25% bupivacaine) and 40 ml of 1% prilocaine (or 80 ml of 0.5% prilocaine). Dosages should be correspondingly less in the elderly, debilitated and young, and basically it should be remembered that the correct dose is the smallest dose required to produce the desired anaesthesia.

8.8 TOXICITY OF LOCAL ANAESTHETICS

The three local anaesthetic agents, lignocaine, prilocaine and upivacaine are remarkably free from side-effects, and in over 20 000 personally administered injections the author has not seen a serious reaction. Occasionally, one sees the vasovagal reaction or faint, but even these are rare if the patient is lying flat.

Nevertheless, toxic reactions have been reported and the doctor should be aware of what might be expected. Two types of reaction can occur, either stimulation or depression of the cerebral cortex and medulla respectively. Where there is stimulation the patient may feel apprehensive or dizzy, and complain of blurred vision, nausea, tremor, convulsions, and respiratory arrest. In depression of the brain, respiratory arrest, cardiovascular collapse and cardiac arrest may occur, often with little warning.

Toxic reactions are most likely to be seen if the technique of intra-venous regional anaesthesia (Bier block) is used and there is a fail-ure of both pneumatic cuffs, allowing a bolus of local anaesthetic agent into the circulation. Prilocaine can cause methaemaglobinaemia.

8.9 NERVE BLOCKS

Any nerve in the body can be 'blocked' by infiltrating local anaesthetic around it. The only caution is to ensure that the local anaesthetic is not injected into the nerve itself, which could result in permanent damage to the nerve. It is, therefore, important, if the patient complains of pain in the distribution of the nerve during injection, that the needle be withdrawn and the injection tried again in a different site.

One of the most useful nerve blocks is the posterior tibial nerve block. As a method of producing anaesthesia of the sole of the foot it is ideal, as in this area the skin is particularly thick, and injections through the horny layer cause intense pain and largely defeat any object of painless surgery. The posterior tibial nerve is a branch of the sciatic nerve; it passes down the back of the calf in company with the posterior tibial vessels to the interval between the heel and the medial malleolus where it ends under the cover of the flexor retinaculum by dividing into the medial and lateral planter nerves, which between them supply the sole of the foot. The posterior tibial nerve may be blocked as it passes behind the medial malleolus, before it divides.

8.10 TECHNIQUE OF POSTERIOR TIBIAL NERVE BLOCK

A point is chosen exactly midway between the medial malleolus and Achilles tendon at the level of the ankle, and the overlying skin painted with povidone–iodine alcoholic solution (Betadine) or similar antiseptic. A sterile syringe with 25swg needle is used to draw in 5 ml of 1% lignocaine with added adrenaline 1:200 000. A small weal of local anaesthetic is raised at the point between the medial malleolus and Achilles tendon, and then the syringe is directed at 45° in a horizontal plane, aiming the needle at the underlying bone. When this is reached, the needle is withdrawn 2 mm and the plunger gently withdrawn to check that the needle is not inside a vein. Then, 2–5 ml local anaesthetic solution is injected around the posterior tibial nerve and the needle is withdrawn (Fig. 8.2b).

Anaesthesia of the sole of the foot gradually develops over the ensuing 10 min and will last for up to 2 h. As the overlying skin at the ankle is so much softer than the horny layers on the sole of the foot, an injection may be given painlessly at this site. The method is particularly useful for suturing lacerations on the sole of the foot or for the treatment of verrucae or other intradermal lesions.

One word of caution: proprioception depends on sensory impulses received from the soles of the feet; therefore it is inadvisable to perform a posterior tibial nerve block on both feet simultaneously otherwise the patient may fall over and be unable to maintain his or her balance.

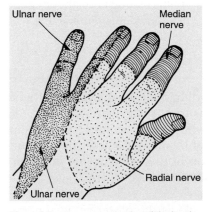

Figure 8.3 Sensory innervation of the hand.

8.11 ULNAR NERVE BLOCK

The sensory distribution of the ulnar nerve in the hand is shown in Fig. 8.3. As can be seen, only the little finger can be totally anaesthetized.

8.11.1 Technique

The ulnar nerve at the wrist lies lateral to the tendon of the flexor carpi ulnaris, which runs down the ulnar border of the arm and is inserted into the pisiform bone. The nerve can usually be palpated as it passes lateral to this tendon proximal to the pisiform bone.

Using 1% lignocaine, a small weal is raised in the overlying skin, and the needle inserted perpendicularly, lateral to the tendon over the nerve (Fig. 8.4). As the needle penetrates the deep fascia it may touch the nerve, causing paraesthesia.

Five millilitres of 1% lignocaine is now injected. The dorsal sensory branch of the ulnar nerve frequently arises proximal to this point, so in order to block this as well, a further 5 ml of 1% lignocaine is injected subcutaneously from the medial side of the level of the ulnar styloid, extending under the skin to the middle of the back of the wrist (Fig. 8.5).

Figure 8.4 Ulnar nerve block first stage (see text).

Figure 8.5 Ulnar nerve block second stage (see text).

As with other nerve blocks, sufficient time should be allowed for the local anaesthetic to be absorbed by the nerve. It is also important not to inject the anaesthetic directly into the nerve; should the patient complain of pain, the needle should be either withdrawn or repositioned and the injection reattempted.

8.12 RADIAL NERVE BLOCK

The radial nerve supplies the sensation at the back of the lateral part of the hand as shown in Fig. 8.3. It accompanies the radial artery in the forearm, and then separates about 7 cm above the wrist, passing deep to the tendon of brachioradialis muscle and subsequently dividing into digital branches.

To block the radial nerve, it is useful to identify the 'anatomical snuff-box' by fully abducting the thumb, revealing a depression over the base of the first metacarpal. This space is bounded anteriorly by the tendons of abductor pollicis longus and extensor pollicis brevis together, and posteriorly by the tendon of extensor pollicis longus.

Figure 8.6 Radial nerve block demonstrating the injection site in the 'anatomical snuff-box'.

8.12.1 Technique

Five millilitres of 1% lignocaine is used. A small weal is raised in the overlying skin and 3 ml injected subcutaneously in the anatomical snuff-box (Fig. 8.6). Then, 2 ml is injected subcutaneously over the lower end of the radius. Sufficient time (10 mins or more) is allowed for the anaesthetic to work.

8.13 MEDIAN NERVE BLOCK

The sensory distribution of the median nerve is shown in Fig. 8.3, where it can be seen to supply the palmar surface of the hand including half of the thumb, the palmar surface of the first and second fingers, and half of the palmar surface of the third finger (ring finger).

At the wrist, the median nerve lies between the flexor carpi radialis tendon laterally and the flexor digitorum sublimis and palmaris longus tendon medially.

8.13.1 Technique

The needle is inserted just lateral to the palmaris longus tendon, a weal raised in the overlying skin, and 5 ml of 1% lignocaine injected around the nerve (Fig. 8.7).

Figure 8.7 Median nerve block. The injection site is identical to that for injection of the carpal tunnel.

Sufficient time is allowed for the local anaesthetic to be absorbed (10–15 min). As with other nerve blocks it is important not to inject directly into the nerve; if pain is experienced by the patient, the doctor should withdraw and change the site of injection.

8.14 DIGITAL NERVE BLOCKS

This technique is used to anaesthetize fingers or toes. With the exception of the thumb and large toe, each digit is supplied with planter or palmer and dorsal digital nerves on each side, all of which will need to be blocked to achieve anaesthesia. The thumb and big toe have additional digital nerve branches, and these also need to be blocked for complete anaesthesia.

8.14.1 Contraindications

Adrenaline must never be used with the local anaesthetic, as vasoconstriction, ischaemia and possible gangrene can occur. Digital nerve block is contraindicated by any condition where there is reduced peripheral circulation, e.g. diabetes, Raynaud's disease, scleroderma and polyarteritis. In addition, local infiltration may only be considered if it can be given at least one phalanx distance away from any infected area.

8.14.2 Technique

Plain lignocaine without added adrenaline is used. After cleaning the skin, a weal is raised over the dorsum of the base of the proximal phalanx. The needle is now advanced, injecting as it proceeds, distributing local anaesthetic under the skin in the direction of the digital nerves. It is now nearly withdrawn and the same procedure followed on the other side.

In the case of the thumb and big toe, a 'ring block' is usually necessary, whereby the digit is encircled with a ring of local anaesthetic.

At this stage it is usual to apply a tourniquet around the base of the digit; this helps to distribute the local anaesthetic around the digital nerves and helps to prolong the action of the drug.

Where there is infection, cellulitis, or suppuration, it is frequently found to be difficult to anaesthetize a digit adequately. In such situations it is necessary to use larger amounts of local anaesthetic and to allow longer for anaesthesia to develop.

8.15 LOCAL INFILTRATION AND BLOODLESS FIELD

Where the doctor requires a bloodless field and anaesthesia in a limb, a safer alternative to a Bier's block is to infiltrate the area with local anaesthesia and then apply an orthopaedic tourniquet

Figure 8.8 Orthopaedic tourniquet applied to the upper arm over a layer of cotton wool.

and Esmarch bandage. This is particularly effective for decompression of the carpal tunnel and release of trigger finger, and exploration for foreign bodies.

8.15.1 Technique for producing anaesthesia and bloodless field in the arm

The following items are required:

- orthopaedic tourniquet
- 3 in. Esmarch bandage
- syringe and needles
- 1% lignocaine.

The orthopaedic tourniquet is applied to the upper arm over a layer of cotton wool (Fig. 8.8). The site of the operation is then anaesthetized using local infiltration of 1% lignocaine. Povidone–iodine in spirit is applied to the operation site and covered with a sterile pad. The 3 in. Esmarch bandage is then applied to the elevated limb, starting at the extremity and working proximally as far as the orthopaedic tourniquet (Fig. 8.9). At this stage the tourniquet is inflated to above arterial pressure and the Esmarch bandage released.

The operation site is now anaesthetized and bloodless.

Caution

Because the application of a tourniquet above arterial pressure can cause discomfort or even pain, it is helpful to give the patient an intravenous premeditation injection of midazolam and fentanyl before applying the tourniquet. For a fit, healthy, young adult the average doses are 4 mg midazolam and 100 µg fentanyl; these doses should be reduced proportionately in the young, elderly or frail.

8.16 ANALGESIA

In this technique the awareness of painful stimuli is reduced and the patient, although appearing to be fully conversant with what is happening, has no recollection of it afterwards. Analgesia is achieved very simply by an intravenous injection of midazolam with or without an added analgesic such as fentanyl. For the average fit, healthy adult,

Figure 8.9 Esmarch bandage applied to the elevated limb.

midazolam 2–6 mg is usually sufficient, with the dosage correspondingly reduced for younger patients and the elderly. This technique is particularly valuable for the patient with malignant ascites who requires paracentesis and who will doze throughout the procedure, and have no recollection of it afterwards. The use of a pulse oximeter will ensure that the patient is not becoming hypoxic during the operation. Where a pulse oximeter is not available, smaller doses of midazolam should be used and the patient's level of conciousness monitored. The ability to answer simple questions should indicate adequate oxygen perfusion to the brain. If there is any doubt, additional oxygen may be administered and the midazolam reversed using an intravenous injection of flumazenil.

If given at the surgery, it is wise to allow the patient to rest for 1 h afterwards and under no circumstances should they drive a car for the next 12 h.

The sedative effects of benzodiazepines can now be reversed with intravenous Flumazenil.

8.17 ENTONOX INHALATION

A mixture of equal parts of oxygen and nitrous oxide is manufactured as Entonox (British Oxygen; Nitronox, USA) and is widely used for obstetric analgesia. The apparatus is patient controlled and exceptionally safe. The giving set attaches to a cylinder of Entonox and the patient can breathe directly via a low-pressure actuating valve in the set (Fig. 8.10). It is a most valuable piece of equipment in the minor operating theatre.

Twenty breaths of the gas will enable the doctor to remove splinters from under finger-nails, incise superficial abscesses, change painful dressings and carry out painful procedures. It may also be used to reduce the pain of giving a local anaesthetic injection, particularly in the sole of the foot, a technique appreciated by children and the nervous.

Furthermore, as recovery is so rapid the patient may leave the surgery as soon as the treatment is completed and no restrictions need be imposed regarding driving or cycling home. Even quite young children can be encouraged to use the Entonox mask (Fig. 8.11).

Figure 8.10 Entonox giving set.

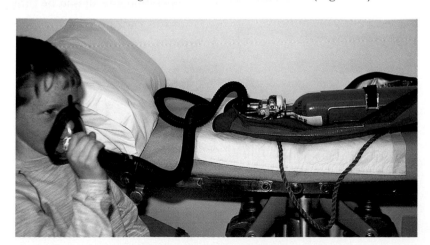

Figure 8.11 Young patient using Entonox prior to removal of a splinter under a finger-nail.

8.18 GENERAL ANAESTHESIA

Few general practitioners now give general anaesthetics outside hospital premises. This contrasts with 50 years ago when chloroform, ether, nitrous oxide and pentothal were all widely used in the patient's home and doctor's surgery. Where a practice has facilities to give general anaesthetics, a doctor with a special interest in anaesthetics, and full recovery and resuscitation equipment, there is no reason why some of the minor operations mentioned should not be done under a general anaesthetic, particularly short-acting intravenous anaesthetics for such conditions as opening abscesses or the removal of toe-nails. On the whole, however, the doctor will find that all of the minor operations described in this book can be very adequately and safely performed under local anaesthesia.

8.19 LOCAL ANAESTHETIC TECHNIQUE IN GENERAL PRACTICE

A frequent cause for discomfort to the patient is not allowing sufficient time for the local anaesthetic to work, and this applies particularly to infiltration anaesthesia and nerve blocks. The doctor can allow time for anaesthesia by giving the local anaesthetic before scrubbing up, and using a sterile, no-touch technique, as follows.

- The area to be anaesthetized is painted with povidone–iodine in spirit (Betadine alcoholic solution).
- Without donning sterile gloves, but using a no-touch technique, the operator draws local anaesthetic into a syringe.
- The needle is changed for the finest gauge consistent with the operation.
- Without touching the exact point of entry of the needle with the fingers, the doctor injects the local anaesthetic.
- The doctor may now scrub up while the assistant repaints the skin with povidone–iodine in spirit and applies any drapes.
- By the time the doctor has scrubbed up, assembled all instruments and sutures, and applied any additional sterile drapes, the operation site should be fully anaesthetized.

CHAPTER 9

Surgical techniques

> And whosoever comes suffering from sores, with wounded limbs, or with wasted bodies, he (Aesculepius) delivers them, different ones from different pains, tending some with kindly incantations, giving some soothing potions, while he set some on their feet again with the knife.
>
> *Pindar, Pythian Ode III*

One aim of each operation will be to achieve as neat a scar as possible. Many patients will expect to end up with no scar at all, and it is perhaps wise to warn them at the first consultation that it is physically not possible to achieve such a result. However, by observing a few simple rules it is possible to obtain a nearly invisible scar in most cases.

Skin is a living tissue, and must be treated gently and with respect. Good healing will only occur if the cut edges are held in exact position and under no tension. Tissues should be cut with a sharp scalpel rather than scissors, which have a shearing action. Dissection should be likewise with a sharp scalpel rather than gauze. Haemostasis should be achieved carefully, although in most minor surgical procedures this is not a major problem.

Sutures should be the finest, consistent with the ability to hold the wound together, and should be removed at the earliest opportunity (Fig. 9.1). Subcutaneous absorbable sutures should be placed as deep as possible, and be as few as possible, and the knots tied in the deeper plane. Absorbable sutures should, in general, not be used for skin where a good cosmetic result is required.

Figure 9.1 The finest gauge sutures, closely spaced together, preferably along the line of a skin crease, are used to obtain the neatest scar.

Many fine, closely positioned sutures are preferable to a few widely spaced stitches. Tissues should be handled as little as possible, and particularly not with any crushing forceps. Single skin-hooks should be used to hold or retract skin flaps. The surgeon who inserts the sutures should be the person who removes them, or at least supervises their removal. Only by personally examining each wound postoperatively can improvements in technique be achieved.

9.1 HAEMOSTASIS

Bleeding may occur from fine capillaries or visible blood vessels, either arteries or veins.

9.1.1 Fine capillaries

When any tissue is cut there is fine capillary oozing. Most of this will stop spontaneously; some will be reduced if adrenaline is included with the local anaesthetic, but in the remainder firm pressure is all that is required. However, pressure needs to be applied for a realistic time (up to 3 min in some cases) and this needs to be timed using a clock or timer. If oozing continues, the application of an alginate dressing (Kaltostat or equivalent) covered by a firm gauze and bandage will usually control the bleeding.

Unusual capillary bleeding may occur where there are coagulation defects or abnormal capillaries, e.g. the patient may be taking anti-coagulant therapy, or there may be a blood dyscrasia, or more rarely vitamin C deficiency or thrombocytopenia.

9.1.2 Visible blood vessels

Bleeding from visible blood vessels is usually more brisk than from capillaries, and often the exact source of bleeding cannot immediately be seen. In this case the application of firm pressure with a swab for 1–3 min whilst spasm of the vessel is occurring will often be all that is required.

If on carefully removing the swab a bleeding source can be identified it should be picked off with a pair of fine artery forceps. As little surrounding tissue as possible should be included in the jaws of the forceps.

Once the blood vessel has been grasped, it must then be secured by tying a fine absorbable suture around it. As the first part of the knot is tied, the forceps are gradually released, at the same time tightening the knot; the forceps are then removed. Alternatively, the vessel may be sealed using a high-frequency electric current in the form of either diathermy or radiosurgery.

If the blood vessel can be seen, and has not been divided, it may be secured by tying two ligatures around it and then dividing between them.

9.2 TISSUE HEALING

Wound healing after surgery can take a year or more to complete and involves three distinct phases: an immediate inflammatory phase taking up to 6 days when damaged blood vessels constrict, and the local immune system activates mediators to attack contaminating bacteria and remove non-viable tissue, an acute proliferative phase lasting between 3 and 24 days when fibroblasts appear and are responsible for the synthesis of collagen, and lastly a chronic remodelling phase lasting from 1 month to 1 year when collagen maturation occurs with contraction and strengthening of the scar.

For good healing to occur each surface must be cleanly cut, have a good blood supply and be in good apposition. Where a surgical incision has been made the above conditions can usually be met; however, where there is a contused traumatic wound, accurate apposition of clean healthy tissues may not be possible, and in this situation it is necessary to trim the traumatized edges with a scalpel. Similarly, any foreign bodies should be carefully removed prior to closure.

In a connective tissue injury, the blood filling the cavity forms a fibrin clot. This becomes replaced by granulation tissue, which then becomes replaced by fibroblast proliferation. Eventually, collagen fibrils form, fibrous tissue develops, and the scar becomes avascular, pale and predominantly collagen. This gradually shrinks over the ensuing months and years.

After 3 weeks, the scar reaches 20% of its ultimate strength, but it should be remembered that scar tissue never exceeds 80% of the strength of normal tissue.

Occasionally the healing process 'overshoots', producing a hypertrophic or keloid scar. This process is not fully understood, but it is known to happen more frequently in pigmented skin and in certain sites of the body, notably over the front of the sternum and shoulder, and in patients of Afro-Caribbean origin.

9.3 SURGICAL TECHNIQUE USING PIGS' TROTTERS

Whilst most doctors will have had more than adequate training in surgical techniques, nevertheless different procedures may be tried using pigs' trotters, obtainable from any butcher's shop or supermarket. The skin texture is very similar to human skin, and incisions, suturing techniques, electrocautery, cryotherapy and various alternative methods of skin closure may be practised (Fig. 9.2). Furthermore, pigs' trotters also provide an ideal medium for teaching suturing techniques to practise nurses and trainees. For radiosurgery, fresh beef-steak is ideal to practice these techniques.

9.4 SURGICAL TECHNIQUE USING SKIN SIMULATORS

Skin simulators designed to simulate conditions met in minor surgery without the use of biological material are now available. They are

Figure 9.2 Pigs' trotters may be used to practise suture technique and other minor surgical procedures.

remarkably realistic, and models of sebaceous cysts, lipoma, perianal haematoma and skin are available from Limbs and Things Ltd (Bristol, UK; Figs 9.3–9.16). Skin simulators are also available from Ethicon (Edinburgh, UK).

Figure 9.3 Model of skin with three layers – epidermis, dermis and subdermis – for practising suturing, undercutting and knot tying (Limbs and Things Ltd, Bristol, UK).

Figure 9.4 (a) Model with several layers representing different tissue planes in which a series of lumps and bumps can be inserted (Limbs and Things Ltd, Bristol, UK). (b) Model with 'lump' situated between layers, simulating a cyst (Limbs and Things Ltd, Bristol, UK)

Figure 9.5 (a) A model face with a variety of different lesions including sebaceous cyst, meibomian cyst, mucous cyst, skin tags, crusty warts, basal cell carcinoma, keratoacanthoma and malignant melanoma (Limbs and Things Ltd, Bristol, UK). (b) A realistic meibomian cyst in the lower eyelid (Limbs and Things Ltd, Bristol, UK).

Figure 9.6 (a) Model to mimic an inflamed ingrowing toe-nail. Detachable toe-ends can be inserted into the 'foot' (Limbs and Things Ltd, Bristol, UK). (b) A selection of 'toe-ends' and the 'master toe'(Limbs and Things Ltd, Bristol, UK). (c) A remarkably realistic inflamed ingrowing toe-nail (Limbs and Things Ltd, Bristol, UK).

Figure 9.7 A sebaceous cyst containing realistically unpleasant-smelling material in the centre. One must beware of puncturing it! (Limbs and Things Ltd, Bristol, UK).

Figure 9.8 A lipoma being dissected (Limbs and Things Ltd, Bristol, UK).

Figure 9.9 A model of the breast containing a simulated fibroadenoma, carcinoma and benign cyst (Limbs and Things Ltd, Bristol, UK).

Figure 9.10 (a) A highly convincing leg with varicose veins containing 'blood' and veins which collapse when the limb is elevated (Limbs and Things Ltd, Bristol, UK). (b) Practising sclerotherapy (Limbs and Things Ltd. Bristol, UK).

Figure 9.11 The use of skin staples in simulated skin (Limbs and Things Ltd, Bristol, UK).

Figure 9.12 Using a skin simulator to practise skin incisions (Limbs and Things Ltd, Bristol, UK).

Figure 9.13 Aspiration of the knee joint (Limbs and Things Ltd, Bristol, UK).

Figure 9.14 Injection of the carpal tunnel (Limbs and Things Ltd, Bristol, UK).

Figure 9.15 Injection of the tennis elbow (Limbs and Things Ltd, Bristol, UK).

Figure 9.16 Injections around the shoulder (Limbs and Things Ltd, Bristol, UK).

Incisions

> There are three ways of opening an abscess so as to give outlet to the matter: by caustic, by incision, or by the introduction of felon. The first is more agreeable to timid patients who are afraid of the pain of incision.
>
> *Encyclopaedia Britannica, 1797*

Patients judge their surgeons by the end result which can be seen, namely. the operation scar. With a little forethought and variation in technique, almost invisible scars can be produced, depending on the knowledge of certain lines on the body, first described by Langer [6] in 1861. Until that time operative incisions were made where they would be most effective to excise the pathological lesion with little regard to the resultant scar. Textbooks of plastic surgery then reproduced pictures of Langer's lines designed to give optimum healing and the neatest scars [7–9] and it was not until 1950 that some doubt was cast on this atlas of lines for incision by Smith [10] and subsequently in 1951 by Kraissl [11], who compared the traditional Langer lines with wrinkle lines or skin creases. Most wrinkle lines run perpendicular to the action of underlying muscles, and it is common experience that incisions made in these wrinkle lines give the neatest scars with minimum disruption of function. Thus, in planning the elective incision the following points should be borne in mind.

- One should look for natural creases and if possible follow these lines (Figs 10.1–10.4).
- Where there is an underlying joint the incision should be placed transversely across it to prevent loss of function.
- To demonstrate some wrinkles, the relaxed skin is gently compressed in different directions to ascertain the line, or the patient asked to contract the underlying muscles.
- In many parts of the body, traditional Langer lines are at variance with natural wrinkle lines; in these situations it is better to use the skin creases.

One of the most important aspects in achieving a neat scar is the avoidance of tension; this may mean careful undercutting to approximate the skin edges, and the placing of many fine sutures rather than widely placed interrupted sutures of inappropriately thick suture material. Tension may also be minimized by subcutaneous absorbable sutures, and externally by the use of Steri-strips in addition to sutures.

Figure 10.1 (a) Wrinkle-lines and optimal sites for incisions on the face. (b) Incisions made in the line of skin creases will give the neatest scars.

Figure 10.2 Langer lines for the forearm, and sites for incisions, across underlying muscles.

Figure 10.3 Langer lines for the lower limb, crossing the direction of the underlying muscles.

Figure 10.4 Langer lines for the upper limb.

Infection is a potent cause of unsightly scars, often as a result of an infected subcutaneous haematoma. The latter can be minimized by careful attention to haemostasis at the time of the operation, the obliteration of any dead spaces and, where appropriate, the insertion of a small drain for 48 h postoperatively.

10.1 TECHNIQUE OF SKIN INCISION

Whichever scalpel blade is used, one paramount principle must be adhered to: the incision through the skin must be at right-angles and never slanted or oblique (Fig. 10.5). Secondly, the scalpel blade should cut completely through the epidermis and dermis in one stroke if at all possible. Thirdly, one should try to estimate the length of the scar at the outset: a neater scar will result if the original scar is not lengthened, and too short a scar will necessitate undue traction on the skin edges and unnecessarily traumatize the tissue. Fourthly, the skin should be under tension while making the incision (Fig. 10.6). This is necessary otherwise the skin will tend to ruck up ahead of the scalpel. Tension is most easily applied using thumb and forefinger as shown.

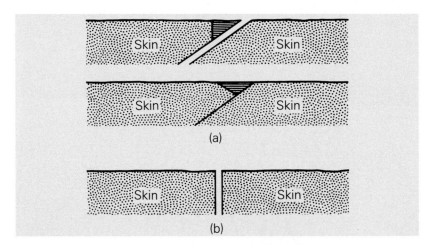

Figure 10.5 Technique for skin incision. (a) Incorrect: oblique incision resulting in a broad scar; (b) correct: vertical incision giving a linear scar.

Figure 10.6 Technique of skin incision keeping the skin under tension with finger and thumb.

10.2 DEEPER DISSECTION

Scalpel dissection and radiowave surgery produce the least tissue trauma. Curved McIndoe scissors have the advantage that they may be used for both blunt and sharp dissection, whilst curved mosquito forceps can be used for blunt dissection by inserting the closed forceps in the wound and opening the blades. Blunt dissection will often reveal underlying vessels and nerves.

At the earliest opportunity, retractors should be inserted in the wound to improve the operator's view. These may be self-retaining, single skin-hooks or combined 'cat's paw' retractors, held by an assistant. A single suture placed in the dermis is a simple effective means of applying traction.

Cutaneous nerves should be divided with a scalpel if they cannot be preserved. This may produce anaesthesia in the distal part of the incision, but with careful closure a high proportion will recover.

10.3 EXCISION

Much of minor surgery entails the excision of a skin lesion, be it a small intradermal naevus or a basal cell carcinoma. This will, of necessity, leave a skin defect to close, and whether an unsightly scar or a near invisible scar ensues will depend on how the excision is planned and how the gap is closed.

If a disc of skin is removed and the edges are pulled together, there is a risk that the centre will have an impaired blood supply and fail to heal, and also a risk of producing a 'dog-ear' at each end of the scar (Fig.10.7a). However, if instead of a disc an elongated ellipse is removed and the edges are undermined, the skin will come together more easily, and there will be no dog-ears (Fig. 10.7b). Next, the direction of the final scar needs to be calculated. This will need to lie along a skin crease or Langer's lines to give the neatest scar. Joining the points of the ellipse will give the line of the final scar (Fig.10.7c, 10.8, 10.9).

As a skin incision heals from side to side, a longer incision with no tension will heal better than a shorter one under tension.

Figure 10.7   Development of 'dog-ear'.
(a) Tension on stitches of circular excision causes dog-ear at either end. (b) Ellipse lengthened so that tension is evened out over the full length of the incision. (c) Scar longer but cosmetically better: no dog ears.

Figure 10.8   Pigmented hairy intradermal melanocytic naevus on face.

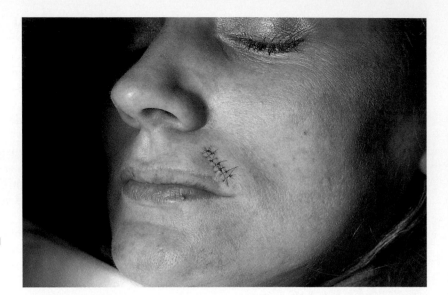

Figure 10.9 Excision by ellipse with the final scar lying along a skin crease. Multiple 6/0 monofilament Prolene sutures were removed after 4 days.

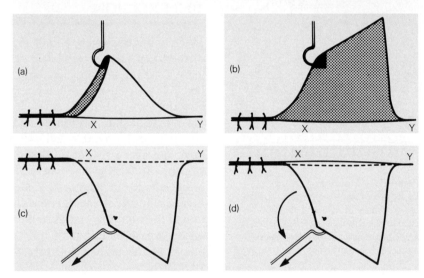

Figure 10.10 Removal of 'dog-ear.' (a) Dog-ear held up with skin hook. Incision at right-angles to skin, *X–Y*. (b) dog-ear after first cut held up. Under surface of skin; skin hook in same place. (c) Flap now lying flat. Underlying skin incision line; skin hook in same place. (d) Flap excised and *X–Y*.

10.4 TECHNIQUE FOR REMOVAL OF A 'DOG-EAR'

If, despite careful planning of the excision, a dog-ear is produced at the end of the scar, it may be eradicated as follows.

- The centre of the incision is sutured as far as possible.
- The remaining dog-ear is lifted up with a single skin hook.
- The base is cut with a scalpel as shown in Fig. 10.10, at right-angles to the skin.
- The flap of skin is now pulled over the same line cut on the opposite side (see Fig. 10.10a–d).

The excess dog-ear is excised, and the wound sutured.

CHAPTER 11

Skin closure

Sutures are best made of soft thread not too hard twisted that it may sit easier on the tissues, nor are too few nor too many of either of them to be put in.

Aulus Cornelius Celsus, 25 BC–AD 50

Following any operation, if skin edges are closely approximated without tension, healing will generally occur in 10 days. Traditionally surgeons have used interrupted sutures to hold the skin edges together, but stitches are not always necessary nor desirable and many alternative methods have been used in an attempt to give as neat a scar as possible.

The simplest method of skin closure is self-adhesive tape; where tension can be avoided, excellent results are obtained and it is particularly suitable for small superficial lacerations on the face and fingers. Ordinary, non-stretch, self-adhesive plaster tape can be used, but better results are obtained with purpose-made sterile strips (Steri-strips 3M) which can be readily applied and have good tensile strength (Figs 11.1 and 11.2).

It is important if using sterile strips that good adhesion is obtained; thus, the skin must be thoroughly dry, and if in an area where increased perspiration occurs, extra adhesion may be obtained by first painting the skin with tinct. benz. co. or collodion before applying the Steri-strips. Additional external support can be given by careful bandaging,

Figure 11.1 Steri-strips may be used both to close a wound and to give additional support for sutures (3M).

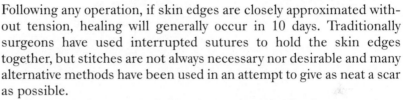

Figure 11.2 Skin closure strips are ideal for small wounds and for giving additional support during healing (*five different sizes*).

Figure 11.3 Simple method of closing a small laceration of the scalp by knotting a few strands of hair on either side of the wound.

and if the original wound is clean, may be left undisturbed for up to 10 days. Most lacerations on fingers and toes can be satisfactorily closed using Steri-strips supplemented with tubular cotton stockinette bandage. It is important that the strip does not completely encircle the digit, in case oedema occurs and the Steri-strip then acts as a tourniquet with ensuing ischaemia or necrosis. In very young children sutures may be preferable to sterile strip closure in case the child inadvertently pulls off the dressing and strips before healing has occurred.

Faced with a small laceration on the scalp, satisfactory skin closure may often be achieved merely by twisting a few strands of hair on either side of the wound and knotting them together over the laceration (Fig. 11.3). Spraying the knot with Nobecutane spray, tinct. benz. co. or collodion will prevent the knot slipping, and the knot may then be cut free after 10 days when healing has occurred. Another 'first-aid' method of skin closure in the absence of suitable suture materials uses hypodermic needles and Nylon fishing line. The needles may be inserted through the skin edges from one side to another, and the Nylon thread passed through the lumen of the needle, which is then withdrawn over the thread, leaving the Nylon ready to be tied. Very satisfactory skin closure may be achieved using this simple procedure (Fig. 11.4).

11.1 SUTURES

The doctor looking through a catalogue of surgical sutures will find a bewildering array of materials in all sizes, colours, absorbability, needle sizes, etc. Basically, the majority of surgical sutures will be either absorbable or non-absorbable. Absorbable sutures, as their name implies, slowly dissolve as the tissues heal, and therefore do not

Figure 11.4 Another simple method of suturing a wound using a hypodermic needle and some Nylon fishing line.

need to be removed; non-absorbable sutures do not dissolve, and need to be removed. The different sutures are described in the following sections.

11.1.1 Interrupted, plain

This is the most common method of suturing. The needle is inserted through the skin, across the subcutaneous part of the wound, through the skin on the opposite side and then knotted, bringing the edges together. As most suture materials have a tendency to slip, a reef knot with one additional throw (surgeon's knot) is used.

11.1.2 Interrupted (mattress)

Where skin edges may not approximate accurately owing to laxity of the tissues or any other reason, good apposition may be achieved by including the skin edges in the suture (vertical mattress). Interrupted sutures give a neat scar but are occasionally quite difficult to remove.

11.1.3 Subcuticular sutures

These are becoming increasingly popular and will give an extremely neat scar providing the skin is not under tension (Fig. 11.5a, b). A straight needle is preferable, although cutting curved needles can be used. The needle is inserted through the skin about 1–2 cm away from, but in line with, the incision. It is passed under the skin to emerge in the subcuticular layer on one side of the wound; it is then passed backwards and forwards across the wound, eventually emerging beyond the other end of the incision corresponding to where the suture commenced. By applying traction to both ends of the suture, the skin edges are approximated neatly and the part of the suture remaining visible is fixed to the skin with either tape, dressings or a single 'button'. Removal is effected by cutting one end flush with the skin, and firmly pulling the other. Subcuticular or intradermal sutures may be either non-absorbable (e.g. Prolene) or absorbable (e.g. coated Vicryl). Many surgeons are now closing wounds using absorbable coated Vicryl as a subcuticular suture. In this case, the suture is knotted beneath the

Figure 11.5 (a) A subcuticular stitch gives a neat scar and takes less time to insert than interrupted sutures. (b) Subcuticular stitch.

skin at both ends and does not need to be removed. However, if inserted too near the epidermis, it may either be rejected or cause a tissue reaction ('Vicrylitis').

11.1.4 Continuous and blanket stitch

These tend to be used for longer scars and are seldom used for minor surgical incisions. As its name implies, a continuous stitch extends from one end of the wound to the other. It is quick to insert, difficult to achieve even tension and even spacing of the stitch, not easy to remove, has an increased risk of infection during removal, and does not allow the removal of individual sutures should fluid collect under the scar and require drainage.

11.2 SUTURE MATERIALS

Every doctor has a personal selection of preferred suture materials; listed in the following sections are the various types available.

11.2.1 Plain catgut

This is made from purified ribbons of animal intestines, which are spun into a strand, electronically gauged and then polished. It is absorbed by body enzymes; originally it was very popular, but has tended to be superseded by synthetic absorbable sutures in recent years.

11.2.2 Chromic catgut

This is made from ribbons of animal intestines, spun into a strand, exactly as plain catgut, but treated so that the strength of the suture is maintained for a considerably longer time than plain catgut. It is still used in obstetrics and for approximating subcutaneous tissues, but is being superseded by synthetic materials.

11.2.3 Braided silk (Mersilk)

The raw silk is treated and de-gummed prior to braiding, resulting in a compact braid which ties easily; it used to be extremely popular but has now been superseded by monofilament Nylon and Prolene sutures.

11.2.4 Monofilament polyamide 6 and 66 (Ethilon)

These are synthetic, monofilament sutures, whose smooth surface does not appear to support bacterial growth. They can be difficult to knot, but are useful for subcuticular sutures.

11.2.5 Monofilament polypropylene (Prolene)

The advantage of polypropylene is that it is supple, ties securely and handles well. As with other monofilament synthetic sutures, knots need to be square ties with additional throws and, in addition, damage from forceps and needle holders should be avoided to prevent fracture of the material. It is extremely smooth and suitable for subcuticular stitches. It is now one of the most popular materials for skin sutures.

11.2.6 Polyglycolic acid synthetic absorbable sutures (Dexon)

These sutures, introduced in recent years, are extremely popular. They appear to cause virtually no tissue reaction as they dissolve, compared with considerable histological tissue reaction with catgut. Their rate of absorption is considerably slower than even chromic catgut, and may take several weeks. Dexon is an ideal suture material for all subcutaneous skin closures.

11.2.7 Coated polyglactin 910 (Vicryl)

Coated Vicryl is a multifilament synthetic absorbable suture, manufactured as a copolymer of glycolide and lactide. Individual filaments are braided together and then treated with an absorbable coating. This coating allows smooth passage of the suture through the skin, and also makes the tying of knots easy. Absorption is by hydrolysis and appears to cause only minimal tissue reaction.

Vicryl is now one of the most popular and widely used sutures for subcutaneous use, with tensile strength lasting for at least 28–40 days.

All suture materials are now graded by metric gauge, which indicates the actual diameter of the suture in tenths of a millimetre, and this gauging has now been adopted by both European and United States Pharmacopoeia, replacing the former system of 0 gauges, thus:

USP/BP	Metric
7/0	0.5
6/0	0.7
5/0	1.0
4/0	1.5
3/0	2.0
2/0	3.0
0	3.5

11.2.8 Polybutester (Novafil)

This is a monofilament suture which is easier to handle and knot than some earlier monofilament sutures.

A selection of the most widely used suture materials is now included in the Drug Tariff and doctors in the UK can prescribe these for use on their National Health Service patients. For minor surgical procedures, the following 'shortlist' will provide a basic treatment set.

■ sterile monofilament polyamide 6 Ethilon 1.5 metric gauge (formerly 4/0) Ref. W 319;. ideal for most skin closures

- sterile braided silk metric 1 (formerly 5/0) Mersilk Ref. W 535; useful for suturing the scalp but gradually being superseded by monofilament Prolene sutures
- sterile coated Vicryl (undyed) 1.5 metric (formerly 4/0) (polyglactin 910) Ref. W 9951; ideal absorbable suture for subcutaneous closure. Good tensile strength for 4 weeks.

11.3 SKIN CLOSURE STRIPS

These are used as an alternative to sutures or to supplement sutures to give additional support. Certain sites such as fingers are better closed with sterile skin closure strips rather than suturing, if possible. When used on digits, care must be taken not to encircle the finger or toe completely with the strip, as a tourniquet effect may result.

Improvised skin closure strips may be made from Sellotape, micropore tape or adhesive zinc oxide plaster.

If applied carefully between sutures at the time of skin closure, they may be left undisturbed when the sutures are removed, thus giving extra strength and support to the wound.

11.4 SKIN CLOSURE CLIPS

These are generally not used for minor surgical procedures, although some surgeons favour their use. The disadvantages are that they

Figure 11.6 Wound closure using skin staples.

Figure 11.7 Use of Proximate skin stapler.

require a special instrument to remove them and they can be uncomfortable for the patient; however, they can give extremely good skin closure and a very neat scar. Most manufacturers now produce sterile disposable packs of clips (Ethicon Proximate disposable skin stapler) (Figs 11.6 and 11.7).

11.5 DRAINS

Although widely used for operations on the neck, breast, thorax and pelvis, drains are generally not necessary when performing minor surgical procedures. Where good haemostasis has been achieved and any dead space closed, haematoma formation is unlikely. If drainage is thought necessary, a small piece of rubber or plastic tubing may be inserted under the sutures and removed after 48 h. Disposable drains with attached vacuum bottles are now available and are excellent where a large lesion, e.g. lipoma, has been removed, leaving a potential dead space.

11.6 STITCHCRAFT AND KNOTS

Practice at tying knots is essential; knots may be formed using two hands as with tying shoe-laces, with one hand, or using instruments.

11.6.1 One-hand tie

The one-hand tie may be practised using a piece of string to tie up a parcel; the instrument tie is most easily practised using surplus sutures and pigs' trotters. In all techniques, the ends of the sutures should be kept taut at all times to avoid slippage (Fig. 11.8). However, correct tightening of the knot is important to avoid eversion of the skin edges and to promote good healing (Fig. 11.9). Where an assistant is

Figure 11.8   One-hand tie.

Figure 11.9 Correct tightening of the knot is important to ensure optimal healing. (a) Correct; (b) incorrect.

Figure 11.10 Placing a skin-hook in each end of the incision helps to align the edges prior to suturing.

available, the use of two single skin-hooks, one at each end of the incision, helps to align the edges and makes accurate approximation easier (Fig. 11.10).

11.6.2 Instrument ties

Instrument ties are more suitable for minor surgery, using less suture material. The suture is passed through both ends of the wound and a short end is left protruding. Holding the needle end of the suture in the left hand, the suture is looped around the end of the needle holder once or twice depending on the type of knot. Still with the loops around the end of the needle holder, the short protruding end is grasped with the tips of the needle holders and pulled back through the loops. By pulling both the end of the suture and the needle holder in opposite directions, the first throw of the knot is tied. The process is then repeated, but on the second throw the suture is looped round the needle-holder in the opposite direction (Fig. 11.11).

11.6.3 Three types of knot are used (Fig. 11.12)

The three types of knot are:

- reef knot
- surgeon's knot
- nylon knot.

For most situations a surgeon's knot comprising two throws followed by one throw as a reef knot is most suitable. Having tied the first throw, it may be 'locked' by pulling the knot to one edge of the wound. This allows the second throw to be formed without the first throw slipping.

In general, when cutting sutures inside a wound the ends should be cut as short as possible. Outside the wound, sufficient length should be left to make removal easy.

Where very fine, smooth sutures have been used, e.g. on the face, and there is a risk of the suture slipping, the wound may be painted with tinct. benz. co. or sprayed with Nobecutane or Opsite (Hydron copolymer 3%), which will not only form a transparent dressing but also glue the knots together. However, although this method is popular with the person inserting the sutures, it is not always popular with the person removing them!

Figure 11.11 Instrument tie, five stages (from B.A. Maurice, *Surgery for General Practitioners*, by permission of Oxford University Press).

Figure 11.12 Different types of knot used in suturing: (a) reef knot, (b) surgeon's knot, (c) nylon knot.

11.6.4 Types of sutures

For minor surgery the three most frequently used sutures are:

- simple interrupted
- vertical mattress interrupted
- subcuticular or intradermal continuous (see Fig. 11.5).

11.6.5 Simple interrupted sutures

To achieve the neatest results the following principles need to be adhered to.

Figure 11.13 Simple interrupted sutures: (a) correct; (b) incorrect.

- The needle should be pushed through the skin at right-angles.
- The exit tract should likewise be at right-angles to the skin.
- The distance of the entry site from the edge of the wound should be equal to the depth of skin through which the suture is passing (Figs 11.13 and 11.14).
- Where deep tissues need to be sutured, a subcutaneous suture of an absorbable material, e.g. 1.5 coated Vicryl, will reduce tension on the skin edges and give a neater scar (Fig. 11.15).
- The doctor should practise on pigs' trotters.

11.6.6 Vertical mattress interrupted suture

This is a very useful stitch when the tissues are lax and the edges tend to invert. It apposes the skin layers accurately, but should not be used if the skin circulation is poor. Tension can be less to take account of any postoperative oedema.
The following principles should be followed.

- The needle tract should be at right-angles to the skin.
- It is a slightly deeper stitch which can incorporate the subcutaneous layer.
- The entry site is judged to be the same distance from the entry site to the point where it comes out of the deep tissue.
- The inner part of the stitch should be made 2 mm from the skin edge and come out half-way through the thickness of skin (Fig. 11.16a, b).
- The doctor should practise on pigs' trotters or skin simulators.

Figure 11.14 Simple suture. (a) The suture is laid evenly across the wound; (b) positioning the knot to one side.

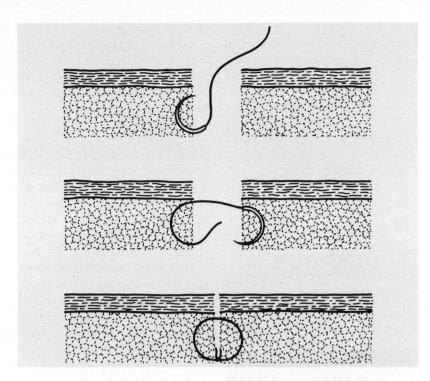

Figure 11.15 Suturing deep tissue (redrawn from B.A. Maurice, *Surgery for General Practitioners*, by permission of Oxford University Press).

Figure 11.16 Vertical mattress suture: (a) stages using straight needle; (b) using curved needle.

11.6.7 Subcuticular or intradermal continuous sutures

Where the edges of the wound can be brought together easily without tension, and where the risk of subcutaneous haematoma formation is slight, a subcuticular or an intradermal continuous suture gives the neatest scar.

Monofilament Nylon, Ethilon or Prolene is used. The stitch starts outside the wound at the end of the incision and passes backwards and forwards under the surface of the skin, emerging outside the end

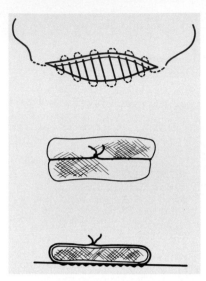

Figure 11.17 Subcuticular suture and method of securing ends by tying over a small gauze swab.

Figure 11.18 Histoacryl blue tissue adhesive; ideal for small lacerations in children.

of the wound at the opposite end. This leaves two ends which need to be secured. One method is to use 'buttons' or split 'lead' shot, but a simpler method is to tie the ends over a gauze swab and then tape the swab to the skin (Fig. 11.17). To remove this suture, one end is divided flush with the skin and traction is applied at the opposite end.

11.7 THE USE OF TISSUE ADHESIVE

Following anecdotal reports of accidental adhesion of skin using 'Superglue', manufacturers have now produced a medical tissue adhesive. It is made as a sterile solution of n-butyl-2-cyanoacrylate monomer sealed in single-dose plastic vials. To help to identify the thickness of adhesive applied, a blue dye is added (Fig. 11.18).

Histoacryl (enbucrilate) blue and Dermabond are especially suitable for the closure of minor skin wounds without suturing, and also for sealing sutured skin wounds. When applied to the skin, they rapidly polymerize into a firm adhesive bond in the presence of anions, especially hydroxyl ions, i.e. when contact is made with water or tissue moisture.

11.7.1 Technique

It is important to clean, dry and check whether the edges of the wound will approximate without tension. Histoacryl blue or Dermabond may then be applied as spots evenly along the length of the wound and the edges held together accurately for 1 min. The correct method of closure of a skin laceration using tissue adhesive is shown in Figs 11.19–11.30.

Caution

It is vital to approximate the edges accurately before applying the adhesive, as polymerization time is only 20 s and mistakes cannot be corrected. It should also be noted that heat is produced during polymerization; thus, the thinnest layer possible should be applied to avoid thermal damage to the skin.

Figure 11.19 Typical wound suitable for tissue adhesive.

Figure 11.20 Cutting off the tip of the nozzle: it must always be held upright and pointed away from the patient.

Figure 11.21 Adhesive is squeezed to the tip of the nozzle, away from the patient, to check flow.

Figure 11.22 Adhesive is applied to the surface of the apposed wound edges, **not** into the wound.

Figure 11.23 Wound edges are apposed with fingers **before** adhesive is applied.

Figure 11.24 Closing a wound on the scalp with finger pressure.

Figure 11.25 Same wound as in Fig. 11.24 immediately after closure with tissue adhesive.

Figure 11.26   Five-year-old child with laceration above eyebrow (photograph taken by Dr David Watson at Lewisham Hospital).

Figure 11.27   Same patient as in Fig. 11.26 6 months later (photograph taken by Dr David Watson at Lewisham Hospital).

Figure 11.28   Four-year-old child with laceration beneath chin (photograph taken by Dr David Watson at Lewisham Hospital).

Figure 11.29   Same patient as in Fig. 11.28 3 months later (photograph taken by Dr David Watson at Lewisham Hospital).

Figure 11.30   Diagram to show the application of adhesive to the surface of a closed wound and not between the wound edges.

Further, Histoacryl should not be applied to blood vessels in case intravascular thrombosis occurs; care should also be taken to avoid contact with the cornea or conjunctive.

Instruments, clothes, swabs, gloves or fingers which come into contact with Histoacryl will adhere to it, so extreme care needs to be taken. Instruments accidentally contaminated with the glue may be cleaned with dimethyl formamide or acetone.

It is recommended that the glue be kept in a refrigerator or freezer and protected from the light. It has a shelf life of 2 years.

Because no local anaesthetic is necessary, this is an ideal method of skin closure for small wounds in young children. In addition, as no sutures need to be removed, follow-up visits are virtually eliminated.

CHAPTER 12

Suturing lacerations

> If thou examinest a man having a wound in his ear, cutting through the flesh, the injury being in the lower part of the ear, and confined to the flesh, thou shouldst draw it together for him with stitching behind the hollow of his ear.
>
> *Edwin Smith, Surgical Papyrus, 3000–2500 BC*

One of the first skills to be acquired by medical students in their clinical training is the suturing of wounds; in the emergency department they meet a variety of injuries and lacerations, and on the maternity wards they learn how to repair perineal tears and episiotomies. House surgeons assist at many surgical procedures and are often responsible for suturing the wound at the end of the operation. Thus, all doctors by the time they qualify are able to suture the majority of wounds likely to be encountered in any minor surgical operation. If it is considered necessary to suture a wound, the following general principles should be borne in mind.

- Healing will occur more readily if the skin edges are accurately and carefully apposed to each other.
- There should be minimum or no tension on the skin edges if at all possible. This may be achieved by careful undercutting of the skin prior to suturing.
- The skin edges should be slightly everted; this is done by applying slight traction to the skin edge and including slightly more of the dermal layer than skin in the stitch.
- Many fine sutures, equally placed close together are preferable to larger sutures spaced further apart.
- Any 'dead space' should be closed either with subcutaneous absorbable sutures, or by including this layer in the skin stitches.
- All stitches should only remain in place as long as they are needed to give support. Thus, stitches on the face may be removed as early as 48 h to 5 days, whereas those on the abdominal wall and foot should remain for 10 days or more.
- All wounds should be as clean as possible.
- There should be the minimum of handling and tissue trauma from forceps.
- Additional support may be given by the use of sterile adhesive strips which can remain in place after the stitches have been removed.
- Practice at different suturing techniques is most easily acquired using pigs' trotters, skin simulation models, or even oranges!

Figure 12.1 Basic instrument set suitable for most suturing.

12.1 INSTRUMENTS REQUIRED

The following 'basic set' is recommended for routine suturing and many simple surgical procedures (Fig. 12.1).

- Kilner needle holder 5 1/4 in. (13.3 cm)
- scalpel handle size 3
- scalpel blades 10 and 15
- pair of standard stitch scissors (sharp/sharp) 5 in. (12.7 cm) pair of toothed dissecting forceps 5 in. (12.7 cm).
- suture material: this is individual preference, but the finer the suture the better, consistent with giving adequate support
- W 319 Ethilon monofilament Nylon 1.5 on curved, reverse-cutting needle
- 507 Ethilon monofilament Nylon 0.7 on slim-blade curved cutting needle
- W 539 Ethicon Prolene 1.5 on slim-blade curved cutting needle.
- syringes and needles and local anaesthesia: the 2 ml syringe is sufficient for small lacerations, 10 ml or even 20 ml for larger. The finest gauge needles should be selected, and a dental syringe with a screw-on 30 swg (0.3 mm) needle is ideal for children.

12.2 TECHNIQUE FOR SUTURING LACERATIONS

The patient should be lying comfortably on a couch or operating-theatre table, this is preferable to the patient sitting or standing as the most unexpected patients faint during a simple suturing procedure; it is also more comfortable for both the patient and doctor. Good illumination is essential, and the wound should first be carefully inspected to determine the extent and nature of the injury, and to ascertain whether any other injury to underlying structures has occurred. Having excluded other injuries, the area should be anaesthetized. This is most conveniently done by infiltration as described in Chapter 8 using first a dental syringe and 30 swg (0.3 mm) needle, changing to a longer needle and larger syringe if necessary, always remembering the maximum dose of anaesthetic which may be given to this particular patient (taking care with the very young and very old).

After allowing a few minutes for anaesthesia to develop, the area may be again inspected, carefully palpated, cleaned thoroughly, and any hairs clipped away from the immediate operative field.

At this stage the doctor will need to decide whether deep tissues will require suturing as well as skin, and if so, catgut, Dexon or preferably coated Vicryl sutures should be inserted. As a general guide, the less deep sutures that are inserted, the better, compatible with achieving haemostasis and closing any 'dead' spaces.

Any bleeding points may be dealt with by electrocautery, diathermy, radiosurgery electrocoagulation, ligature, clipping, or just firm pressure for a few minutes. Next, an attempt should be made to bring the edges of the wound together to see whether undue tension will be created. If this is likely, the skin should be widely undercut to help to approximate the edges. Any ragged edges should be carefully trimmed and dead tissue excised.

Using the toothed dissecting forceps to hold the skin edges, interrupted sutures are inserted, tying the knots on the same side and avoiding any tension, taking into account the fact that tissues may swell during the first 2 days following injury.

If an assistant is available, two Gillies skin-hooks can be used, one at either end of the wound, applying traction, which aligns the wound neatly, and makes insertion of sutures easier (see Fig. 11.10). A dry dressing may now be applied, with or without a covering of Nobecutane or Opsite spray on the skin.

Deep, dirty, penetrating wounds should be cleaned as thoroughly as possible, and the patient given prophylactic antibiotics and a reinforcing tetanus immunization if not up-to-date. Dirty contaminated grazes can be scrubbed using chlorhexidine in detergent (Hibiscrub) after first anaesthetizing the area with infiltration anaesthetic.

12.3 TECHNIQUE FOR CLOSURE WITH 'GLUE'

Where the edges of the wound can be brought together easily, it may be appropriate to consider one of the cyanoacrylate glues (Histoacryl Blue, Dermabond or Indermil). After drying the edges with absorbent gauze, the glue is applied using a glass rod. The edges are then held firmly together for 2 min. Care must be taken not to stick the operator's fingers to the patient's skin.

Figure 12.2 A common injury.

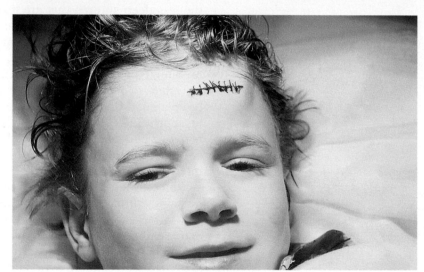

Figure 12.3 'No hard feelings!'.

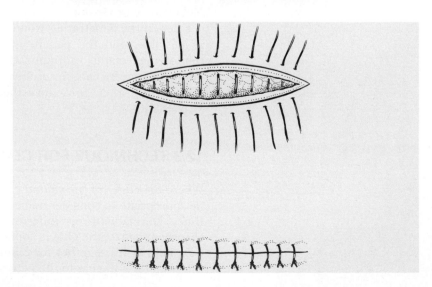

Figure 12.4 Skin closure with interrupted sutures.

Figure 12.5 (a,b) A laceration from a sharp knife is easily closed using interrupted non-absorbable sutures, preferably monofilament Prolene or subcuticular Vicryl.

Figure 12.6 (a,b) Where the edges of the wound can be approximated without tension and the site splinted afterwards, a subcuticular suture may give a neater scar.

Figure 12.7 (a,b) Wounds may extend deeper than appears at first sight.

Figure 12.8 Small lacerations on the tongue often heal without any attention. Deeper cuts require suturing, using an absorbable material.

Figure 12.9 Lacerations over the anterior surface of the tibia, particularly in elderly women, are difficult to heal. Any tension in the wound must be avoided. In this wound the skin flap should be carefully stretched back to its original position and taped in position using Steristrips. The wound should then be covered with a sterile pad and a firm compression bandage. This will give better results than suturing.

Normally, no anaesthetic is needed, and no further follow-up required.

12.4 CHOICE OF SKIN CLOSURE

Mention has already been made about alternative closures to sutures, and these should always be borne in mind when faced with a laceration. It may be more appropriate to use a subcuticular stitch, sterile self-adhesive strips, clips or just a firm dressing.

Figure 12.10 Before excising any lesion the doctor decides whether the edges can be brought together without undue tension. This wound will need undercutting, subcutaneous supporting sutures and many fine sutures, supported with large self-adhesive skin closure strips, kept on for several weeks after the sutures have been removed.

CHAPTER 13

Dressings

> Now, after thou hast stitched it, thou shouldst bind it with fresh meat the first day. Thou shouldst treat it afterwards with grease and honey every day until he recovers.
>
> *Edwin Smith, Surgical Papyrus, 3000–2500 BC*

It has been suggested that dressings on surgical wounds are unnecessary, that they merely prevent the doctor and patient observing what is happening underneath, and this is certainly true on many occasions. Every doctor will have observed how well incisions heal on the scalp and face, where no dressings are used.

13.1 REASONS FOR USING DRESSINGS

Where dressings are used, they probably help in four ways:

- absorption of any secretions
- protection from contamination
- additional support during the healing phase
- limitation of excessive movements during healing.

13.1.1 Absorption of secretions

Any wound which is discharging or oozing will be helped by the application of an absorbent, sterile, dry dressing, which must be changed frequently.

13.1.2 Protection from contamination

If a surgical operation has been performed under sterile conditions and primary skin closure is expected, a sterile dry dressing firmly applied at the end of the operation should be left undisturbed until the sutures are removed. Peeping under the dressing 'to see how it is healing' is to be condemned as this only increases the chances of cross-infection. Only if there is a definite indication such as unexpected pain, swelling fever, or signs of infection should the original dressing be disturbed; in every other case it should be left well alone.

13.1.3 Additional support

Sutures alone may not give adequate support to a healing wound, and in this case a dressing firmly bandaged in place will give additional external support, reduce tension on the stitches and promote healing.

13.1.4 Limitation of movement

Wounds on the limbs may be subjected to excessive forces during healing, for example transverse wounds near the knee joint may tend to pull apart during walking and kneeling. By applying a thick layer of bandage, limitation of movements of the joint will be achieved, and promote healing. Similarly, on the hand or fingers where sterile strips may have been used in preference to sutures, but by themselves are not strong enough to withstand full movements, supportive bandaging will supplement the Steri-strips and avoid the need for suturing.

13.2 TYPES OF DRESSING

13.2.1 Non-adherent dressings

Where there is considerable discharge from either an ulcer, burns, blisters or sinuses, ordinary dry dressings may become adherent and difficult to remove. In such cases non-adherent dressings may be used, such as Melolin X-A, Johnsons N.A. dressing, Mepore, Vaseline-impregnated gauze or similar preparations.

13.2.2 Antibacterial dressings

These consist of *tulle-gras* dressings impregnated with antibacterial substances. They are of limited use and carry the risk of causing skin sensitization. In certain situations such as ingrowing toe-nail operations where there is known to be heavy infection, the routine use of such dressings appears to accelerate healing, e.g. Inadine (povidone–iodine).

13.2.3 Acrylic resin aerosol dressings (Nobecutane or Opsite)

These consist of acrylic resin dissolved in a mixture of acetate esters in aerosol containers. By spraying on the skin from a distance of 20 cm a protective film is produced. This is useful on sites where conventional dressings would be difficult to keep in place, e.g. the scalp; in other sites it may be used instead of a dry gauze dressing, particularly after sutures have been removed.

13.2.4 Cotton conforming bandages (Kling, Crinx, Easifix and Kurlex)

These lightweight bandages are so designed that they will bandage irregular surfaces and maintain even tension. They are cheap, efficient and widely used.

13.2.5 Elastic bandages

Where firm external elastic support is required, for example on the legs to control varicose veins, elastic web bandages are ideal. Wounds and ulcers on the lower leg tend to heal more slowly, the more so when oedema is present. The early application of firm elastic bandages reduces oedema and accelerates healing. They are frequently used in the treatment of varicose veins and varicose ulceration.

13.2.6 Elasticated net stockinette (Netelast)

This elastic tubular dressing is designed to hold dressings in place in sites such as the axilla, breast, perineum, buttock and scalp. It is manufactured in different widths, and with ingenuity all parts of the body can be covered. It has the advantage of being extremely comfortable but does not give much compression.

13.2.7 Elasticated tubular stockinette (Tubigrip)

For additional elastic support, elasticated tubular stockinette is used; particularly for wounds on arms and legs. As with the elastic net stockinette it is manufactured in various sizes to suit most parts of the body. It is used to give compression for sclerotherapy for varicose veins.

13.2.8 Cotton surgical tubular stockinette (Tubegauz)

This is a non-elastic, cotton stockinette, which is ideal for bandaging fingers and toes. It is manufactured in various widths, and is applied with a special tubular applicator using a twisting action to increase compression if required (Fig. 13.1a, b).

Figure 13.1 (a, b) Application of a cotton tubular stockinette bandage to the finger: ideal for gentle compression. Multiple layers will give additional splintage to the digit, thus often making suturing unnecessary. *Continued over page.*

Figure 13.1 Continued. (a, b) Application of a cotton tubular stockinette bandage to the finger: ideal for gentle compression. Multiple layers will give additional splintage to the digit, thus often making suturing unnecessary.

13.2.9 Alginate dressings

Where there is troublesome oozing of blood, the application of an alginate dressing (Kaltostat or similar) will cause coagulation and control most simple bleeding. This is particularly useful in ingrowing toe-nail operations.

CHAPTER
14

Suture removal

The shorter the time sutures are *in situ,* the neater the scar. However, if they are removed too soon, there is a risk of the wound gaping; consequently, a compromise has to be reached, and the optimum time will vary in different sites on the body. Thus, the majority of sutures are removed on the 10th postoperative day, but on the face it is preferable to remove them very much earlier, and on the foot it might be advisable to leave them for a day or two longer. It is also possible to remove alternate sutures one or two days before the remainder, and this improves the appearance of the final scar. Where it is desirable to remove sutures early, but the practitioner feels that the wound may not be firmly adherent, additional external support may be given using sterile self-adhesive strips.

14.1 TECHNIQUE OF SUTURE AND CLIP REMOVAL

Unfortunately, a wound which has healed well may be contaminated by poor suture removal technique, resulting in stitch abscesses and an infected scar. Where possible, the sterile dressings applied at the time of the operation should be left undisturbed until the sutures are to be removed. A sterile dressing pack should be used and a no-touch technique employed, using sterile instruments. The doctor or nurse should either wear a mask or not talk during the procedure to reduce droplet cross-infection.

Fine sutures are best removed using a pair of iris scissors and dissecting forceps; most other sutures may be removed using either standard pointed stitch scissors or prepacked disposable stitch cutters and forceps. To minimize any risks of contamination, the knot should be picked up with forceps and one side of the suture cut flush with the skin; it may then be removed by carefully pulling on the knot (Fig. 14.1).

14.1.1 Subcuticular stitch removal

One end of the subcuticular stitch is cut flush with the skin, while the other end is grasped with artery forceps and traction applied.

Figure 14.1 Removal of stitches. (a) Cut under knot; (b) as the stitch is pulled out, the edges are drawn together.

Additional support may be given by the application of sterile self-adhesive strips, which can be applied either at the time of the original operation or at the time of suture removal.

14.1.2 Removal of skin clips

Skin clips require a small pair of clip removers, which bend the clip open and cause minimum trauma to the skin. The blade is inserted under the clip and by applying pressure with the second blade, the clip opens (Fig. 14.2).

Skin stapling can result in minimal scarring (Fig. 14.3).

 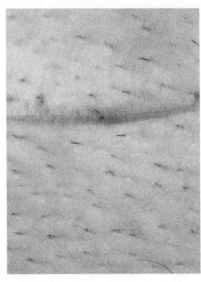

Figure 14.2 The Proximate skin staple remover in use.

Figure 14.3 Typical scar following skin stapling.

CHAPTER 15

Chemical cauterization

> Warts . . . They may be removed also by the knife and the parts from whence they are cut afterwards touched with lunar caustic (silver nitrate) to prevent them from returning. But when this method is practised the operator ought to be certain that he has removed the wart entirely, for where part has been left, the most formidable symptoms have sometimes ensued.
>
> *Encyclopaedia Britannica, 1797*

The application of caustic chemicals to the tissues can be used to advantage to treat certain lesions; they are cheap, easily obtainable, effective and quick to apply and no special instruments are required. The two disadvantages of using chemicals are difficulty in controlling the exact area treated and the fact that only superficial lesions can be treated. Nevertheless, three substances are used commonly in medical practice: silver nitrate, liquefied phenol and monochloroacetic acid.

15.1 SILVER NITRATE

This has been used for centuries and is well known to most doctors: When applied to moist tissues, it causes them to turn white owing to the formation of silver chloride; this then gradually turns black when exposed to light. Unless both patient and operator are particularly careful, accidental touching of the skin with the silver nitrate will result in stubborn, unsightly, black stains which are extremely difficult to remove. Similarly, if left on plastic work surfaces in the surgery, silver nitrate will cause permanent black staining.

It is produced as a solid pointed stick which may be fixed in a holder, or more recently, individual wooden applicators with a small, hard bead at the tip containing 75% silver nitrate. These are disposable, avoid any risks of cross-infection, and are easier and cleaner to handle. Finally, silver nitrate is made as a solution of any desired strength for topical application.

15.1.1 Granulations

These respond well to the application of silver nitrate, often being cured with just one application. Following separation of the umbilical cord in the newborn infant, occasionally messy granulations occur; one or two applications of silver nitrate and a dry dressing are all that is required.

15.1.2 Vaginal vault granulations

Vaginal vault granulations following hysterectomy are easily treated with topical silver nitrate, rarely needing more than two applications.

15.1.3 Small granuloma pyogenicum

If curette and electrocautery are not available or inappropriate, the application of silver nitrate may result in a cure.

15.1.4 Epistaxis

Repeated nose-bleeds in children and young adults frequently occur from the small leash of blood vessels in 'Little's area' which are readily visible. The application of silver nitrate directly to this area often results in cure; it is slightly uncomfortable at the time of application and causes reflex watering of the eyes, but is usually acceptable to children (Chapter 32). No anaesthesia is necessary for this procedure.

15.1.5 Cervical erosions

Many cervical erosions are asymptomatic and need no treatment; where the patient is experiencing an increased discharge or has symptoms of pain suggesting infection or cervicitis, cauterization of the cervix with silver nitrate may be tried. Using the applicator, the whole of the erosion including the external cervical os is treated with silver nitrate; the area so treated becoming white. The patient is warned to expect an increased, watery vaginal discharge for 1 or 2 weeks during healing. Some doctors like the patient to use an antiseptic vaginal cream (e.g. Sultrin – triple-sulpha cream) twice daily during this healing phase.

15.1.6 Ingrowing toe-nails

A silver nitrate caustic applicator has been traditionally used for ingrowing toe-nails for years; it is suitable for the treatment of any granulations which occur, but the black staining is a disadvantage and alternative methods may be more appropriate (Chapter 30).

15.1.7 Chronic sinus or fistula

Long-standing suppuration and discharge through a skin sinus or fistula may result in the formation of fleshy polyp and/or heaped-up granulations. Both may be helped by the application of silver nitrate, often on more than one occasion. Where possible, the underlying cause of the fistula or sinus should be treated.

15.1.8 Chronic conjunctivitis

A weak aqueous solution of silver nitrate may be used to treat patients with chronic inflammation of the eyelids. This is known as 'silvering of the eyelids'. Benoxinate drops are instilled prior to the application of 1% silver nitrate, which is then washed out with normal saline.

15.2 PHENOL (CARBOLIC ACID)

Phenol crystals or pure liquefied phenol containing 80–90% w/w in water may be used for cauterization, while weaker solutions may be used for injection into hydrocele cavities (Chapter 22) or for the injection of haemorrhoids (Chapter 36). In each case the treatment relies on the irritant effect of the phenol on the tissues. Used as a 5% solution in glycerin, phenol may also be used for intrathecal and superficial nerve blocksThe main use of liquefied phenol in general practitioner minor surgery is for ingrowing toe-nails, where it is used to cauterize and destroy the nail matrix (Chapter 30). In this situation, its threefold action of cauterization, destruction of nerve endings and sterilization makes it an ideal agent.

15.2.1 Granulations

The application of liquefied phenol is often an effective treatment for granulation tissue. More than one treatment may be necessary, and a delayed 'phenol reaction' may be seen on the 8th–10th day with increased inflammation and discharge.

15.2.2 Molluscum contagiosum

This condition is caused by a viral infection, and is typified by small, pearly, hard papules with an umbilicated centre. It may be treated with liquefied phenol by dipping a sharpened wooden applicator in phenol and then piercing each individual papule, transferring a minute quantity of phenol inside each spot.

15.2.3 Chronic paronychia

Following loss of the nail 'quick' and subsequent infection, often with yeasts, chronic paronychiae may be treated with phenol applied directly with a small wooden applicator sharpened in the shape of a chisel, dipped in phenol. This treatment may be supplemented with topical and occasional systemic antimycotics.

15.2.4 Ear-lobe cysts

Small infected cysts, particularly those occurring in the lobes of the ears may be treated effectively by incision, evacuation of any contents, and the application of pure liquefied phenol on a small wooden applicator and cotton wool.

15.2.5 Hydrocele and epididymal cysts (Chapter 22)

Aspiration alone rarely cures either of these conditions, but aspiration followed by the injection of 2.5–6% aqueous phenol results in 90–100% cure; the treatment needs to be repeated more than once.

15.2.6 Injection of haemorrhoids

Despite many alternative and more sophisticated treatments for haemorrhoids, 5% oily phenol still remains the treatment of choice for many doctors for their patients with haemorrhoids. The injection is given submucosally in doses of 1–10 ml (Chapter 36).

15.3 MONOCHLOROACETIC ACID

This is a simple, effective treatment for small warts, xanthelasmata and superficial skin lesions.

15.3.1 Warts

Monochloroacetic acid may be pricked into a wart using a pointed wooden applicator. The concentrated 'saturated' solution should be used. It will be noticed that initially the acid is rapidly absorbed by the wart. More is applied and pricked in until no more is absorbed. Any surplus acid is mopped off the wart, which is then left exposed to the air and kept dry. Healing occurs in 8–14 days and the treatment may be repeated if necessary (Chapter 27).

15.3.2 Xanthelasma (xanthoma)

This is a deposit of excess lipids in the skin, commonly found on the medial side of upper and lower eyelids. Biochemical abnormalities are often not demonstrated and if treatment is requested they may be removed by surgery, electrocautery, cryotherapy, radiosurgery or the very careful application of monochloroacetic acid on a small wooden applicator.

15.3.3 Superficial skin lesions

Small naevi, plane warts, superficial keratoses, etc., may all be treated by the careful application of monochloroacetic acid as an alternative to radiosurgery, electrocautery, diathermy or cryotherapy.

Electrocautery

> Put an assortment of olivary cauteries on the fire, large and small, and blow on them until they are well heated. Take one, large or small, apply the cautery to the artery itself after having quickly removed the finger, and keep it there until bleeding is arrested.
>
> *Albucasis, AD 936*

From the earliest times, physicians have used instruments heated to red heat and applied to wounds to control haemorrhage and destroy diseased tissues. The use of an electric current instead of a fire to heat the instrument enabled much greater control of the cauterization to be achieved, and in practice today most electrocauteries comprise a handle incorporating a switch, and a platinum wire electrode which can be heated to red heat by the passage of an electric current through it.

Early instruments used a dry battery and rheostat to control the current and, therefore, the temperature of the wire. These were not entirely satisfactory as the current drain was considerable and the batteries soon became exhausted, often in the middle of a surgical procedure.

With the advent of domestic electricity supplies, lead-acid accumulators were used which could be recharged at a convenient time and were still portable enough to be taken to a patient's home or doctor's treatment room. Furthermore, they could withstand heavy current drain for several hours. As most domestic electricity supplies were direct current, transformers could not be used, and the only means of producing a low voltage and high current necessary for an electrocautery was by means of a heavy-duty variable resistor or rheostat, a method which was wasteful of electricity and not particularly safe for the patient.

The invention of the step-down transformer, whereby the domestic electricity supply of 110 V (or subsequently 240 V) alternating current could be transformed to any chosen voltage, now enabled equipment previously run from batteries to be used on domestic supplies, with no worry about unexpected battery failure. In addition, the low-voltage winding of the transformer could be isolated completely from the primary, high-voltage winding, thus ensuring complete electrical safety for the patient and doctor.

Modern cautery transformers still employ this same principle, incorporating a rheostat to vary the output current (Figs 16.1 and 16.2). Unlike many electronic components the electrocautery works equally

Figure 16.1 A cautery-light transformer with pistol-grip and Mark Hovell handles.

Figure 16.2 A cautery designed for ophthalmic use but very suitable for minor surgical procedures (Keeler Instruments, London).

well on direct current or alternating current; thus, there is no need to rectify the alternating output from the transformer.

More recently, nickel–cadmium rechargeable batteries have been introduced. They have the ability to withstand a heavy current drain, are light in weight, and a completely portable instrument can be produced with no attached wires (Figs 16.3 and 16.4). However, unless regularly recharged, the batteries can fail suddenly, more so than conventional dry cells, so some form of stand-by is desirable. In addition, after several hundred recharges, the batteries lose their ability to retain a charge and need to be replaced.

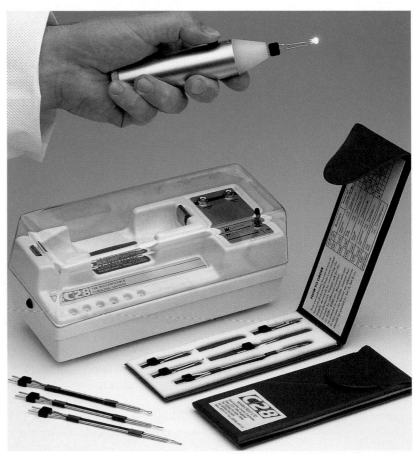

Figure 16.3 Model C282 cordless rechargeable battery cautery; quick and simple to use (Warecrest Ltd).

Figure 16.4 Five cautery burners for use with the C282 rechargeable cordless electrocautery.

Figure 16.5 Disposable electrocautery (Aaron Medical Industries, USA; Cardiokinetics Ltd, UK).

Finally, small, lightweight, disposable cauteries have been introduced, incorporating dry-cell, non-rechargeable batteries. These are extremely light, very portable and most useful for fine cauterization (Fig. 16.5).

The doctor purchasing an electrocautery will be faced with a bewildering array of burners, handles and transformers (Fig. 16.6). For the majority of minor surgical procedures, a portable rechargeable cautery will give the best results. There are no trailing wires, the instrument may be taken between consulting rooms and also to the patient's home, and the risk of inadvertently putting too high a voltage across the burner is eliminated.

Burners come in two lengths, long and short. For the majority of cases the short burner is easier to handle and gives better control. The longer burners are mainly for use in cauterizing the cervix through a vaginal speculum.

A few basic instruments plus an electrocautery will enable a doctor to perform much simple skin surgery (Figs 16.7 and 16.8). Of the many differently shaped burners, the following will be found to be most useful.

- Cutting electrode: this may be used for dividing skin tags and papillomata as well as removing some intradermal naevi (Figs 16.4 and 16.9).
- Ball-ended coagulating electrode. This is one of the most useful burners for sealing small bleeding points: although more expensive than the other burners, it will be found to be the most frequently used (Figs 16.4 and 16.10).

Figure 16.6 A selection of cautery burners, together with Mark Hovell's cautery handle.

Figure 16.7 C282 rechargeable cautery with Volkmann double-ended sharp-spoon curette; two of the most useful instruments for skin surgery.

Figure 16.8 Rechargeable cautery and holder, curettes, dental syringe and local anaesthetic, plus fine-toothed dissecting forceps, selection of cautery burners and histology pots.

Figure 16.9 Small skin tags being removed with a cutting burner. Small lesions need no local anaesthetic.

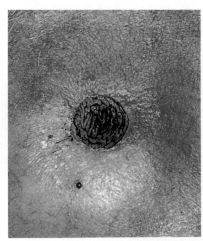

Figure 16.10 Appearance of the base of a lesion removed with the curette and cauterized using the ball-ended platinum burner.

■ 'Cold-point' burner: instead of the heat being produced directly by the platinum wire as in other burners, the 'cold-point' has a central needle-like electrode, around which is wound a heating element. Heat is transferred by conduction to the tip. It is ideal for releasing subungual haematomata, and especially for treating spider naevi, where the needle tip is pressed against the feeding arteriole and effectively seals it (Figs 16.11 and 16.12).

■ Simple ∧-shaped burner: this is useful for a variety of lesions and can be used both to cut and to coagulate (Figs 16.13–16.16).

Figure 16.11 The cold-point cautery burner; ideal for subungual haematoma and spider naevi.

Figure 16.12 The cold-point burner being used to treat a spider naevus.

Figure 16.13   Papilloma on scalp; base infiltrated with local anaesthetic.

Figure 16.14   The papilloma is picked up with forceps and separated with the electrocautery.

Figure 16.15   Papilloma nearly separated from its base; notice the absence of bleeding.

Figure 16.16   The end result immediately after removing the papilloma. No dressing is required.

16.1 USES OF ELECTROCAUTERY

16.1.1 Haemostasis

Small bleeding vessels can be readily sealed by the application of the electrocautery burner. The operator will soon discover the optimum temperature of the wire; generally a dull cherry-red is about right. If not hot enough, the wire will adhere to the tissues; if too hot, it will burn through bleeding vessels without sealing them. An adjustment on the rheostat is all that is required.

16.1.2 Skin tags (Chapter 26)

These may be picked up with fine-toothed forceps and divided easily with the electrocautery. No pressure is required; a repeated small movement of the red-hot wire will neatly separate the lesion from the base, with no bleeding.

16.1.3 Subungual haematoma (Chapter 42)

Resting the electrocautery tip against the nail and switching on the current results in a small, painless hole in the nail with immediate release of blood. The cold-point electrode gives the neatest result.

16.1.4 Accessory digits (Chapter 42)

Where there is no underlying bony connection, accessory digits may be easily separated at birth using the electrocautery alone.

16.1.5 Basal cell carcinoma (Chapter 25)

Many small basal cell tumours of the skin may be curetted and the bases extensively cauterized with the electrocautery, with very good results. By repeating the curettage and cautery twice or three times, even better results may be obtained.

16.1.6 Cauterization of the cervix (Chapter 38)

Cervical erosions are easily treated with the electrocautery; generally no anaesthetic is necessary and the results are good.

16.1.7 Condylomata (Chapter 38)

Individual condylomata may be destroyed using the electrocautery, small lesions will not require anaesthesia, while larger ones can be infiltrated prior to treatment.

16.1.8 Entropion (Chapter 31)

Spot burns with the cautery help to produce fibrosis in the skin/muscle operation for entropion.

16.1.9 Epistaxis (Chapter 32)

Mild epistaxes are best treated with silver nitrate cauterization, but stubborn epistaxes may be treated with electrocautery to Little's area after preliminary topical anaesthesia. Care must be taken not to perforate the nasal septum.

16.1.10 Granuloma pyogenicum (Chapter 25)

These vascular lesions are ideally treated with curette and electrocautery; however, bleeding can be profuse and require several applications of the cautery There is a low recurrence rate.

16.1.11 Haemangioma of the lip (Chapter 45)

After infiltrating with local anaesthetic, a haemangioma on the lip can be treated very effectively by inserting the electrocautery into the centre of the lesion.

16.1.12 Intradermal lesions (Chapter 25)

Small intradermal lesions may be destroyed by the application of the electrocautery alone, while larger lesions may be curetted followed by electrocautery to the base.

16.1.13 Keratoacanthoma (Chapter 25)

Curettage followed by cauterization of the base is a simple and effective method of treating this rapidly growing tumour.

16.1.14 Molluscum contagiosum (Chapter 25)

Small lesions are better destroyed with phenol or iodine pricked into each spot, but equally good results may be obtained using the cautery.

16.1.15 Solar keratoses (Chapter 25)

Most solar keratoses may be removed with a sharp curette and the base cauterized using an electrocautery.

16.1.16 Spider naevi (Chapter 25)

If the central vessel of a spider naevus is touched with the electrocautery, rapid cure results.

16.1.17 Squamous celled carcinoma (Chapter 25)

Small squamous celled tumours may be curetted, followed by liberal cauterization of the base. As with basal cell carcinoma, better results are obtained by repeating the curettage and cauterization two or three times.

16.1.18 Warts and verrucae (Chapter 27)

Almost all warts and verrucae can be removed with a sharp-spoon curette, cauterizing the base afterwards.

16.1.19 Xanthelasmata (Chapter 43.4)

Used with care, the electrocautery may be a suitable treatment for small xanthelasmata.

16.2 COMPARISON BETWEEN INSTRUMENTS

16.2.1 Mains-operated cauteries

The design of mains-operated electrocauteries has changed little over the last 50 years. Basically, they consist of a mains transformer with a lead to a switched handle. Mains-operated instruments have the advantage that higher currents and therefore higher temperatures may be obtained. This can be useful if a large lesion is being removed. A second advantage is that the instrument is always immediately ready for use and does not need prior recharging.

The main disadvantage of mains-operated electrocauteries is the trailing wires to the handle and burner, which makes a completely sterile technique difficult unless the connecting wires and handles are sterilized each time they are used. They are also not as portable as the disposable or rechargeable cauteries.

Because the current and voltage may be increased by using the rheostat, although higher temperatures may be achieved, there is also the risk of overheating and destroying the burners accidentally.

16.2.2 Rechargeable cauteries

The advantages of rechargeable cauteries are:

- the absence of any trailing wires
- greater portability, enabling the doctor to take it easily between consulting rooms, and even to the patient's home
- they may be used where there is no electricity supply
- there is no risk of accidentally destroying the burners by overheating
- the handle may be enclosed in a sterile plastic sheath if a sterile operating field is required.

The disadvantages of rechargeable cauteries are:

- the battery may fail without warning: this may generally be prevented by adequately charging prior to use
- the heat at the tip is less easily controllable than with a rheostat, and may be insufficient to deal with large, vascular lesions.

16.2.3 Disposable cauteries

The advantages of disposable cauteries are:

- they are cheaper to buy at the outset but more expensive in the long run

- there are no trailing wires
- they are very portable.

The disadvantages are similar to those of the rechargeable cauteries, i.e.:

- battery may fail without much warning
- insufficient heat may be generated for large vascular lesions
- the burners are generally more fragile and there is less choice of burner.

16.3 HAZARDS WITH INFLAMMABLE ANTISEPTICS

Spirit-based skin antiseptics or any other inflammable skin application should never be used with the electrocautery or diathermy because of the risk of burns to the patient. In fact, it is unnecessary to use any antiseptic as the heat of the platinum burner is self-sterilizing.

CHAPTER 17

The unipolar diathermy

An ailment I will treat . . . with the fire-drill.

Edwin Smith, Surgical Papyrus, 3000–2500 BC

High-frequency electric currents have been used for minor surgical procedures for 200 years. Early machines used rotating mica discs to generate static electricity which was stored in large Leyden jar condensers, connected to a spark gap and electrodes which were applied to the patient [12]. By the beginning of the twentieth century, portable machines were in production (Fig. 17.1) which used batteries or domestic electricity supplies. The spark gap was still utilized and is still used in some machines today, being superseded by solid-state electronic circuitry (Fig. 17.2a, b).

The bipolar diathermy machine is a standard item of equipment in almost every operating theatre in the world. A low current at very high

Figure 17.1 A domestic high-frequency machine which belonged to the author's grandfather; 1910 approx. This produced similar currents to the modern Hyfrecator.

Figure 17.2 (a) The Birtcher Hyfrecator Plus 7-797. (b) Finger-switch electrode holder.

Figure 17.3   Needle electrode of the unipolar diathermy being used to treat a wart on the fingertip.

frequency and high voltage is passed through the patient. Two electrodes are needed to complete the circuit: one is large in area and is usually strapped to the patient's thigh, while the other is usually connected to diathermy forceps or an electrode. If this latter electrode is placed in contact with the patient, a current sufficient to heat the tissues is generated. By varying the waveform and intensity of the current, tissues may be coagulated or cut.

The unipolar diathermy uses a similar principle: it generates a very high voltage, at very high frequency but relatively low current, but unlike the bipolar diathermy does not require a large second electrode to be connected to the patient. This makes it more suitable for use in minor surgery where large currents are not needed. A high-frequency current may be used in one of three ways, viz: desiccation, fulguration and coagulation.

In desiccation the electrode is inserted into the lesion to be treated to the depth at which the tissue is to be destroyed. The heat generated in the electrode dries out and thus destroys the tissue, which separates in a few days (Figs 17.3 and 17.4).

Fulguration is achieved by holding the electrode just above the surface to be treated and drawing a stream of sparks from the electrode to the point of treatment. The tissues are charred and destroyed, being rejected in a few days (Fig. 17.5). Tissue damage is fairly superficial, which may be an advantage.

Figure 17.4   Desiccation of a wart by inserting a needle electrode into the lesion and passing a current through it. This generates heat within the wart and destroys it.

Figure 17.5   Fulguration of a wart by holding the electrode just above the lesion and allowing a stream of sparks to pass from the electrode to the wart, thus generating heat and destroying it.

Figure 17.6 Coagulation using a bipolar electrode pressed against the skin. Tissue destruction is confined to the area between the electrodes.

Figure 17.7 Bipolar forceps for coagulating bleeding vessels; used with Hyfrecator or diathermy.

In coagulation a bipolar electrode is used which is connected to a separate winding on the transformer. It is placed on the surface to be treated and an electric current flows between the two poles of the electrode, generating heat and thus destroying the tissues (Fig. 17.6). Similarly, bipolar forceps may be used to coagulate small bleeding vessels (Fig. 17.7).

As individual machines vary, the doctor who has not used a Hyfrecator before can experiment using a piece of raw meat held in the hand and applying different electrodes: desiccation, fulguration and coagulation. The depth and extent of treatment can then be assessed by cutting through the meat and examining the lesions produced.

Small cutaneous lesions and those affecting the cervix, vagina and bowel can be treated without the need for a local anaesthetic. For the majority of other lesions, however, it is more comfortable to infiltrate with local anaesthetic prior to treatment.

17.1 ADVANTAGES OF HIGH-FREQUENCY CURRENTS

The advantages are:

- quick, effective destruction of lesions with no blood loss
- accuracy – most lesions can be destroyed with minimal damage to adjacent tissues.

■ the treated area is left sterile
■ good cosmetic results with little postoperative pain
■ excellent for vascular lesions.

17.2 DISADVANTAGE OF HIGH-FREQUENCY CURRENTS

As with the electrocautery the lesion is destroyed and cannot be examined histologically, except by taking a preliminary biopsy.

17.3 SOME APPLICATIONS OF HIGH-FREQUENCY TREATMENT

17.3.1 Warts

The base of the wart is infiltrated with local anaesthetic and desiccated with a fine-needle electrode inserted to the base of wart.

17.3.2 Verrucae

The technique is similar to that for warts.

17.3.3 Haemangiomata

As with warts a method of desiccation is used. Haemangiomata may require more than one treatment, depending on their size.

17.3.4 Large haemangiomata

The base is infiltrated with local anaesthetic and bipolar coagulation is used. Treatment may need to be repeated.

17.3.5 Spider naevus

Local anaesthesia is not used. The needle electrode should be inserted into the main blood vessel, usually in the centre.

17.3.6 Xanthelasma

The treatment is light fulguration with or without local anaesthesia.

17.3.7 Solar keratosis

Local anaesthetic is infiltrated; then curettage followed by fulguration to the base is carried out.

17.3.8 Cervical erosions

These may be treated with fulguration without local anaesthesia.

17.3.9 Papillomata

Small papillomata may be desiccated or fulgurized without anaesthesia. Larger lesions should have the base anaesthetized first.

17.3.10 Naevi

Large naevi may be better excised, but small naevi can be easily destroyed by desiccation. If pigmented, the area desiccated should include a narrow area of healthy adjacent skin.

As can be seen, almost any skin lesion can be effectively treated with a high-frequency current. As the tissue immediately following treatment is sterile, healing may be promoted by the application of a sterile dry dressing, and advising the patient to keep the area dry until healing is complete.

CHAPTER
18

Cryotherapy

> Thou shalt make for him cool applications of ice and salt for drawing out the inflammation from the mouth of the wound.
>
> *Edwin Smith, Surgical Papyrus, 3000–2500 BC*

The first recorded use of cold for medical treatment was in the Edwin Smith Surgical Papyrus (3000 BC). Hippocrates describes the use of snow and ice for relieving pain and arresting haemorrhage (400 BC), but it is only in the last 100 years that freezing as a recognized treatment has achieved popularity.

Liquid air, liquid oxygen and carbon dioxide snow were used at the beginning of the twentieth century [13–14, 15], and in 1950 liquid nitrogen was used successfully to treat a variety of skin lesions [16–20]. More recently, nitrous oxide has been used as a cryogen, using the Joule–Thompson effect to cool a probe applied to the lesion.

The boiling points of gases found in the atmosphere are shown in Table 18.1. As can be seen, nitrogen has the most advantages in that it is freely available (78% of the air in the atmosphere is nitrogen), is often a waste product in industry, is not inflammable, is chemically inert and has the fourth lowest freezing point. Because of these features, liquid nitrogen is now the cryogen of choice in medicine.

18.1 MECHANISM OF ACTION

If human tissue is cooled to −25°C partial destruction occurs, and if cooled to −50°C total destruction takes place. Modern needle thermocouples now enable accurate observation of the effects of freezing and the relationship between probe temperature and depth of tissue destruction.

The result of freezing is the formation of ice crystals in the intracellular and extracellular fluids, resulting in cell dehydration, shrinkage, abnormal concentrates of electrolytes within the cells, thermal 'shock' and denaturation of lipid-protein complexes, and cell death.

It is found in practice that better results are obtained with a quick freeze and a slow thaw cycle, and it also seems better to give the lesion a second freeze immediately after the first freeze has thawed. This double freeze–thaw cycle is common to all freezing agents, whether spray or probe.

Following cryosurgery, a blister may develop, which dries to a scab in about 1 week and eventually separates. Occasionally, a blood-filled blister results which, although looking alarming, heals quickly.

Table 18.1 Boiling points of various gases

Gas	% in atmosphere	Boiling point
Nitrogen	78.1	− 196
Oxygen	20.9	− 183
Argon	0.93	− 186
Carbon dioxide	0.30	− 79
Neon	0.018	− 246
Helium	0.005	− 269
Freon 12	—	− 30
Nitrous oxide	—	− 89

Liquid nitrogen cryoprobe (−196°)

Skin

Intermediate zone of freezing
Reversible tissue damage if
less than −50°C

Ice ball forming in tissue (−150°C to −50°C)
Irreversible damage if > −50°C

Figure 18.1 Cross-section of lesion treated by freezing.

(a)

(b)

Figure 18.2 (a) The hemisphere of ice must extend beyond the lesion in order to include the whole volume. (b) Insufficient area of freezing leaves the base of the lesion still active.

Table 18.2 Relationship of tissue temperature and survival

Tissue temperature	Percentage survival
0 - −10°C	100%
−11- −20°C	67%
−21 - −30°C	38%
−31 - −40°C	14%
−41 - −50°C	3%
−51 - −60°C	0%

During the healing phase, which is usually surprisingly free from pain, depigmentation may occur in the treated skin and a narrow area surrounding it: this should be explained to the patient, particularly if they are dark-skinned. The pigment normally returns after several months.

Most lesions do not require additional local anaesthesia, although freezing of lesions on the digits may cause pain, and this may preclude its use in young children.

It is still possible to infiltrate the base of a lesion with local anaesthetic prior to freezing if the doctor judges that the procedure may give unacceptable discomfort to the patient, but the effects of freezing in this case may not be quite as predictable.

Whichever method of freezing is employed, the object is to produce a subcutaneous hemisphere of ice, in which is included the lesion to be destroyed (Fig. 18.1). Thus, the circumference of ice needs to extend beyond the edge of the lesion (Fig. 18.2).

A good way of demonstrating this is to practise on a pig's trotter, freezing an imaginary lesion and then bisecting the skin with a scalpel to observe the depth of frozen tissue. Tissue destruction is directly proportional to the degree of freezing, as shown in Table 18.2.

18.2 INDICATIONS FOR CRYOSURGERY

Most superficial skin lesions may be treated with cryosurgery, with the exception of melanoma and certain intradermal naevi. Shallow lesions such as solar keratoses and seborrhoeic warts are ideal for treatment and will respond to any of the different freezing agents.

The most widely used application for cryosurgery is in the treatment of warts, common warts, verrucae and genital warts. In this

Figure 18.3 A carbon dioxide pencil which can be made from a J-size CO$_2$ cylinder.

situation, in addition to tissue destruction it is thought that the release of the wart virus into surrounding tissue may stimulate the immune mechanism and thus accelerate the clearance of warts in other areas of the body as well. Liquid nitrogen is probably the freezing agent of choice, as carbon dioxide and nitrous oxide rarely produce sufficient depth of cell destruction.

With experience, the doctor may also consider treating small basal cell carcinomata, small squamous cell carcinomata and kerato-acanthomata. These will require liquid nitrogen, an adequate freeze and meticulous follow-up, and confirmation of diagnosis by means of a cryobiopsy. Occasionally, other factors such as the age of the patient may determine the size and site of the lesion to be treated (Fig. 18.24).

Pigmented lesions, and particularly melanomata, are not suitable for cryosurgery. Certain vascular lesions and haemorrhoids have been treated with cryosurgery; although successful, the postoperative phase is often prolonged, with blood-stained discharges, and is generally not well accepted by the patient.

18.3 CRYOSURGICAL EQUIPMENT

Three main freezing agents are commonly employed for cryosurgery: carbon dioxide snow, nitrous oxide and liquid nitrogen.

18.3.1 Carbon dioxide snow

This is produced from a cylinder of compressed gas, and employs the Joule–Thompson effect, whereby cooling occurs on expansion of the gas within a confined chamber. The snow is then compacted into a pencil applicator (Fig. 18.3), which is pressed against the lesion. Temperatures of −78.5°C are achieved. Carbon dioxide snow may also be mixed with acetone to produce a freezing sludge for treating larger areas of skin.

It is the least effective freezing agent, but is simple, cheap, readily available, and suitable for treating superficial lesions such as solar keratoses and seborrhoeic warts.

18.3.2 Nitrous oxide

Figure 18.4 The Wallach LL50X nitrous oxide cryosurgical instrument with a selection of probes and 'instant thaw' trigger (Prospect Medical Ltd).

Nitrous oxide is supplied under a pressure of 800 lb/in^2 in cylinders. A nitrous oxide cryoprobe consists of a reducing valve which attaches to the cylinder, and a length of connecting tube to a handle on which is screwed a cryoprobe (Fig. 18.4). A control tap on the handle causes cold nitrous oxide to reach the probe tip, resulting in freezing, or stops the flow of nitrous oxide, which builds up pressure and consequently warms, resulting in thawing.

This freezing–thawing facility is a great advantage and enables the probe to be disconnected easily from the skin after treatment. Nitrous oxide cannot be sprayed on the skin, so only a probe can be used with

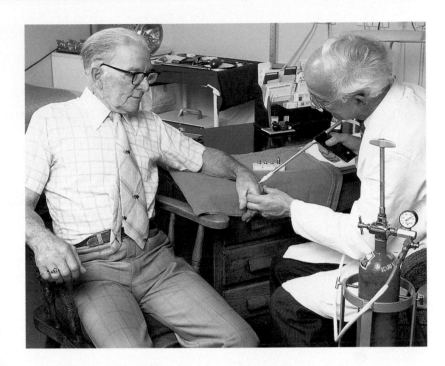

Figure 18.5 The nitrous oxide cryoprobe applied to a solar keratosis on the back of the hand.

Figure 18.6 The nitrous oxide cryoprobe in the surgery; treatment is quick and effective.

this method of cryosurgery. In general practice, nitrous oxide has the advantage that it is always immediately available for use, unlike liquid nitrogen, which may have to be collected from an outside source.

Technique of using the nitrous oxide cryoprobe

Cryoprobes are available in various shapes and sizes; the one approximating most closely to the lesion to be treated is chosen and fitted to the handle (Figs 18.5 and 18.6).

Any hard skin overlying the lesion (e.g. wart) is pared down with a scalpel (Figs 18.7 and 18.8), and a small quantity of water-soluble jelly (e.g. K-Y jelly) is applied either to the skin or to the probe, which is then pressed against the lesion and freezing commenced (Fig. 18.9).

Figure 18.7 Hard skin overlying a wart or verruca should be pared down with a scalpel prior to freezing.

Figure 18.8 Hard skin pared away exposing verrucae.

Figure 18.9 Using a cryoprobe, a small quantity of water-soluble jelly (e.g. K-Y jelly) is applied to the lesion and the probe pressed against it; freezing then causes the probe to adhere to the lesion.

(a)   (b)

Figure 18.10 The cryoprobe is applied to the lesion, which has been smeared with water-soluble jelly to help adhesion.

Figure 18.11 Once the probe is adherent to the skin, it may be gently withdrawn as shown.

Figure 18.12   The Fern cryoprobe; this uses liquid nitrogen and has a thawing facility. A spray attachment is also available (Medinox International Ltd).

Within a short time, ice forms at the probe tip and causes the probe to adhere to the lesion. At this stage, by applying slight traction to the probe, the skin may be lifted away from underlying structures, thus reducing the likelihood of damage (Figs 18.10 and 18.11). Freezing is continued until a rim of ice 1–2 mm around the outer edge of the lesion is seen.

By switching off the nitrous oxide and pressing the 'thaw' switch, the probe tip warms up and detaches itself from the skin. The frozen area is now allowed to thaw, the probe reapplied and a second freeze given, followed by a second thaw.

The patient is warned to expect some throbbing or discomfort over the next few hours: no dressing is necessary, but if a marked inflammatory reaction is expected, for example a large area frozen in an area of thin skin, it may be reduced by an application of a potent fluorinated steroid cream (e.g. Dermovate) under a dressing on completion of freezing.

There is a risk of cross-infection using the same cryoprobe. Although this seems to be minimal, nevertheless it should be borne in mind when treating several patients, and the probes either autoclaved or wiped with a suitable antiseptic solution.

18.3.3 Liquid nitrogen

Liquid nitrogen is now the most widely used freezing agent, and in recent years a variety of liquid nitrogen cryosurgery instruments has been introduced (Figs 18.12–18.14).

Liquid nitrogen is a waste product from industry and is relatively cheap. It boils at −196°C and needs to be kept in a Thermos-type

Figure 18.13   (a) The Cryo-jet (liquid nitrogen) with spray attachment (Cryomedical Instruments Ltd). (b) The Wallach liquid nitrogen ultrafreeze CY-6500 (Prospect Medical Ltd).

Figure 18.14 The CS-76 liquid nitrogen cryosurgical unit, which is self-pressurizing, portable and non-electric. It may be used with spray needles and closed-end probes (Frigitronics Ltd, Downs Surgical plc).

container; even then it is continually evaporating and gradually reverts to nitrogen gas.

Where a doctor or practice considers using liquid nitrogen, a decision needs to be made either to collect small quantities from a nearby source at regular intervals, or to invest in a large Dewar-type flask which will store up to 3 months' supply of liquid nitrogen at one filling, and from which small quantities may be drawn off when needed.

The disadvantage of collecting quantities from an outside source is that patients need to be called back a second time and a special clinic arranged at which all patients may be treated at one session.

18.3.4 Methods of using liquid nitrogen

Four techniques of freezing using liquid nitrogen are available:

- cryospray
- cryoprobe
- individual probe
- cotton-wool swab applicator.

18.3.5 Cryospray

Most instruments designed for cryospray consist of a double-insulated Thermos-type flask, with a screw-on lid and pressure safety valve, with a finger-operated on/off valve which delivers liquid nitrogen under moderate pressure to a spray-tip with a variable diameter hole. Liquid nitrogen is then sprayed as a fine jet on the lesion to be treated, with the nozzle held about 1 cm away from the lesion (Figs 18.15–18.19).

As with other cryotherapy techniques, best results are obtained with two freeze–thaw cycles. Furthermore, evidence suggests that better results are also obtained with a relatively quick freeze and a relatively slow thaw.

Figure 18.15 Liquid nitrogen cryospray. The spray nozzle is held about 1 cm away from the lesion.

Figure 18.16 Freezing occurring over the surface of the lesion. Two freeze–thaw cycles are recommended.

Figure 18.17 Small warts are easily treated with a fine-aperture cryospray nozzle.

Figure 18.18 Large solitary wart over the fifth interphalangeal joint.

Figure 18.19 Treatment of a large wart with liquid nitrogen cryospray. Caution is needed to avoid damage to underlying structures, in this case extensor tendons and joint.

Having received two freezes, the patient is warned to expect some discomfort, and if a marked inflammatory reaction is expected, a potent fluorinated steroid cream is applied under a dressing.

Cryospray treatment is remarkably simple to apply but has inherent dangers, the main one being the risk of damage to underlying structures such as digital nerves and tendons. It is not a treatment to be undertaken lightly or delegated to an untrained assistant.

Figure 18.20 Cryoprobe for use with liquid nitrogen or nitrous oxide.

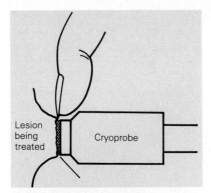

Figure 18.21 Method of separating the cryoprobe from a lesion using a finger-nail to snap off the line of adherence.

18.3.6 Cryoprobe

As with nitrous oxide, cryoprobe attachments are available to screw to the liquid nitrogen outlet in place of the spray applicator. They consist of hollow metal probes of different diameters through which the liquid nitrogen is passed (Fig. 18.20). Here it evaporates and cools the tip of the probe to −196°C, and the nitrogen gas is then taken away through a flexible exhaust tube attached to the side of the probe.

18.3.7 Technique for liquid nitrogen cryoprobe

This is similar in some respects to that used with nitrous oxide. The probe nearest in size to the lesion is chosen. Any hard skin overlying the lesion (e.g. wart) is pared down, and a small quantity of water-soluble jelly (e.g. K-Y) is applied either to the lesion or to the tip of the probe, which is then pressed against the lesion and freezing commenced.

As soon as a rim of ice is seen forming at the tip of the probe, gentle traction is applied to the probe, thus pulling the skin away from underlying structures and reducing the risk of damage.

Freezing is continued until a rim of ice 1–2 mm wide is seen surrounding the lesion. At this stage, freezing is discontinued, and with the majority of liquid nitrogen cryoprobes it will be necessary to separate the probe from the skin using pressure with the finger-nail in order to snap off the probe from the lesion (Fig. 18.21).

Where the doctor treats large numbers of patients with liquid nitrogen, it is worth investing in one of the machines which has a built-in heating cable to thaw the probe-end and also to keep the transfer tube supple (Fig. 18.12).

As with the nitrous oxide cryoprobe, two freeze–thaw cycles are recommended for best results. The possibility of cross-infection can be prevented by sterilizing the probe-tip between patients.

18.3.8 Individual probe

A simple, cheap, metal probe can be used successfully for cryotherapy using the same method as is used for cotton-wool applicators (Fig. 18.22).

Figure 18.22 (a) Simple, inexpensive probes for use with liquid nitrogen, made from aluminium or copper. (b) Individual probe being used to treat a digital wart.

Figure 18.23 Rowmed probe.

Figure 18.24 Liquid nitrogen cryospray used to treat basal cell carcinoma on scalp of patient aged 98. Complete healing in 10 weeks.

Liquid nitrogen is poured into an insulated polystyrene cup, and the metal probe dipped in until boiling stops, indicating that the probe is at −196°C. It is removed, the tip wiped clean with a dry swab and applied to the skin lesion, which has been pared down if necessary and covered with a thin film of water-soluble jelly (Fig. 18.22). The mass of the metal probe is such that quick freezing occurs, followed by a slow thaw, and separation occurs without difficulty as the probe warms up.

All the advantages of a cryoprobe accrue, without the need to purchase expensive equipment.

18.3.9 Cotton-wool applicator

One of the earliest methods of applying liquid nitrogen was by means of a cotton-wool swab, dipped in liquid nitrogen and pressed against the lesion. Treatment is quick, simple, cheap and effective. Swabs should not be reinserted in the liquid nitrogen as it has been shown

Figure 18.25 Cotton-wool swab dipped in liquid nitrogen and applied to the lesion.

that the human wart virus can remain alive in liquid nitrogen and there is the risk of cross-infection. Cotton-wool swabs are not as precise or as effective as the purpose-designed cryoprobe (Fig. 18.25).

18.3.10 Use of the auriscope speculum for accurate freezing

Small cutaneous lesions may be frozen very precisely by choosing an appropriately sized auriscope speculum, placing it over the lesion and spraying liquid nitrogen into the open end (Fig. 18.26).

18.3.11 Use of adhesive putty

This is normally used for sticking posters to walls, but can be used in cryotherapy for treating irregularly shaped lesions, particularly if

Figure 18.26 (a, b) Precise freezing may be achieved using an auriscope speculum.

near the eye, ear or mouth. The edge of the lesion is first identified using a marker pen and the putty is applied around it. When the spray is applied, the putty freezes to the skin and protects it. A narrow margin under the edge of the putty will also be frozen.

18.3.12 Thermoelectric coolers (TEC)

These devices date back to 1821 when Thomas Seebeck discovered that if two dissimilar metals were joined together to form a circuit, and the junctions were maintained at different temperatures, a current would flow in the circuit. In the reverse situation, where a current is passed across a junction of two dissimilar metals, a temperature difference could be maintained between these junctions. This was known as the Peltier heat, and depending which way the current flowed, the junctions would either warm or cool. This effect has been used to produce a portable, electric, cryoprobe and has the advantage that supplies of carbon dioxide, nitrous oxide or liquid nitrogen are not necessary – only a supply of electricity. Probe temperatures of −50°C can be obtained, which are sufficient to treat many superficial lesions (Fig. 18.23).

18.4 CONTRAINDICATIONS AND DANGERS OF CRYOSURGERY

18.4.1 Contraindications

Because cryosurgery is now so widely used, it is sometimes forgotten that there may be conditions where freezing may be contraindicated.

The doctor or nurse should consider the following as possible reasons for not using freezing agents on the skin:

- any known intolerance to cold
- Raynaud's disease
- cold urticaria
- cryoglobulinaemia
- pyoderma gangrenosa
- autoimmune diseases
- agammaglobulinaemia;
- poorly controlled diabetes mellitus;
- dark skin where hypopigmentation following treatment would be unacceptable.

18.4.2 Dangers of cryosurgery

Because cryosurgery looks so easy, it is often forgotten that liquid nitrogen causes tissue death. Thus underlying structures may be irreparably damaged, e.g. cutaneous nerves and tendons [21]. It is therefore vital to be aware of the exact anatomy and avoid damage to underlying structures. The doctor should be particularly wary of treating warts on the sides of fingers.

Liquid nitrogen must be transported in a proper flask with a safety release valve for gas. A domestic vacuum flask is not the most suitable container and if it is used, under no circumstances should the lid be screwed down, otherwise it will explode because of the build-up of pressure.

Similarly, when transferring liquid nitrogen from one container to another, one should wear goggles and use protective gloves if at all possible. Splashes of liquid nitrogen on the hand, do not generally cause burns.

When carrying a full flask of liquid nitrogen one must ensure that it remains upright and does not tip over. This applies particularly when transporting a container in a motor vehicle. Adequate ventilation must be provided when transporting by car, preferably placing the container in the boot.

18.5 CRYOBIOPSY

One major advantage of cryotherapy is the ability to take a cryobiopsy to establish a diagnosis. This is done while the tissues are frozen, with

Figure 18.27 A cryobiopsy may easily be taken with a sharp-spoon curette.

Figure 18.28 If necessary, the base may also be cauterized with the electrocautery.

Figure 18.29 The cryoprobe applied to a wart on the foot.

Figure 18.30 Once the probe is adherent to the wart, gentle traction may be applied.

Figure 18.31 A cryobiopsy may easily be performed, or the wart removed completely using a sharp-spoon curette.

either a punch biopsy forceps or curette (Figs 18.27 and 18.28). A small piece of alginate dressing is placed in the wound to check bleeding as thawing occurs, covered by a dry, sterile dressing. Unlike cauterization with heat, freezing does not damage the histology of the cells, and the cryobiopsy may therefore be placed directly in 10% formol-saline and sent for routine histology exactly as any other specimen (Figs 18.29–18.31).

Freezing also produces thrombosis in the microcirculation after 24 h, so that provided the diameter of the vessels involved is small enough, many vascular lesions can be treated. Intradermal haemangiomata, particularly on the face, may be given repeated short freezes every 6 weeks, which will result in a gradual regression and total cure.

Following treatment of any lesion, the area should be kept as dry as possible and if necessary covered with a dry, sterile dressing.

18.6 SUCCESS RATES FOR CURING LESIONS

The success rates for curing various lesions are shown in Table 18.3.

Table 18.3 Success rates for various lesions

Lesion	Cure rate
Viral warts (hands)	75% if treated at 2–3 week intervals
Verrucae	60% if treated at 2–3 week intervals
Molluscum contagiosum	Similar to hand warts
Actinic keratoses	Nearly 100%
Seborrhoeic warts	Nearly 100%
Dermatofibroma	85% when treated at 2–3 week intervals
Tattoos	50% for small tattoos but high morbidity
Ingrowing toe-nails	50–60%
Labial mucoid cysts	85%
Synovial cysts	60%

Figure 18.32 Small ganglion over distal inter-phalangeal joint often disperses after cryosurgery.

Figure 18.33 Ganglion frozen with liquid nitrogen. Care needs to be taken to avoid damaging underlying structures.

Postoperative instructions following liquid nitrogen treatment

1   Liquid nitrogen destroys tissues by freezing to $-196°C$. This results in ice forming inside the cells, and as this thaws, it causes cell death.

2.   Immediately following treatment, apart from a slight discomfort, it will look as if nothing has happened to the skin.

3   Gradually, over the next few days, swelling, reddening, and sometimes blistering will occur.

4   Following this stage, healing occurs, which is usually remarkably pain-free, and leaves only a very slight scar, or none at all.

5   In dark skins, there is usually an area of depigmentation following cryotherapy; this normally recovers over the next year.

6   Reaction to liquid nitrogen is very variable; in some patients quite alarming looking blistering can occur, together with swelling of the surrounding tissues. Despite this, satisfactory healing still occurs.

7   Keep the treated area dry for 6 days if at all possible; it does not need any dressing unless blistering has occurred, in which case a simple non-stick dressing may be applied.

8   It is important to check with your doctor whether you need to be seen again, as more than one session is occasionally needed to cure some lesions.

9   If you have any queries, please do not hesitate to contact the surgery.

Figure 18.34   Information leaflet given to each patient receiving cryotherapy.

CHAPTER 19

Histology

Although many skin lesions have characteristic or virtually diagnostic clinical appearances, histological examination of excised lesions is essential in ensuring a precise pathological diagnosis.

As a general guide, therefore, it is advisable to send all specimens for routine histological examination. Even quite innocent-looking skin lesions can occasionally turn out to be early neoplasms. The doctor is then in difficulties if the original specimen has been thrown away and a further lesion appears at the site of the first excision. Another advantage of sending all specimens for routine histology is to increase the doctor's diagnostic acumen. Only by comparing the histological report with the original clinical diagnosis can the accuracy of the latter be improved.

One point which is often overlooked is the importance of giving the histopathologist all relevant information about the specimen in order to obtain an accurate diagnosis. In many cases precise diagnosis involves interpretation of the histological changes seen in a tissue section in the light of the clinical circumstances; for example, squamous cell carcinoma and keratoacanthoma look alike histologically, but can be more readily differentiated if the history about the length of time for which the lesion has been present is given on the request form.

Most pathologists would like the following minimum clinical information with every specimen:

- name
- address
- age
- sex
- history, including duration
- site of lesion
- size of lesion
- method of removal (e.g. excision, biopsy or curettage)
- clinical diagnosis.

19.1 HISTOLOGICAL APPEARANCES OF COMMON LESIONS (Figs 19.1–19.16)

For a more comprehensive account of histology, the reader is referred to one of the many histopathology textbooks. However, it is helpful to have a little knowledge of the histological appearances of the commonly encountered skin lesions seen in minor surgery, and the following have been chosen as being representative. They have been grouped into epidermal lesions of increasing severity, followed by dermal lesions.

Figure 19.1 (a) Histological appearance of normal skin showing the keratinizing stratified squamous epithelium of the epidermis overlying the connective tissue structure of the dermis. Scattered pale-staining melanocytes are present in the basal layer of the epidermis. (b) Section of normal skin including sweat glands in the lower dermis. (c) Diagrammatic appearance of normal skin histology. (d) Evolution of naevi showing histology.

Figure 19.2 (a) Sebaceous cyst (pilar cyst). These common, benign cysts may grow to a very large size. Note the central punctum. (b) Histological appearance: note that the cyst lining corresponds to the hair follicle outer sheath with no granular layer. Amorphous eosinophilic content. (c) Epidermoid or inclusion cyst being removed from the ear-lobe. (d) Epidermoid cyst: note that the cyst lining corresponds to the epidermis including the granular layer. The content is keratin.

Figure 19.3 (a) Viral wart (verruca vulgaris). Usually multiple, raised, hyperkeratotic and commonly found on the hands and feet. (b) Histology: note the papillomatous structure with surface hyperkeratosis, acanthosis and cytoplasmic vacuolation in scattered cells in the upper Malpighian and granular layers, indicating viral aetiology.

Figure 19.4 (a) Molluscum contagiosum. Multiple, umbilicated lesions are commonly found in children under 5 years. Solitary, large lesions are seen in adults, similar in appearance to warts. (b) Histological appearance: note surface parakeratosis and acanthotic epidermis with numerous molluscum bodies, granular eosinophilic cytoplasmic masses in the cells of the Malpighian, granular and horny layers. (c) Higher magnification of epidermal cells distended by intracytoplasmic, eosinophilic, virus-containing molluscum bodies.

Figure 19.5 (a) Benign melanocytic naevus (junctional naevus stage). Dark, discrete lesion with smooth edges and even colour. (Photograph by courtesy of Dr. R.J. Cairns). (b) Histological appearance; note nests of proliferating melanocytes in the basal layer of the epidermis at the epidermodermal junction. No dermal involvement.

Figure 19.6   (a) Benign melanocytic naevus (compound naevus stage) (Photograph by courtesy of Dr. R.J. Cairns). (b) Continuing junctional activity with epidermal melanocytic nests associated with dermal migration of cords of naevus cells.

Figure 19.7   (a) Intradermal naevus. Lightly pigmented, raised skin papilloma. (b) Benign melanocytic naevis (intradermal naevus stage). Residual cords and nests of naevus cells in the dermis. No residual junctional activity.

Figure 19.8   (a,b) Seborrhoeic wart (basal cell papilloma) Note raised, multiple brown–black lesions with stuck-on appearance. (c) Note epidermal thickening featuring basal-cell proliferation, horn cysts and surface keratosis.

- normal skin
- sebaceous cysts (pilar, tricholemmal, andepidermoid)
- viral wart
- molluscum contagiosum
- melanocytic naevus (junctional naevus stage)
- melanocytic naevus (compound naevus stage)
- melanocytic naevus (intradermal naevus stage)
- seborrhoeic wart (basal cell papilloma)
- keratoacanthoma
- basal cell carcinoma (rodent ulcer)

- squamous cell carcinoma
- malignant melanoma
- keloid scar
- haemangioma
- blue naevus (benign dermal melanocytoma)
- histiocytoma.

Sebaceous cysts are rarely of 'sebaceous gland' origin. They are usually either pilar (tricholemmal) or epidermoid (implantation) cysts.

Figure 19.9 (a,b) Keratoacanthoma. Rapidly growing, spontaneously resolving lesion, with central ulceration and keratin plug. (c) Low-power magnification: part of keratin cup of keratoacanthoma with underlying squamous cell proliferation. (d) High-power magnification: note base of lesion showing irregular squamous cell proliferation. Note also close similarity to squamous cell carcinoma; therefore, length of history is important.

Figure 19.10 (a,b) Basal cell carcinoma (rodent ulcer). Common, slowly growing, non-metastasizing lesion, locally destructive and on exposed sites. Note surface capillaries and pearly appearance. Eventual ulceration and rolled-over edges. (c) Histological appearance showing clumps of neoplastic epidermal basal cells infiltrating the dermis. Surface ulceration.

Figure 19.11   (a) Squamous cell carcinoma of lower lip. Note hyperkeratotic, ulcerated, rapidly growing lesion, which can metastasize. (b) Histological appearance; note irregular proliferation of neoplastic squamous cells, ulceration and underlying infiltration of the dermis. Horn pearls present.

Figure 19.12   (a) Malignant melanoma. Note irregular margin and variations in colour (black/brown/red). Prognosis depends on the thickness and depth of infiltration of the lesion. Can metastasize and be very aggressive. (Photograph by courtesy of Dr. R.J. Cairns). (b) Polypoid malignant melanoma showing surface ulceration and infiltration of upper one-third of the dermis. (The Breslow thickness was 4.2 mm.) (c) Histological appearance. Irregular groups of variably pigmented malignant cells infiltrating the epidermis and dermis.

Figure 19.13   (a) Keloid scar. Note pale, hypertrophied area. (b) Note coarsely thickened hyalinized collagen bundles in the dermis.

Figure 19.14 (a) Haemangioma. (b) Histological appearance: note numerous small vascular channels, mainly of capillary structure, in the dermis.

Figure 19.15 (a) Blue naevus (benign dermal melanocytoma). May be mistaken for a melanoma. Uniform colour, blue–black, smooth, raised lesion, which is benign. (b) Histological appearance: note deeply pigmented melanocytes in the dermis. The overlying epidermis is normal.

Figure 19.16 (a) Histiocytoma (dermatofibroma). Firm, pale, fibrous nodule commonly on the lower limbs following trauma. Benign. (b) Histological appearance: note fibroblastic and histiocytic proliferation in the dermis in variable proportions in different lesions.

Figure 19.17 A histological specimen being put into formol-saline. It is good practice to send every specimen for routine histological examination.

19.1.1 Evolution of the naevus (Fig. 19.1d)

Melanoblasts migrate in fetal life from the neural crest to the junction between the dermis and epidermis. An arrest of this migration in the dermis may form a blue naevus. In childhood, junctional activity is usual and the naevus is termed a **junctional** naevus. In early adulthood, melanocytes may also migrate into the dermis as well as the dermoepidermal junction to form nests and columns of cells. This is now a **compound** naevus. In late adulthood through to old age all of the activity is now in the dermis. Schwann cells may appear with the melanocytes and there may be less pigmentation as the naevus matures. This is now an **intradermal** naevus.

19.1.2 Benign melanocytic naevus

The common pigmented mole or naevus, also known as a benign melanocytic naevus, progresses through three evolutionary stages before ultimate involution. Commonly arising in adolescence, the earliest stage is that of junctional naevus, followed by compound and intra-dermal naevus stages.

19.2 THE HISTOLOGY BOOK

For medicolegal reasons as well as audit it is important not only to send specimens off for histology (Fig. 19.17), but also to have personally seen every report when they return. One way of ensuring that no reports are lost is to use a histology book (Fig. 19.18). In this are recorded the date, patient's name and address and clinical diagnosis, and, when received, the final histological diagnosis. Any missing reports are easily spotted and action is taken.

Figure 19.18 Sample page from histology book. Note that the histology report for Lee Black has not been returned or noted by the doctor, and will need to be followed up.

Date	Name	Address	Diagnosis	Histology	Received
1.1.96	John Smith Senior	12 South St London	Sebaceous cyst	Sebaceous cyst	✔ ✔
1.1.96	Alice Green (Mrs)	Southcot 23a High St	Intradermal naevus	Intradermal naevus	✔ ✔
8.1.96	Christopher Braston	24 Acorn Rd E. Hosting	?Melanoma ?Naevus	Junctional naevus (benign)	✔
8.1.96	Lee Black (12.10.04)	Rose Cott 12 West St	?B.C.C.		
15.1.96	Ann Gray (23.5.21)	245 High Rd Larkhill	Seborrhoeic wart	Seborrhoeic wart	✔
15.1.96	Dr. Philip Hoaking	The Mount E. Bradshaw	?Fibroma R. thigh	Histiocytoma	✔

CHAPTER 20

Statistical analysis

> You know, my children, that Surgical Operations are divided into two classes: those that benefit the patient, and those that more often kill . . . abstain from undertaking dangerous and difficult treatments
>
> *Albucasis, 1013–1106 AD*

By keeping simple records of every operation performed, valuable statistical analysis is possible, which in turn may be of help in planning future requirements for the practice. A register of operations may be compiled using a hardback book in which is entered the date, patient's name, address, age and sex, together with the type of operation. This list may be numbered chronologically or include a code for additional data retrieval or computer storage. At the end of each year, a breakdown of the year's operations is made, from which can be compiled a summary and analysis (Table 20.1).

20.1 RECORD-KEEPING

The importance of keeping accurate comprehensive and legible records of every operation cannot be emphasized enough. Details should be written down immediately the operation is finished and not committed to memory; such details as which digit, whether left or right, which joint, whether infected or not, size, situation and extent of the lesion, history, signs and symptoms, findings at operation, method of anaesthesia, dose of anaesthetic used, skin preparation, method of excision, whether histology was requested, haemostasis, closure, type and number of sutures used, type of dressings used, estimated date of suture removal and subsequent management should all be entered on the patient's notes, signed and dated. At this stage the doctor should personally check that any specimen which is being sent for histology is correctly labelled and corresponds to the histology request form.

20.1.1 Information leaflets

Preprinted information leaflets may be given to the patients after their operations (see Chapter 50 for full list):

- liquid nitrogen
- ingrowing toe-nails
- injection ganglion
- injection varicose veins
- electrocautery
- meibomian cysts.

Table 20.1 Analysis of minor operations performed over 5 years by the author.

20.2 ORGANIZING A MINOR OPERATING LIST

It is much better to set aside a time each week for a minor operating list than to perform each operation as it arises. Not only can the patient make preparations, but the surgery staff and nurses can prepare instruments, equipment and forms in advance, clean the room and generally anticipate what will be needed. It is also a more efficient use of everyone's time. The only disadvantage of arranging a list is the risk of cross-infection, particularly if an unsuspected abscess or a heavily infected lesion is treated at the beginning of the list before the remaining 'clean' cases. With scrupulous attention to aseptic technique, and the use of central sterile supplies department (CSSD) packs, cross-infection should not occur; nevertheless, it is good practice to put 'clean' operations such as vasectomy or excision of ganglion, where infection could be disastrous, first on the list, and arrange 'dirty' cases such as infected ingrowing toenails and abscesses at the end.

Having decided to reserve a set time regularly for minor operations, an appointment book should be made (Fig. 20. 1), giving time and date, details of the patient's name and address, nature of operation and estimated time allowed. Initially, the doctor should keep this appointment book personally, and personally see every patient. With experience, an accurate estimate of the time that each operation takes will be learned and at this stage the appointment book may be taken over by a receptionist or secretary, with clear instructions from the doctor about arrangements for transport and subsequent follow-up. Telephone numbers of patients should be recorded in case it is necessary to change the order of the list and contact the patient at short notice.

A typewritten list of the operations should be prepared, with copies for the treatment room, nurses, receptionists, filing clerks and doctor. By so doing, appropriate patient notes may be prepared, histology forms and containers labelled, and necessary instruments and dressings prepared.

20.3 INFORMING THE PATIENT

The doctor should personally discuss with the patient every detail of the operation: what is involved, the type of anaesthetic, the site and

Table 20.1   Analysis of minor operations performed over 5 years by the author

Category	Operation	Year 1	Year 2	Year 3	Year 4	Year 5
Injections	Tennis elbow	52	56	45	45	54
	Intra-articular	23	38	38	41	41
	Carpal tunnel	22	18	23	42	53
	Piles	26	27	48	22	36
	Hormone implant	37	30	47	51	68
	Others	6	2	9	21	29
Aspirations	Cysts and bursae	24	23	48	33	25
	Hydrocele	5	6	5	8	15
	Abdominal paracentesis	1	4	2	3	3
	Breast cysts	10	18	19	13	27
	Bartholin's cysts	3	3	3	3	2
	Aspirate and sclerose ganglion	14	22	22	16	16
	Others	5	5	2	3	8
Incisions	Abscesses	39	38	32	30	37
	Meibomian cysts	11	16	13	25	19
	Thrombosed external piles	33	29	17	9	20
	Others	2	2	7	9	5
Excisions	Suture lacerations	58	50	41	31	27
	Sebaceous cysts	44	51	68	76	69
	Intradermal naevi	93	67	97	131	165
	Lipoma	6	6	9	13	20
	Basal cell carcinoma	14	6	17	12	10
	Others	15	12	25	15	17
Curette	Warts and verrucae	115	136	98	81	93
	Others	66	48	35	29	17
Toes	Ingrowing toe-nails	45	34	48	57	42
	Removal of toe-nails	9	5	6	12	2
	Others	0	2	0	0	0
Tourniquet	Decompression carpal tunnel	2	3	12	22	21
	Release trigger finger	0	2	2	1	0
	Others	0	2	0	0	0
Diagnostic	Protoscopy	98	137	192	187	259
	Sigmoidoscopy	85	77	154	137	172
	Needle biopsy	6	7	3	6	20
	Skin biopsy	14	4	8	17	14
	Rectal biopsy	3	3	5	3	2
	Others	1	1	2	8	12
Miscellaneous	Pinch graft to ulcer	3	3	2	2	3
	Varicose veins	11	8	24	42	44
	Cervical erosions	7	4	1	7	8
	Cryocautery	280	215	416	428	604
	Others	5	21	25	14	26
Totals for the year		1295	1244	1644	1721	2108

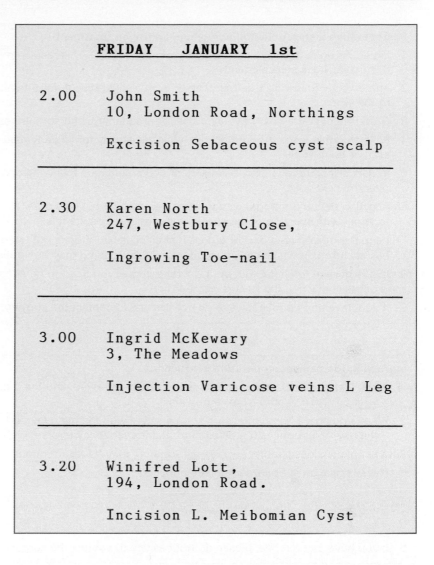

FRIDAY   JANUARY   1st

2.00   John Smith
10, London Road, Northings

Excision Sebaceous cyst scalp

2.30   Karen North
247, Westbury Close,

Ingrowing Toe-nail

3.00   Ingrid McKewary
3, The Meadows

Injection Varicose veins L Leg

3.20   Winifred Lott,
194, London Road.

Incision L. Meibomian Cyst

Figure 20.1 An appointment book can also be used for the 'operating list' each week.

size of any scar, the removal of any sutures, how long the procedure will take, whether transport will be required to take the patient home or whether they will be able to drive or walk home, alone or accompanied. It is important to give an estimate of how long the patient may need to be away from school or work, and any risks of the operations should be carefully explained. It is also important to advise patients whether the operation will be 100% curative (e.g. excision of simple naevus or cyst) or whether recurrence may be expected and what proportion can be expected to recur (e.g. varicose vein sclerotherapy, excision of ganglia, ingrowing toe-nails). It is well known that much of the information given to patients is not remembered; consequently, it is helpful to have preprinted leaflets to give to the patients to take away with simplified details of their operation, appointment times and any necessary arrangements. These leaflets may also act as an *aide-mémoire* for the doctor and staff (Fig. 20.1).

Postoperative instructions following liquid nitrogen treatment

1 Liquid nitrogen destroys tissues by freezing to −196˚C. This results in ice forming inside the cells, and as this thaws, it causes cell death.

2 Immediately following treatment, apart from a slight discomfort, it will look as if nothing has happened to the skin.

3 Gradually over the next few days, swelling, reddening, and sometimes blistering will occur.

4 Following this stage, healing occurs, which is usually remarkably pain-free, and leaves only a very slight scar, or none at all.

5 In dark skins, there is usually an area of depigmentation following cryotherapy; this normally recovers over the next year.

6 Reaction to liquid nitrogen is very variable; in some patients quite alarming looking blistering can occur, together with swelling of the surrounding tissues. Despite this, satisfactory healing still occurs.

7 Keep the treated area dry for 6 days if at all possible; it does not need any dressing unless blistering has occurred, in which case a simple non-stick dressing may be applied.

8 It is important to check with your doctor whether you need to be seen again, as more than one session is occasionally needed to cure some lesions.

9 If you have any queries, please do not hesitate to contact the surgery.

Ingrowing toe nails postoperative instructions

1 A small strip of nail, including the nail has been removed, and the base treated with pure phenol to prevent this narrow strip from regrowing.

2 When you arrive home, please rest on a settee with the feet elevated on a cushion for the remainder of the day; this reduces the discomfort and the tendency to bleeding.

3 A simple analgesic tablet such as paracetamol may be taken for any postoperative discomfort.

4 Please make an appointment to see nurse on

. . . . at . . . .

and a second appointment to see nurse on

. . . . at . . . .

5 If you have any queries, please do not hesitate to contact the surgery.

Injection treatment for ganglion

A ganglion is a cyst tilled with clear jelly; it is often situated near a joint, and may cause pain, and slowly increase in size. Some eventually rupture spontaneously and disappear, but this may not happen for up to 3 years.

1. Injection treatment consists of drawing off the jelly from the ganglion, and then injecting an irritant fluid into the empty cyst.

2. This causes an inflammation within the ganglion. A pressure bandage is then applied with the object of compressing the inflamed surfaces and thus obliterating the cyst.

3. Please keep the bandage in place for 2 weeks.

4. If it works loose, you may reapply it firmly, but do not disturb the pressure-pad overlying the ganglion.

5. At the end of 2 weeks, you may remove the pad and bandage, and normally no further follow-up visits are required.

6. If, however, you have any queries, please do not hesitate to contact the surgery.

Figure 20.2 Preprinted information leaflets which may be given to the patients after their operation. (See Chapter 53 for full list.)

Injection treatment for varicose veins

Injection treatment for varicose veins consists of injecting an irritant fluid into the vein and applying a firm dressing over the injection site. The object of the treatment is to create an inflammation inside the vein, and then by compressing the inflamed surfaces together, hope that they will adhere to each other, thus obliterating the lumen of the vein.

The following simple instructions should be followed:

1. The bandages should be left on (day and night) for 3 weeks. Some discomfort should be expected during the first few days; in a small number of patients it is very painful, in which case you should take any simple analgesic tablets such as paracetamol, aspirin, or codeine at regular intervals until the pain subsides.

2. If the outer layers of bandage work loose or begin to dig into the skin, it is helpful to carefully remove the outer bandage whilst lying down, and to then reapply it firmly from the toes up to the knees, making sure not to disturb the pressure pads overlying the injection sites in the veins.

3. Walk at least three miles every day.

4. If you wish to have a bath, the bandaged leg may be kept dry by putting it inside a large watertight polythene bag (e.g. a bin-liner) with two elastic bands around the top.

5. After 3 weeks, please make an appointment to see the doctor to have the bandages removed.

6. If you have any queries, please do not hesitate to contact the surgery.

Postoperative instructions – Electrocautery

1. Many warts, moles, naevi, and keratoses can be removed by planing off with a sharp blade or curette.

2. Following removal, the base of the lesion is treated with either the electrocautery or diathermy.

3. This seals any bleeding vessels and leaves a dried crust on the surface.

4. Healing will occur over the next 2-4 weeks on average.

5. It is helpful to keep the area completely dry for at least 2 days, and preferably longer.

6. If you have any queries, please do not hesitate to contact the surgery.

Meibomian cysts – Postoperative instructions

1. A Meibomian cyst occurs in the eyelid and is caused by a blockage of the little lubricating duct inside the eyelid.

2. Treatment consists of incising the cyst under a local anaesthetic.

3. This is done from inside the eyelid, so you will not have a visible scar.

4. After the operation, eye ointment is applied, and a pad and bandage put on; this is to protect the eye against dust, etc. on the way home, as the eye is still anaesthetized.

5. The pad and bandage may be removed after 4 hours.

6. Do not be alarmed when you remove the pad – there will be a mixture of ointment, secretions and blood, which can look alarming!

7. Gently clean the eyelids with warm water.

8. Thereafter, apply the eye-drops three times a day for 1 week.

9. It is not normally necessary to see you again, but if you have any queries, please do not hesitate to contact the surgery.

20.4 COMPLICATIONS

With careful selection, good operating technique and the provision of sterile instruments and dressings, complications from minor surgical procedures are rare. The most common complication is sepsis; this may be unavoidable if the lesion is already infected (e.g. ingrowing - toe-nails, infected sebaceous cysts and abscesses) or may occur as a result of cross-infection during the operation or postoperative period.

Tissues should be handled as little as possible, a no-touch technique developed by doctor and assistant, breathing and coughing over the wound avoided, sterile drapes used to keep the operating field as free from contamination as possible, and careful application of skin antiseptics should be made, making sure not to miss any areas. The widespread use of powerful antibiotics as a 'cover' is unnecessary and should be condemned as bad practice; however, the judicious use of antibiotics in a few carefully selected patients is justified and may result in healing by first intention. These may be given orally, by injection or directly into the lesion (e.g. Fucidin inserted in abscess cavities prior to closure).

20.4.1 Haemorrhage

This is rarely a problem; most is venous and can be controlled by firm pressure and the use of diathermy or electrocautery. Small arteries can be clipped with curved mosquito artery forceps and tied if necessary, but most can be controlled by skin sutures alone.

20.4.2 Damage to nerves, tendons and arteries

Again, these complications are extremely rare. Knowledge of the underlying anatomy is essential, and the awareness of variations from normal and the use of bloodless operating fields for such operations as carpal tunnel decompression are mandatory. Should damage occur to any nerve, tendon or artery, this fact should be carefully recorded, accurate measurements taken and a decision taken whether to attempt repair or refer to a specialist colleague. Provided the blood supply to the affected part is adequate, closure and referral at a later date are recommended unless immediate help is available. It is wise that the patient be informed and any action to be taken discussed with him or her (Chapter 51).

20.5 BRAVERY CERTIFICATES

Some procedures inevitably will be uncomfortable or even painful despite all measures aimed at pain relief. Where children are involved, a 'bravery certificate' (Fig. 20.3) signed by the doctor and staff and given to young patients at the end of the procedure helps to take their mind off the discomfort, restores trust, and often makes a return visit less traumatic to parents, child and doctor.

Figure 20.3 'Bravery certificates', which are popular with young patients.

CHAPTER 21

Audit

Minor surgery lends itself admirably to audit, i.e. the monitoring and appraisal of care against predetermined standards, with the aim of improving overall standards of care. It is a valuable exercise for the surgeon, as without regular assessment even the best doctor has only an anecdotal impression of what his or her results are as far as the patients are concerned.

We should be saying to ourselves: 'Is what I think I am doing what really gets done, and if not, why not?'

It is very simple to count the numbers and types of minor operations done each year and to analyse these in groups. The following questions also need to be examined.

- Am I getting it right?
- Are my diagnoses accurate?
- What is my success rate?
- What is my failure rate?
- What is my infection rate?
- How many patients do I then refer to specialist colleagues?
- Is what I am doing cost-effective?
- What are my scars like?
- Am I offering a good service; is it better than the local hospital service?
- Are my patients satisfied with the service?
- What are the waiting times?
- Am I satisfied with methods of pain relief?
- Are all histology reports seen, noted and acted upon?
- Am I becoming a specialist in complications?
- Is there always a trail of blood to the waiting room from my treatment room?
- Should I give up minor surgery?

It is helpful to consider a series of criteria to be satisfied before any audit process is undertaken [22, 23]:

- There should be potential benefits in terms of better care.
- It should be ethically acceptable to both patient and doctor.
- There should be a willingness to make changes in the light of the results of an audit.
- Standards should be set and aims agreed by the participants.
- There should be an appropriate sample size and selection.
- Data collection must be accurate and honest.
- The results must be confidential to the participants unless agreed otherwise.

Audit of minor operations in general practice may conveniently be divided into the following groups.

- Method: what was actually done?
- Results: was the histological report the same as the clinical diagnosis?
- Follow-up: infection, histology, etc.
- Cost: comparison of results with other centres.
- Outcome: patient satisfaction.
- Implementation of changes.
- Then reaudit to analyse improvements.

For those doctors considering introducing some form of audit for their minor operations, a start can be made by counting and analysing the types of operation done over 1 year. Secondly, a histology book (Chapter 14) may be introduced to compare clinical diagnosis with histological diagnosis. Thirdly, a patient questionnaire may be introduced to evaluate patient satisfaction. Fourthly, an 'infection and outcome' book may be kept recording both satisfactory and unsatisfactory outcomes.

By such means it is possible not only to monitor what one is doing, but also to identify areas where there are problems, and ultimately improve the service to patients, as well as increasing job satisfaction and enjoyment.

PART 2

Routine minor surgery

CHAPTER 22

Injections and aspirations

> In the cure of ascitic hydropsy proceed thus: after having placed the patient on his back, draw the skin upward. Then take a knife and pierce as far as siphac [peritoneum]. Have to hand a cannula and place it in the puncture and draw away as much of the watery matter as the patient may endure. But bear ever in mind that it were better to take too little than empty wholly for the loss of strength that cometh thereby.
>
> *Mundinus, Abdominal Paracentesis, AD 1275–1326*

With the availability of steroid and local anaesthetic injections the doctor now has a very effective treatment for many musculoskeletal and articular problems. Even when the exact diagnosis is in doubt, e.g. 'fibrositis' or 'lumbago', a carefully placed injection of steroid with local anaesthetic may dramatically relieve all of the patient's pain. Similarly, an acutely inflamed joint in rheumatoid arthritis will respond very well to aspiration and injection of steroid.

22.1 CHOICE OF STEROID

There are many different steroid preparations available and nearly as many differing views on which is the most suitable. There is probably little to choose between the different preparations, but as a general guide, if a weaker preparation will give as good results as a stronger steroid, the weaker one should be used.

Similarly, if an exact point of tenderness can be identified it may be preferable to inject a small quantity of potent steroid into the lesion, but if a more diffuse area is involved it may be helpful to inject a larger volume of a more dilute preparation. Thus most soft-tissue lesions will respond adequately to hydrocortisone mixed with a larger volume of lignocaine, whereas most intra-articular injections seem to respond better to the smaller volume potent steroids. Three preparations are commonly used:

- hydrocortisone acetate (Hydrocortistab) 25 mg/ml
- methylprednisolone acetate (Depo-Medrone) 40 mg/ml
- triamcinolone hexacetonide (Lederspan) 20 mg/ml.

Hydrocortisone and triamcinolone may be mixed with lignocaine, but methylprednisolone tends to flocculate in the syringe. It is, however, manufactured premixed as Depo-Medrone plus Lidocaine. Triamcinolone is relatively insoluble (0.0003% at 25°C) and consequently stays in the tissues for several weeks or months.

22.2 LANDMARKS

A good knowledge of surface anatomy is essential for accurate positioning of soft-tissue steroid injections, particularly to avoid damage to underlying structures such as nerves and tendons. Where possible, as accurate a diagnosis as possible is desirable, and will improve overall results.

22.3 INDICATIONS FOR USE

Steroid injections are useful in the treatment of the following conditions:

- rheumatoid arthritis
- osteoarthritis
- traumatic arthritis
- gouty arthritis
- synovitis and bursitis
- 'fibrositis'
- tendinitis
- epicondylitis
- intermittent hydrarthrosis.

22.4 CONTRAINDICATIONS FOR THE USE OF STEROIDS

Because of the relative insolubility and the limitation of systemic activity of steroids, there are not many absolute contraindications, but the following situations should be considered carefully:

- active or recently healed tuberculosis
- ocular herpes simplex
- in the presence of infection
- acute psychoses
- where there is a history of known hypersensitivity
- where previous injections have produced atrophy.
- Immunization procedures are better avoided in patients on high-dose steroids, because of the possibility of neurological complications.
- It is advisable not to inject more than three joints at one session.
- Too many repeated injections in one joint are inadvisable.

Following steroid injections the patient should be asked to rest the affected limb for 24–48 hours where possible.

22.5 TENNIS ELBOW (LATERAL EPICONDYLITIS)

This is one of the easier lesions to inject, but the results are often disappointing inasmuch that many recur after an apparently successful injection.

It is also worth noting that the natural history of lateral epicondylitis or tennis elbow is almost complete resolution in 2 or 3 years even without any treatment; therefore the doctor is dealing with a self-limiting condition and the effect of any injection is, hopefully, to accelerate healing. In the first instance it is important to establish a correct diagnosis, as cervical nerve root entrapment can cause similar pain, particularly C6 lesions referred to the lateral epicondyle. The patient usually complains of pain in the elbow, worse on attempting to pick up wide objects, and can usually localize the point of maximum tenderness. Gripping causes pain, but flexion and extension of the elbow is usually painless. On examination, there is marked tenderness on palpating the extensor insertion into the external (lateral) epicondyle, and pain on resisted dorsiflexion of the wrist. As would be expected, the right elbow is affected much more than the left.

22.5.1 Technique

With the patient sitting comfortably facing the doctor and the elbow flexed to a right-angle, the point of maximum tenderness is identified (Fig. 22.1). The overlying skin is painted with povidone–iodine in alcohol (Betadine alcoholic solution) or similar antiseptic. A mixture of steroid and local anaesthetic is now drawn into a sterile 2 ml syringe using a no-touch technique. Three preparations are commonly used:

- methylprednisolone and lignocaine, marketed as Depo-Medrone 40 mg with Lidocaine 10 mg premixed in a 1 ml or 2 ml single-use vial; it should not be mixed with any other injection
- triamcinolone hexacetonide, marketed as Lederspan 20 mg in 1 ml single-use vials; this may be mixed with saline or lignocaine as required
- hydrocortisone acetate, marketed as Hydrocortistab 25 mg/ml in all-glass single-use ampoules; this too may be mixed with saline or lignocaine as required.

Figure 22.1 Injection for tennis elbow (lateral epicondylitis), palpating the most tender spot.

Having drawn the solution into the syringe, the doctor carefully removes the needle and replaces it with a new sterile 25 swg × 5/8 in. (0.5 mm × 10 mm) needle, fixing it very firmly; this reduces still further any risks of cross-infection. The patient and doctor should not talk or cough over the exposed needle, and for the same reason it is a good idea routinely to wear a mask.

Without touching the site of the injection or touching the needle, the point of maximum tenderness is located, and the injection made directly into it. Considerable pressure is needed, hence the reason for fixing the needle firmly to the syringe; the object is to distribute the injection around the bone interface where most of the pain nerve endings are found. The remainder of the injection is placed in the tissues adjacent to the epicondyle (Fig. 22.2).

Having received the injection, the patient is asked to 'work it in' during the next few hours by repeatedly extending the elbow joint pronating the wrist and at the same time palmar flexing the joint. It is also worth warning the patient that the injection site may be extremely painful during the first 24 h, and thereafter relief may be expected. With meticulous technique there should be no danger of infection, but one of the most common side-effects to be seen is atrophy of tissues beneath the injection site, resulting in a small depression in the skin; this is seen in other situations where subcutaneous steroid injections are given, and is not confined to tennis elbow.

Aftercare is equally important, it is not a good idea to exercise the hand and fingers strenuously, 'to see if it has worked'; on the contrary, the lesion must be rested for several days to allow sound healing.

Despite this, recurrences are common, and the question of a second injection arises. This is unlikely to be as successful as the first, and most doctors therefore limit the number of injections to two or three, preferring to let the condition cure itself spontaneously thereafter.

Figure 22.2 Injection of steroid and local anaesthetic being given into the most tender spot for tennis elbow.

22.5.2 Alternative treatments

Relief may also be obtained from analgesics, physiotherapy in the form of friction and ultrasonics, and the application of a firm, non-stretch bandage or splint around the body of the forearm muscles just distal to the painful insertion.

22.6 GOLFER'S ELBOW (MEDIAL EPICONDYLITIS)

This has the same signs and symptoms as a tennis elbow except that the tenderness is over the medial epicondyle and is reproduced by resisted palmar flexion of the wrist. Treatment is exactly the same as that for tennis elbow, but the volume of injection may be slightly less. The most tender spot is located by extending the elbow and externally rotating the wrist; the overlying area is painted with povidone–iodine in spirit (Betadine alcoholic solution) and the injection made from the anterior surface. It must be remembered that the ulnar nerve lies in a groove just behind the medial epicondyle and any injection should be accurately placed to avoid damage to this nerve. Likewise, it is important to look for any operation scars around the elbow joint in case the patient has had a transposition of the ulnar nerve from behind the epicondyle to in front, for previous nerve entrapment. Putting the patient's arm behind their back gives better access to the medial epicondyle.

22.7 OLECRANON BURSITIS

This is commonly due to repeated trauma: most cases will resolve with firm support, but where the condition is giving discomfort or the bursa is unusually large, aspiration may be attempted, followed by the injection of one of the three steroid preparations, e.g. 1 ml Depo-Medrone, 1 ml Lederspan or 1 ml Hydrocortistab. Infection is not uncommon and extreme care needs to be taken to avoid introducing infection at the time of aspiration (Fig. 22.3).

22.8 INTRA-ARTICULAR INJECTIONS

Any joint in the body may become inflamed or develop an effusion or arthritis, and the majority may be entered with a sterile needle either to withdraw fluid or to inject steroids, or both.

Certain points need to be borne in mind.

- An absolute sterile technique is mandatory as septic arthritis is a disaster.
- A knowledge of the anatomy of the joint is essential, together with the best method of approach.
- It should always be remembered that steroid injections rarely cure the underlying pathology: they merely suppress the active inflammation.
- Repeated injections in any one joint are inadvisable unless all other measures have failed.

Figure 22.3 Olecranon bursitis.

Figure 22.4 Injection sites at the elbow.

22.8.1 The elbow

Pain can arise at either the true elbow joint or the radiohumeral joint. Injection of the true elbow joint is performed with the elbow flexed and the needle inserted posteriorly, whereas the radiohumeral joint is approached laterally (Fig. 22.4).

22.9 THE PAINFUL SHOULDER

This is a common complaint and accurate diagnosis of the exact cause is often difficult. Many are due to referred pain from the cervical spine, and others from inflamed bursae, tendons or capsule, and it is in this latter group that steroid injections offer much relief.

The six common lesions are supraspinatus tendinitis, subacromial bursitis, infraspinatus tendinitis, subscapularis tendinitis, 'capsulitis' and arthritis. Fortunately each can be treated by a common approach, namely the posterior aspect of the shoulder.

22.9.1 Technique

With the patient sitting with his or her back to the doctor, the spine of the scapula is palpated and followed laterally until it becomes the acromial process; using the index finger, the coracoid process is located anteriorly. The line joining these two points gives the direction of injection. The overlying skin is painted with povidone–iodine in spirit (Betadine alcoholic solution) and 2 ml methylprednisolone 40 mg with lignocaine 10 mg (Depo-Medrone with Lidocaine) drawn into a 2 ml syringe. The needle is discarded and replaced with a new 21 swg × 1½ in. (0.8 × 40 mm) needle. The needle is inserted about 1 in. (2½ cm) so that it runs below the acromial process towards the coracoid process. There should be no resistance to injection as the needle is in the upper recess of the shoulder joint (Fig. 22.5).

Figure 22.5 Injection sites for the painful shoulder.

As with tennis and golfer's elbows, the patient should rest the joint for 1 or 2 days, then gently exercise; likewise, he or she should be warned that the pain may be exacerbated during the first 24 h before relief is obtained. Injection may be combined with physiotherapy to achieve maximum benefit.

22.9.2 Acromioclavicular joint

Injury to this joint is common in sportsmen and women, and sub-luxation or dislocation can occur, as can degenerative arthritis and even a 'spur'. The joint is of the plane variety, and it is possible to enter it with care from the front, centrally. Using a fine-gauge needle (25 or 23 swg), up to 0.5 ml may be injected.

22.9.3 Glenohumeral joint

This is the true shoulder joint. Signs of disease in this joint are limitation of external rotation and pain. The joint is best approached by the posterior approach as described in Section 22.9.1, and the ease of injection usually indicates that the needle is in the right place.

22.9.4 Bicipital tendinitis

This is due to an inflammation of the synovial sheath surrounding the tendon of the long head of the biceps in the bicipital groove. It can be successfully treated by injection.

Technique

The tender area is palpated with the patient reclining and the palm externally rotated and facing upwards. The overlying skin is cleaned using povidone–iodine in spirit. The needle is introduced alongside the tendon in the bicipital groove and the injection made. If there is doubt, some local anaesthetic may be injected first, which should relieve the pain. Care should be taken not to inject into the tendon as this could cause it to rupture.

22.10 INJECTION OF THE CARPAL TUNNEL

Symptoms from compression of the median nerve in the carpal tunnel are very common and consist of numbness or pain over the middle three fingers, which is worse at night when the patient typically hangs the arm out of bed or shakes the hand in an attempt to alleviate the discomfort. Pain may also radiate from the wrist proximally to the elbow. Eventually, wasting of the thenar muscles occurs (Fig. 22.6). The injection of steroids into the carpal tunnel often relieves all symptoms permanently, and even if the symptoms recur following injection, at least the doctor will know that the original diagnosis was correct and that surgical decompression will be successful.

22.10.1 Establishing the diagnosis

The typical history is paraesthesia affecting the middle three fingers, but occasionally paraesthesia occurs in the whole hand, which suggests that the superficial branch of the ulnar is also involved. It is more common in pregnancy, myxoedema, rheumatoid arthritis, acromegaly, osteoarthritis and obesity.

The following tests may be used:

- Tinel's test: percussion over the flexor retinaculum reproduces the symptoms
- Phelan's sign: forcibly flexing the wrist for up to 1 min reproduces the symptoms
- electrophysiological tests: if there is still doubt, electromyography can be done, which will give an accurate diagnosis.

Figure 22.6 Untreated, compression of the median nerve may result in severe wasting of the thenar muscles.

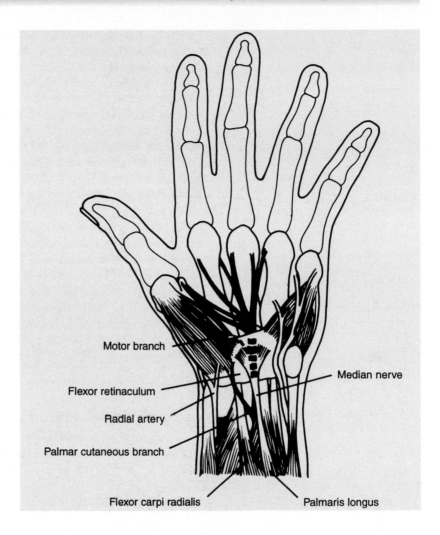

Figure 22.7   Anatomy of the wrist and median nerve in relation to the carpal tunnel.

22.10.2 Technique

The injection site is on the palmar surface of the hand, just lateral to the midline in the line of the skin crease dividing the forearm and hand. The median nerve lies just beneath the tendon of the palmaris longus muscle (Figs 22.7 and 22.8).

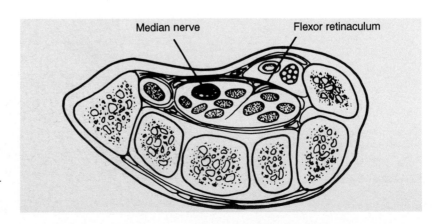

Figure 22.8   Cross-section of the wrist showing the median nerve in the carpal tunnel surrounded by tendons.

With the patient sitting by the side of the doctor, his or her hand is placed palm upwards on a sterile sheet from a sterile dressing pack. The overlying area is liberally painted with povidone–iodine in spirit (Betadine alcoholic solution). Neither patient nor doctor should speak or cough over the injection site.

A 2 ml sterile syringe is used to draw in 1 ml of methylprednisolone acetate (Depo-Medrone); the needle is then discarded and replaced with a new, sterile 25 swg × 5/8 in. (0.5 × 16 mm) needle. Lignocaine is not added on this occasion as local anaesthetics injected around the median nerve would produce unacceptable anaesthesia of the fingers and in most cases the injection of steroid alone is not painful.

The patient is told to flex the wrist against the resistance of the doctor's hand. This will demonstrate the palmaris longus tendon (present in over 60% of the population). The doctor makes a mark with a pencil tip or your thumb-nail just lateral to the tendon at a level of the distal palmar crease. This is the site of the injection. The patient is asked to relax the wrist, and the needle is inserted at an angle of approximately 45° pointing towards the fingers. The needle tip should now be lying behind the flexor retinaculum. Aspiration is done to check that the needle is not inside a blood vessel, then up to 0.5 ml steroid is slowly injected (Figs 22.9 and 22.10). Normally, there is little

Figure 22.9 Injection of the carpal tunnel showing the angle of the needle and bevel in relation to the median nerve.

Figure 22.10 Injection of the carpal tunnel, facing away from the patient. The entry point of needle is in the thinner skin of the wrist.

Figure 22.11 The median nerve is considerably larger than is generally realized. This figure shows the flexor retinaculum divided at operation.

resistance and only slight discomfort to the patient. Any severe pain or 'electric shocks' in the fingers which might indicate irritation of the median nerve should be reported. Should this occur, the needle is withdrawn slightly and repositioned more laterally, away from the nerve. The patient should be warned that the symptoms may be aggravated for 24–48 h and told to take a mild analgesic such as paracetamol. For those doctors who feel uneasy about injecting directly into the carpal tunnel, it has been recently shown that an injection of steroid placed 4 cm proximal to the wrist crease gives equally good results and carries less risk of injury to the median nerve (Fig. 22.11) [24].

22.11 INJECTION OF TRIGGER FINGER

Trigger finger is due to a tenosynovitis of the flexor tendons of the fingers with a nodular expansion of the tendon which catches in the tendon sheath. The patient complains of locking of one finger or thumb in flexion, which then gives a click when forcibly extended. Treatment by injection is often very successful; the injection is made into the tendon sheath and not the tendon itself.

22.11.1 Technique

The fourth finger is commonly affected and is injected as follows. The patient sits facing the doctor with the hand, palm upwards, resting on a sterile sheet on the desk. Povidone–iodine in spirit (Betadine alcoholic solution) is applied, and 1 ml of methylprednisolone acetate (DepoMedrone) drawn into a 1 or 2 ml syringe. The needle is discarded and a new, sterile, 25 swg × 5/8 in. (0.5 × 16 mm) needle attached. An even better method is to use a disposable 1 ml insulin syringe and 30 swg needle. The injection is made over the site of the triggering, which is commonly in line with the flexor tendon where it crosses the distal palmar crease (Fig. 22.12). As with carpal tunnel injection, the needle should be inserted at an angle with the bevel pointing downwards, parallel to the underlying tendon, applying gentle pressure to the syringe plunger as the needle is advanced. By palpating the tendon sheath with the fingers of the opposite hand, the doctor can usually feel when the injection fluid has entered the tendon sheath. An injection of 0.5 ml of solution is made, the needle is withdrawn, and the patient asked to exercise all of the fingers for 1 min to distribute the steroid evenly. Improvement usually occurs after 48 h and may be permanent. Where triggering recurs, surgical division of the sheath is recommended.

Figure 22.12 Injection site for trigger finger.

22.12 INJECTION FOR DEQUERVAIN'S DISEASE

DeQuervain's disease (stenosing tenosynovitis of the short extensor and long abductor thumb tendons) is a common cause of wrist pain. It is often due to overuse of the fingers and thumb, resulting in pain on using the wrist and on gripping, and in a few patients can be very resistant to treatment and cause much discomfort. Often there is visible swelling over the line of the tendons, and palpable crepitus can be elicited in many cases.

22.12.1 Technique of injection

The skin is cleaned using povidone–iodine in spirit. The needle is inserted tangentially alongside the tendon, into the tendon sheath. Injection should offer no resistance, and the fluid may be felt or seen to travel along the tendon sheath. If doubt exists about the placing of the needle, the doctor should disconnect the syringe and ask the patient to move his or her thumb. If the needle tip is in the tendon, movement of the thumb will cause tilting of the needle.

Ten milligrams of hydrocortisone in 2 ml 1% lignocaine is injected; alternatively, 4 mg triamcinoline in 2 ml 1% lignocaine, or 1 ml Depo-Medrone plus Lidocaine may be used.

It is preferable to offer injection earlier rather than later, as the longer the condition has existed the less effective is steroid injection. In fact, if it has existed for longer than 6 months, surgical decompression is usually required.

22.13 RADIOCARPAL JOINT

This joint is commonly involved in early rheumatoid arthritis and often responds well to a carefully placed steroid injection. The easiest site for injection is over the dorsum of the wrist, in the gap between the end of the radius and the lunate and scaphoid bones (Fig. 22.13). Gentle palmar flexion opens up the joint and assists injection. If the needle is in the correct space, it enters easily and injection may be done easily. With advanced rheumatoid arthritis, normal surface landmarks are lost and entry into the joint space may be more difficult. After cleaning the skin with povidone–iodine in spirit, 10 mg hydrocortisone acetate in 5 ml of 1% lignocaine may usually be injected. As an alternative, 4 mg triamcinolone in 5 ml 1% lignocaine or 1 ml DepoMedrone plus Lidocaine may be used.

22.14 FIRST CARPOMETACARPAL JOINT (THUMB BASE)

This joint is commonly involved in both osteoarthritis and rheumatoid arthritis. It is also unusual in that steroid injections in this joint are equally effective whether the diagnosis is osteoarthrosis or rheumatoid arthritis. The reason for this is not clear.

Figure 22.13   Site of injection for the radiocarpal joint.

Figure 22.14 Injecting the first carpometacarpal joint.

The diagnosis may usually be made by pressing over the joint in the 'anatomical snuff-box' and by forced adduction of the thumb into the palm.

22.14.1 Technique of injection

The doctor feels for the joint line with the tip of the index finger, and marks it with a felt-tip pen. By applying countertraction, the joint space is opened up and the needle inserted into the joint space, after the skin has been cleaned with povidone–iodine in spirit (Fig. 22.14).

Only a very small volume can be accommodated, i.e. 0.5 ml or less of Depo-Medrone with Lidocaine.

22.15 METACARPOPHALANGEAL JOINTS

The metacarpophalangeal joints are less easy to inject, but respond well to intra-articular steroid injections, particularly in rheumatoid arthritis.

The line of the joint needs to be identified. This is normally about 1 cm distal to the crest of the knuckle, and may be made more obvious by gentle subluxation of the joint (Fig. 22.15).

22.15.1 Technique of injection

The doctor applies traction to the patient's finger with one hand while injecting with the other. By putting an index finger on the opposite side of the joint, the doctor can feel the distension of the joint as the injection is being made. The skin is cleaned with povidone–iodine in spirit.

About 0.25–0.5 ml Depo-Medrone with Lidocaine is all that the average metacarpophalangeal joint will take.

Figure 22.15 Site for injection of the metacarpophalangeal joint.

22.16 INTERPHALANGEAL JOINTS

Again commonly affected by rheumatoid arthritis, the interphalangeal joints may be helped by carefully placed steroid injections. The method is similar to that used for injecting metacarpophalangeal joints, but a lateral approach is preferable and the needle just inserted at the joint line. It is not possible to insert it further owing to the shape of the joint. Countertraction helps to open the space. An injection of 0.1–0.3 ml Depo-Medrone and Lidocaine is used.

As with all steroid injections, the patient is advised to rest the joint for 24–48 hours after injection.

22.17 INJECTION OF TENDON SHEATHS IN THE HAND

The indications for injections in the tendon sheaths are triggering of nodules, effusion or recent adhesion formation. (See Section 22.11, Trigger finger.) The tendon sheaths are arranged as shown in Fig. 22.16.

Figure 22.16 Arrangement of the tendon sheaths in the hand.

22.17.1 Technique

First, the overlying skin is cleaned with povidone–iodine in spirit. Where there are palpable nodules, these may be infiltrated with a mixture of steroid and local anaesthetic, e.g. Depo-Medrone and Lidocaine. Where the whole of the tendon sheath is distended, it is preferable to inject directly into the sheath itself.

With the patient seated or lying down with the palm of the hand uppermost, the needle is inserted over the tendon sheath and slowly advanced until a space is found where little resistance to injection is encountered. If in doubt, the syringe can be disconnected and the needle gently pushed until it is in the tendon itself, as shown by tilting of the needle on movement of the finger. The needle is then slightly withdrawn, the syringe reattached and the injection made.

22.18 INJECTION OF SMALL GANGLIA

Ganglia are jelly-filled cysts lying adjacent to joints or attached to tendon sheaths. They often appear to be connected to the joint by a valve mechanism, which allows fluid to enter but not leave the cyst. The fluid in the ganglion therefore gradually builds up.

Small ganglia may often respond to a steroid injection placed directly in the cyst. Larger ganglia should either be excised surgically, or more easily aspirated and sclerosed (Chapter 43).

22.19 INJECTIONS AROUND THE HIP JOINT

Steroid injections into the hip joint are beyond the scope of this book, but periarticular soft-tissue injections in the structures adjacent to the hip joint give very rewarding results.

22.19.1 Subtrochanteric bursitis

This condition is more common than realized. The patient, and sometimes the doctor, ascribe the pain in the 'hip' to be due to osteoarthritis. The patient complains of pain, worse when lying on the affected side in bed, and a point of tenderness can usually be found by asking the patient to lie on the couch, painful side uppermost, hip flexed, and identifying the most tender area along side the greater trochanter.

The spot is marked, the skin cleaned with povidone–iodine in spirit, and inject a large volume (10–15 ml) of 1% lignocaine containing 50 mg hydrocortisone or the equivalent amount of triamcinolone 10–15 mg is injected using a 21 swg needle. In obese patients it may be necessary to use a 3 in. (7.7 cm) spinal needle to reach bone.

The needle is advanced until it touches the greater trochanter, slightly withdrawn and injection made into the area of the tough fibrous insertion of the gluteal fascia.

22.20 MERALGIA PARAESTHETICA

This is a superficial entrapment neuropathy due to compression of the lateral cutaneous nerve of the thigh as it passes through the deep fascia about 4 in. (10 cm) below and medial to the anterior superior iliac spine. Classically, the patient complains of pain and paraesthesia over the anterolateral area of the thigh.

If the patient's symptoms have lasted for less than 2 weeks, it is worth waiting to exclude a diagnosis of herpes zoster. Having identified a local tender spot at the site of the penetration of the nerve, local anaesthetic and steroid are infiltrated around the area, e.g. 5 ml 1% lignocaine with 5–10 mg hydrocortisone.

22.21 ASPIRATION AND INJECTION OF THE KNEE

Generally, an effusion will be present. The best approach to the knee is laterally at the junction of the upper pole of the patella and the patellar tendon.

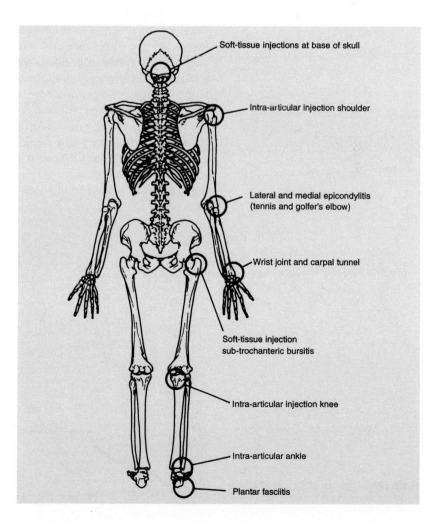

Figure 22.17 Sites of the most common soft-tissue and intra-articular steroid injections.

Figure 22.18 Intra-articular steroid injection – the knee.

Povidone–iodine in spirit (Betadine alcoholic solution) is liberally applied and three separate syringes are prepared: the first is a 2 ml syringe loaded with 2% lignocaine and 25 swg × 5/8 in. (0.5 × 16 mm) needle with which to infiltrate local anaesthetic; the second is a 20 ml sterile syringe with 21 swg × 1½ in. (0.8 × 40 mm) needle for aspirating the effusion; and the third is a 2 ml syringe loaded with 2 ml triamcinolone hexacetonide 20 mg/ml (Lederspan). The needle on this third syringe is disconnected.

The skin is painted with antiseptic, then the skin and subcutaneous tissues down to the joint are infiltrated with lignocaine (Fig. 22.18). Using the same track and the 20 ml syringe, any effusion is aspirated, put in a container for laboratory examination and the colour noted: it may be clear, cloudy or blood-stained. If clear, this suggests osteoarthritis, and if bloodstained, a recent haemarthrosis; in both

Figure 22.19 Injection of the knee joint; relationship of the needle to underlying structures.

cases it is safe to inject steroids. This may be done simply by disconnecting the 20 ml syringe from the needle and connecting the loaded 2 ml syringe. Gentle aspiration to confirm that the needle is still inside the joint is followed by injection of steroid. The needle is then withdrawn and a sterile dressing applied together with a firm compression bandage. If the aspirate is cloudy, it is not safe to inject steroids before excluding a septic arthritis; the fluid should be examined by Gram stain and culture, and by polarized light for birefringent crystals found in gout.

It is a good idea routinely to send any fluid aspirated for culture; not only can the unsuspected infection be diagnosed but, if any infection subsequently occurs, it is helpful to know that it was there at the time of the injection and not introduced by the operator.

22.22 SEMIMEMBRANOSUS BURSITIS (POPLITEAL OR BAKER'S CYST)

This is a distension of the semimembranosus gastrocnemius bursa, and usually occurs whenever there is disease within the knee joint causing an effusion. Owing to a one-way valve mechanism, fluid can track from the knee to the bursa, but not back again.

Treatment of a semimembranosus bursitis is therefore treatment of the underlying knee problem. There is no point in injecting the cyst with steroids, but a judiciously placed injection in the knee joint, by reducing the effusion, will often cure the cyst.

22.23 PREPATELLAR BURSITIS

This is a common condition caused by trauma to the prepatellar area as a result of excessive kneeling. It is also known as housemaid's knee, clergyman's knee, coalminer's beat-knee, carpet-layer's knee, etc.

Most cases resolve spontaneously and give little trouble. If, however, it is judged necessary to treat the condition, an injection of Depo-Medrone 1 ml usually results in a rapid resolution.

22.24 THE FOOT

The main indications for steroid injections at the ankle are rheumatoid arthritis and seronegative arthritis. It is always important to exclude any infection as a cause of swelling and pain and, particularly in the foot, gout.

22.24.1 The ankle

The ankle is relatively easy to inject. By asking the patient to dorsiflex the foot, the tendon of tibialis anterior can be identified and the needle introduced just lateral to this, in the space between the tibia and the talus.

Figure 22.20 Injecting the skin over the ankle joint with local anaesthetic prior to aspiration and injection of the joint.

Calcaneal spur   Site of injection

Figure 22.21 Plantar fasciitis; site of injection.

Insertion of a needle directly into the ankle joint can be very painful; therefore, an advance injection of local anaesthetic is given (Fig. 22.20).

When the needle is in the joint, it is often possible to aspirate fluid, confirming that the needle is in the correct place, and also enabling a sample of fluid to be sent for bacteriology and biochemical examination. Injections of 20 mg triamcinolone (1 ml), 100 mg hydrocortisone acetate or 40 mg Methylprednisolone may now be given.

Scrupulous aseptic technique is mandatory to avoid any possibility of introducing infection, and the overlying skin should be thoroughly painted with povidone–iodine in spirit before any injection is given.

22.24.2 Plantar fasciitis

This is a common condition, causing extreme pain under the calcaneum. A localized tender spot can always be found, and X-rays frequently show the presence of a calcaneal spur, which is correctly more a transverse ridge rather than a spur. The presence or otherwise of a spur on radiological examination does not alter the decision to inject a planter fasciitis, particularly as the results of any surgical treatment for calcaneal spurs are not good.

Technique

With the patient lying on the couch, the point of maximum tenderness is identified and marked (Fig. 22.21). The overlying skin is painted with povidone–iodine in spirit, and the injection made either from the medial side of the foot, or directly through the sole of the foot. Because the exact site of pain is not always easy to identify accurately, it is preferable to use a larger volume of a dilute solution of hydrocortisone or triamcinolone in 1% lignocaine than a small volume of stronger steroid. Having said this, it is not always possible to inject more than 1 ml because of discomfort. If the injection has been made in the correct site, the local anaesthetic causes rapid relief of pain.

22.24.3 Tendo achilles tendinitis

This is mentioned largely to advise **against** injection. Although pain and swelling around the Achilles tendon are common, steroid injections have been known to cause rupture of the tendon, with disastrous consequences. It is, therefore, not recommended to be carried out by the general practitioner (GP).

22.24.4 First metatarsophalangeal joint

The first metatarsophalangeal (MTP) joint is commonly affected by crystal synovitis of gout, and by osteoarthrosis and rheumatoid arthritis.

The joint is best injected from the medial side, siting the point of entry in the joint line, below the extensor tendon.

Technique

The overlying skin is painted with povidone–iodine in spirit and the injection given using either 1 ml Depo-Medrone with Lidocaine, 2–5 mg triamcinolone in 1 ml 1% lignocaine or 5–10 mg hydrocortisone, also in 1% lignocaine 1–2 ml.

22.25 MISCELLANEOUS JOINT INJECTIONS

22.25.1 Temporomandibular joint

Pain in the temporomandibular joint may frequently be relieved by a carefully placed steroid injection using a 25 swg needle. Failing this, a temporary 'denture' may be made to alter the angle of bite.

22.25.2 Sternomanubrial joint

This joint may cause pain and be palpably swollen. The patient will experience sternal pain and be worried that they have heart disease. If a localized tender spot can be found and pressure reproduces the pain, it may be helpful to inject a small quantity (2–5 mg triamcinolone) directly into the joint.

22.25.3 Tietze's syndrome (costochondritis)

This is a common finding, particularly in women between the ages of 30 and 65 years. Steroid injections are disappointing, but worth attempting if the patient is in much pain. Better results may be expected when there is visible and palpable swelling over the joint. Great care must be taken not to insert the needle too deeply and cause damage to the pleura, lungs or pericardium.

22.26 MISCELLANEOUS SOFT-TISSUE INJECTIONS

Injection of steroids, with or without local anaesthetic, is often a valuable treatment even when the exact diagnosis is unsure. Up to 10 ml of 1% lignocaine with added hydrocortisone 25 mg is used, and infiltrated widely around the most tender spot [25].

22.27 ABDOMINAL ASCITES

By far the most common cause of ascites seen by the GP is intra-abdominal malignancy. By this stage of their illness, such patients are ill, weak, nauseated and breathless. It is therefore very much kinder to 'bring the mountain to Mohammed' by taking the instruments and equipment to the patient's bedside, rather than transporting an already terminally ill patient to the surgery or hospital, particularly as the procedure will weaken the patient still further. In addition, by draining the ascites in the patient's own bedroom, an intravenous 'premedication' injection of fentanyl 100 μg and midazolam 2–6 mg may be given so that the patient sleeps throughout the procedure and has no recollection of it afterwards; consequently, the patient will have no apprehension should it need to be repeated at another date subsequently.

With modern diuretics, abdominal paracentesis is not performed as frequently as formerly; nevertheless, there are significant numbers of patients who obtain good relief of their symptoms by judicious aspiration. It is neither necessary nor desirable to draw off all the ascites, as such a manoeuvre would be likely to precipitate a severe hypotensive reaction and would rapidly deplete the patient of large quantities of protein; the aim should be to remove enough fluid to make the abdomen feel soft and to alleviate dyspnoea, vomiting and discomfort. If doubt exists about the exact cause of the ascites, a diagnostic aspiration is easily performed, and the fluid sent for analysis, culture and cytology. If this reveals malignant cells, the diagnosis may be easier and the need for an exploratory laparotomy avoided. Where an ovarian neoplasm is suspected, the CA-125 blood test may give an answer.

In addition to aspiration, cytotoxic drugs may be injected into the peritoneal cavity through the same cannula.

The following instruments are required for abdominal paracentesis:

- 1 5 ml syringe with 23 swg × 1 in. (0.6 × 25 mm) needle with fentanyl 100 μg and midazolam 2–6 mg
- 1 5 ml syringe with 25 swg × 5/8 in. (0.5 × 16 mm) needle loaded with lignocaine 1% and adrenaline 1:200 000 needle 21 swg × 1/2in. (0.8 mm × 40 mm)
- sterile dressing pack
- abdominal paracentesis pack (comprising trocar and cannula or intravenous cannula, connecting tubing, connector, adjustable screw clamp)
- self-adhesive tape 1 in. (25 mm)
- povidone–iodine in spirit (Betadine alcoholic solution)
- 1 standard sterile urine collecting bag with drainage tap
- sterile universal containers if required for culture, examination and cytology
- 1 many-tailed bandage (optional)
- four large safety pins.

22.27.1 Technique for abdominal paracentesis

The patient will already be in bed and preferably with three or four pillows so that he or she is semirecumbent. A premedication intravenous injection of fentanyl 100 μg and midazolam 2–6 mg may be offered; some patients will appreciate being asleep for the aspiration, while others will prefer to remain awake. Certainly, with careful attention to detail while infiltrating with local anaesthetic, the procedure is totally without discomfort.

Depending on the underlying intra-abdominal pathology, a site is chosen away from any masses, usually in the lower abdomen towards the flank. The diagnosis of ascites is verified by gentle percussion, and the patient turned very gently towards the chosen side. Repeat percussion should confirm the presence of shifting dullness. A waterproof dressing sheet (Inco-sheets are ideal) is placed under the patient to protect the lower sheet, and the area chosen liberally painted with povidone-iodine in spirit (Betadine alcoholic solution). Using the 25 swg × 5/8 in. (0.5 × 16 mm) needle on the 5 ml syringe with lignocaine and adrenaline, a small bleb of local anaesthetic is raised in the skin. Very gradually, the needle is advanced through the skin and underlying tissues, injecting all the time. If the 25 swg needle is not long enough to reach the peritoneal cavity, it is exchanged for a 23 swg × 1 in. (0.6 × 25 mm) or 21 swg × $1^1/_2$ in. (0.8 × 40 mm) needle and the injection continued (Fig. 22.22). The peritoneum is particularly sensitive, and great care should be used to infiltrate and advance the needle very slowly, allowing adequate time for anaesthesia to develop before advancing the needle. As this is the only part of the procedure which can be uncomfortable if poor technique is used, it is worth spending time to ensure that it is completely painless. This will also increase the patient's confidence and help to allay any anxiety. If the first paracentesis has been painless, the patient will not mind any subsequent aspirations.

Having completely anaesthetized the track from skin to peritoneum, the abdominal trocar and cannula are inserted exactly through the same track (Fig. 22.23). A little pressure is usually necessary, accompanied by a rotating action. Once the peritoneal cavity is entered, the trocar is withdrawn 1 cm and the blunt cannula pushed into its hub. The trocar is now withdrawn and ascitic fluid spurts from the cannula, which should be rapidly connected via the thin rubber tubing and connector directly to a sterile urine drainage bag with drainage tap (Figs 22.24 and 22.25); this in turn can be attached to the patient's mattress with two large safety pins. The volume of ascites can be easily measured by reading the quantity on the marks on the urine drainage

Figure 22.22 Abdominal paracentesis; after preliminary skin antisepsis, local anaesthetic is infiltrated through the skin, down to the peritoneum.

Figure 22.23 Inserting the trocar and cannula.

Figure 22.24 The trocar is withdrawn and the cannula connected by rubber tubing to a drainage bag.

Figure 22.25 Rubber tubing is connected to urine-drainage bag.

bag. When full, the bag can be emptied merely by opening the drainage tap into a basin beneath. If the rate of flow via the cannula is too rapid, it may be slowed by the application of an adjustable screw clamp to the rubber tubing (Fig. 22.26). Throughout the procedure, regular checks on the patient's pulse and blood pressure should be made.

Once sufficient fluid has been withdrawn to alleviate pressure effects, nausea, dyspnoea, discomfort and tightness, the cannula should be withdrawn, a self-adhesive dressing applied and, if thought necessary, a many-tailed abdominal bandage applied. Unless an excessive volume of fluid has been withdrawn this is probably unnecessary.

The patient should then remain in bed for the next 12 h to allow the circulation and blood pressure to reach equilibrium; should the patient need to get out of bed for any reason he or she should be

Figure 22.26 Abdominal paracentesis. A procedure that may readily be performed in the patient's home.

accompanied. The immediate relief of symptoms is generally followed by a gradual weakening of the patient, and on average it is rarely necessary to have to repeat an abdominal paracentesis more than three times.

The procedure for diagnostic 'tap' is exactly the same as for paracentesis, except that a 20 ml syringe attached to a 21 swg × 1½ in. (0.8 mm × 40 mm) needle is used instead of the trocar and cannula (Fig. 22.27).

Figure 22.27 Abdominal paracentesis; diagnostic aspiration. Fluid may then be sent for analysis and cytology.

If preferred, a size 14 swg (2 mm) intravenous cannula (Abbocath T) 14 may be used in place of the traditional trocar and cannula; this gives equally good results and is probably slightly easier to insert, but a Luer type adaptor is necessary to connect to the tubing.

22.28 ASPIRATION OF PLEURAL EFFUSIONS

The majority of GPs will probably not need to aspirate pleural effusions. The main indication is diagnostic cytology. Carcinoma of the lung is now replacing tuberculosis and empyema as the main indication for aspiration. A chest X-ray is desirable whenever possible and this will help to decide the best side for aspiration. With modern chemotherapeutic agents, radiotherapy, diuretics and surgery, the need for large volume aspiration is far less than in previous years. The following instruments are required:

■ 10 ml syringe filled with 1% lignocaine and 1:200 000 adrenaline
■ 25 swg × 5/8 in. (0.5 × 16 mm) needle
■ two-way tap with Luer connectors
■ 21 swg × 2$^1/_2$ in. (0.8 mm × 63 mm) needle
■ sterile universal containers.

Careful clinical examination and a recent chest X-ray will determine the best site for aspiration; this will usually be an intercostal space towards the back. As the intercostal blood vessels run along the underside of each rib, it is important to insert the needle just above the rib to avoid them.

A preliminary intravenous injection of fentanyl 100 μg and midazolam 2–6 mg may be offered if the patient is unduly apprehensive. The overlying skin is painted with povidone–iodine in spirit (Betadine alcoholic solution) and a small amount of lignocaine injected intradermally with the 25 swg (0.5 mm) needle to raise a weal. The needle is then changed for the longer 21 swg (0.8 mm) needle and two-way tap, and the subcutaneous tissues, intercostal muscles and pleura are infiltrated with local anaesthetic. As with abdominal paracentesis, the local anaesthetic should be given very slowly, injecting a little before advancing the needle and allowing time for the area to become anaesthetized. The doctor should be fully conversant with the working of the two-way tap and should test it before use. It should be possible to inject local anaesthetic through the needle, aspirate fluid back and, by turning the tap, isolate the needle in the pleural cavity while injecting the aspirated fluid into the universal container. It is essential that air is not accidentally allowed into the chest.

Normally, the practitioner can feel the various layers through which the aspirating needle is passing; as soon as the pleural cavity is entered, fluid should be withdrawn into the syringe and transferred to the universal container (Fig. 22.28). If it is intended only to withdraw a small quantity of effusion for cytology, the two-way tap may be omitted and a 20 ml sterile syringe with 21 swg × 2$^1/_2$ in. (0.8 × 63 mm) needle used instead. In this case, just 20 ml of fluid is taken and the needle and syringe are withdrawn. A collodion dressing is immediately applied.

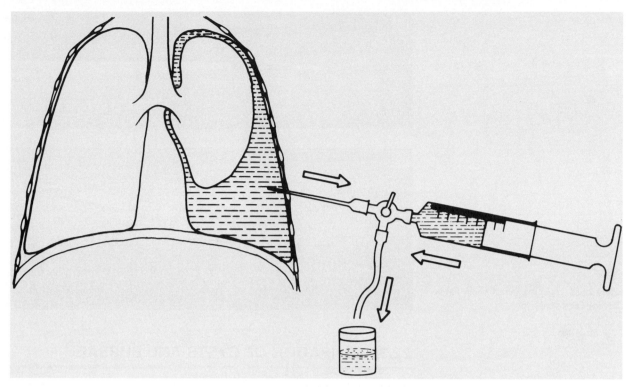

Figure 22.28 Aspiration of pleural effusion. The needle should be inserted above a rib to avoid intercostal blood vessels.

Figure 22.29 Needle aspiration of a breast lump: blowing contents on to a microscope slide.

22.29 NEEDLE BIOPSY

Histological diagnosis of certain tumours may be obtained by needle biopsy. Its use in general practice is limited, but it has a particular place for swellings in the breast which the practitioner feels are probably cystic and which, when aspiration is attempted, produce no fluid and feel hard, indicating the possibility of a tumour. By applying strong traction to the syringe plunger to create a vacuum and at the same time rotating the syringe and needle in a clockwise and anticlockwise direction as the needle is slowly withdrawn, a small piece of tissue will be left in the needle (Fig. 22.29).

By carefully 'blowing' the contents of the needle on to a microscope slide and fixing with preservative (the fixative used for cervical cytology is suitable), a sample may be sent for histological or cytological examination. Although not giving 100% positive accuracy, nevertheless a diagnosis may be made correctly in about 90% of needle biopsies. A swelling with a negative needle biopsy should still be referred to the surgeons for excision, but a swelling with a positive diagnosis on needle biopsy enables the patient and surgeon to plan the most appropriate treatment. Biopsy specimens may also be taken using a Tru-cut biopsy needle (Fig. 22.30), which is manufactured as a sterile disposable unit in various lengths and diameters.

Figure 22.30 (a,b) The Tru-cut biopsy needle (Travenol Laboratories, Inc.).

22.30 ASPIRATION OF CYSTS AND BURSAE

Simple cysts may occur anywhere in the body. They may contain watery fluid which can be easily aspirated with a needle or thick semisolid material which is quite impossible to aspirate through any needle. The two most commonly encountered cysts occur in the breast and thyroid, and aspiration in these situations affords immense relief to patient and doctor alike and is often curative. As with all injection techniques, scrupulous asepsis must be observed, the minimum of trauma inflicted by the selection of the finest needle consistent with aspiration, and all fluid aspirated should be sent for cytological examination. Where any possibility of infection exists, the fluid should also be sent for bacterial culture.

22.30.1 Aspiration of breast cysts

The typical breast cyst is smooth, round, very mobile, slightly tender, and not adherent to skin or deep structures. Diagnosis may be helped by the use of ultrasonography and mammography, but ultimately the only way to establish an accurate diagnosis is by aspiration. It follows that there will be occasions when a 'typical' breast cyst is found on aspiration to be solid, and in this situation, the needle should not be immediately withdrawn, but used for needle biopsy.

To carry out the aspiration it is more comfortable for the patient to be lying down. The skin overlying the cyst is liberally painted with povidone–iodine in spirit (Betadine alcoholic solution) and the injection site anaesthetized using lignocaine and a fine 25 swg × 5/8 in. (0.5 × 16 mm) needle. A 20 ml sterile syringe with a 19 swg × 1½ in. (1.1 × 38 mm) needle is used for aspiration. The cyst should first be fixed with the finger and thumb of the left hand, and the aspirating needle pointed towards the centre of the cyst. By applying gentle traction to the syringe plunger as the needle is advanced, the practitioner will know when the cyst has been entered. Typically, the fluid aspirated is a dark green colour. As much as possible should be removed, hopefully emptying the cyst, and sent for cytology. Even if a negative cytology is obtained, the patient should be seen again in 4 weeks to check that the cyst has not re-formed and referred to a consultant if any doubt exists.

22.30.2 Thyroid cysts

Although not as common as breast cysts, thyroid cysts are just as easy to aspirate. It is advisable to confirm the diagnosis by ultrasonography or scan, and the technique, precautions, cytological examination and follow-up are identical to those for breast cysts.

22.30.3 Aspiration and injection of hydrocele

A primary hydrocele is an excessive collection of serous fluid in the tunica vaginalis within the scrotum; it occurs at any age, but most commonly in adult life. The diagnosis is usually straightforward, particularly if the swelling transilluminates, but it must be remembered that a hernia in an infant also transilluminates.

Aspiration alone rarely cures a hydrocele, but aspiration and the injection of dilute aqueous phenol on two or three separate occasions can offer up to 90% cure [26]; failing this, surgical treatment of the tunica vaginalis is recommended.

A secondary hydrocele occurs as a result of infection or inflammation within the scrotum; thus, it is always important to first examine the testis, epididymis and cord to exclude any disease in these orders. The treatment of a secondary hydrocele is the treatment of its cause.

The following instruments are required:

- 2 ml syringe with 25 swg × 5/8 in. (0.5 × 16 mm) needle
- 2 ml 1% lignocaine
- 18 swg (0.9 mm) intravenous cannula, e.g. Abbocath T18
- 10 ml ampoules of $2\frac{1}{2}$% aqueous sterile phenol
- 20 ml syringes for aspiration and injection.

An injection of $2\frac{1}{2}$% aqueous phenol is not a standard preparation and therefore it needs to be ordered specially; however, it has a good shelf life and a small amount may be kept in store ready for use.

The technique for aspiration and injection of hydrocele is as follows. The patient should lie on the couch or operating table. Good illumination is important, and a sterile sheet should be placed under the scrotum and between the legs. Povidone–iodine in spirit (Betadine alcoholic solution) is applied to the scrotum, which may cause a slight stinging sensation, and a point is chosen for aspiration. This point should be on the lower side, away from the testicle and avoiding any blood vessels on the surface of the scrotum. Local anaesthetic is carefully injected through the scrotal wall and underlying tissues, down to the hydrocele sac. This may be confirmed by gently withdrawing the syringe plunger and noting straw-coloured fluid entering the syringe. In a relatively small hydrocele it helps to hold the neck of the hydrocele, this makes it tense and prevents it extending into the inguinal canal. It also ensures that the operator has not missed an inguinoscrotal hernia.

The local anaesthetic needle is now withdrawn and the 18 swg (0.9 mm) intravenous cannula inserted through the same needle track. By removing the central cannula needle, a soft, pliable catheter is now situated within the hydrocele sac. This is far less traumatic than the old steel trocar and cannula, and gives equally good results. The serous fluid may be either allowed to run out freely into a container, or aspirated by connecting a 20 ml syringe to the cannula, with or without a three-way tap. As the hydrocele empties, the sac is gently compressed with the left hand to remove most of the fluid, and the volume noted. If any doubt exists about the underlying pathology, the fluid should be sent for culture and cytology.

Keeping the cannula in place, a calculated volume of 2.5% sterile aqueous phenol is now injected according to the following formula:

Volume aspirated	Volume injected 2.5% phenol
Up to 50 ml	5 ml
Up to 200 ml	10 ml
Up to 400 ml	15 ml
Over 400 ml	20 ml

The cannula is now withdrawn and a simple collodion dressing applied.

After 6 weeks the procedure is repeated. Most of the hydrocele will have recurred and it is important to have warned the patient that this is likely. At the second aspiration, if it is noticed that the fluid appears darker or even blood-stained, success can be anticipated.

The patient is seen a third time 6 weeks later, and on this occasion the volume of fluid should be considerably smaller, or may not have re-collected at all. For the elderly patient who would be a poor general anaesthetic and surgical risk, this is undoubtedly the treatment of choice, offering over 90% chance of complete cure.

22.30.4 Epididymal cysts

These are not as common as a primary hydrocele; nevertheless, they can be aspirated and injected with 2.5% aqueous phenol exactly as described for hydrocele. Success is even higher, offering nearly 100% cure, provided the cyst is not multiloculated, in which case surgical excision is probably the treatment of choice. Aspiration and sclerosant injection should not be offered to men who intend to have a family, as reductions in sperm counts have been reported following this treatment.

CHAPTER 23

Incision of abscesses

Recent wounds if inflammation has set in, will result in fever with chills and throbbing. One should induce suppuration as soon as possible and not let the pus be blocked up. The flesh should be lacerated by the weapon. After that new tissue sprouts up

Hippocrates, 460–377 BC

The instruments required for the incision of an abscess are as follows:

- scalpel handle size 3
- scalpel blade no. 11
- 1 malleable probe
- 1 pair sinus forceps
- assorted small drains
- Fucidin gel
- sterile dressings
- wide-bore aspirating needle and syringe.

It is only within one generation that we have witnessed a dramatic reduction in the numbers of bacterial infections, largely thanks to antibiotics. The image of the family doctor taking out his 'lancet' from his pocket to open a 'boil' is still in living memory. Large necrotic abscesses, so familiar in the nineteenth century, are now fortunately rarer, and in one year, the general practitioner will need to open only a few. Common sites for abscesses are the perineum, infected operation scars and fingers. Small abscesses probably require little other than a dry dressing.

Spreading cellulitis and induration with lymphangitis is best treated with antibiotics, but once pus has collected it should be released, usually by incision. If the abscess is superficial and distending the overlying skin which has become thinned, incision using a pointed no. 11 scalpel blade on no. 3 handle is all that is necessary (Figs 23.1 and 23.2). Deeper abscesses, recognized by fluctuation, pain, fever and rigors with leucocytosis, will require incision, but because of the pain, will require some form of anaesthetic; this may best be managed with a general anaesthetic, but occasionally, where a general anaesthetic is considered inappropriate, careful local anaesthesia or Entonox inhalation may suffice. However, even this causes pain, is not always effective, and increases the risk of spreading the infection.

Once the abscess has been incised, the pus should be expelled by pressure, a bacterial swab taken for culture of the organisms and a suitable drain inserted to prevent premature closure of the wound.

Figure 23.1 Paronychia on the thumb; simple incision and dressing are all that is required.

Figure 23.2 Web-space abscess; incision and dressing are required.

Recently, good results have been obtained by incising the abscess, curetting the lining and instilling Fucidin gel. No drain is necessary, a dry dressing is applied, healing occurs rapidly and recurrence is rare. In some cases, even primary closure is possible.

Aspiration alone, using a wide-bore needle, often results in a cure, particularly with Bartholin's abscesses (Chapter 38), and may avoid the need for more radical surgery.

Dermatological minor surgery

24.1 NORMAL SKIN

As the majority of minor surgical operations is performed on skin, it is helpful to have a knowledge of simple skin biology and histology.

24.1.1 Anatomy (see Fig. 19.1)

The skin comprises epidermis, dermis, and skin appendages such as pilosebaceous follicles, eccrine and apocrine sweat glands.

In the epidermis the basal or germinative layer is made up of small keratinocytes which gradually migrate to the surface over approximately 4 weeks. With the keratinocytes are smaller numbers of melanocytes whose function is to produce melanin pigment, which in turn finds its way to the keratinocytes and ultimately protects the cells against the effects of ultraviolet irradiation, which is known to damage nuclear DNA.

Naevus cells, found in pigmented naevi, are similar to melanocytes, and there is some evidence that melanocytes can differentiate into naevus cells.

Between the epidermis and the dermis is the basement membrane, which effectively cements the two layers together. Collagen is the main component of the dermis, with fibroblasts being the predominant cell, responsible for producing the three dermal proteins: elastin, reticulin and ground substance.

Congenital capillary abnormalities may present as vascular naevi.

24.1.2 The pilosebaceous unit

This traverses both the dermis and epidermis and comprises the hair follicle, sebaceous glands, and erector pili muscle. The sebaceous glands produce sebum by disintegration of the glandular cells. Blockage of sebum in teenage adults results in acne.

Epidermal cysts occur following implantation of epidermis or from the lining of pilosebaceous follicles, and are filled with macerated keratin. The cysts seen commonly on the scalp are tricholemmal (pilar) cysts derived from the hair follicle; they occur in families, being inherited as an autosomal dominant gene, and are often multiple.

24.1.3 The nail

Nails are formed from epidermal invagination. The nail plate grows from the nail matrix and lies on the nail bed. The proximal part of the nail is the lunula, and the protective membrane covering the proximal part of the lunula is the cuticle. Damage to the cuticle may result in chronic infection around the nail bed. Ingrowing nails are a result of lateral pressure, chafing and infection along the edge of the nail.

24.2 LESIONS SUITABLE FOR TREATMENT

24.2.1 Skin tags and papillomata

These are some of the easiest and most common conditions to treat. Small ones may merely be snipped off with scissors and the base cauterized either chemically or with heat (Fig. 24.1) or removed with a radiosurgery wire loop (Chapter 42).

24.2.2 Intradermal naevi

These are also extremely common and may be removed by either curette and cautery excision, radiosurgery or destruction by cryotherapy.

24.2.3 'Sebaceous cysts' (tricholemmal, pilar, epidermal)

These lend themselves admirably to minor surgery. Whichever method is used to treat them, the important point is to be sure that the whole capsule has been removed, otherwise recurrence is likely.

24.2.4 Viral infections (warts and molluscum contagiosum)

Surgery has a limited role in the treatment of these troublesome conditions. Medical measures should always be tried first, but where these fail, and particularly where there are solitary lesions, treatment may be curette, radiosurgery, cautery, cryotherapy, or excision.

24.2.5 Vascular lesions

Certain vascular haemangiomata may be destroyed by electrocautery, diathermy, or cryotherapy. The granuloma pyogenicum is easily treated by curette and cautery; spider naevi are easily destroyed by cold-point electrocautery, but strawberry naevi and port-wine naevi are generally not suitable for minor surgical treatment.

24.2.6 Hypertrophic and neoplastic lesions

Solar keratoses, seborrhoeic warts, keratoacanthoma and small basal cell carcinomata, histiocytomata and other small neoplastic lesions may

Figure 24.1 Skin tags in axilla; easily removed by electrocautery.

be removed by either curette and cautery, radiosurgery, cryotherapy or excision, depending on the experience and confidence of the operator.

24.3 LESIONS TO AVOID

24.3.1 Site

The doctor should avoid operating on the face, posterior triangle in the neck, axilla and femoral triangle unless he or she is absolutely sure of the anatomy and can anticipate and deal with unexpected problems (Figs 24.2 and 24.3). Similarly, surgery to all but very superficial lesions in the breast should be avoided, as good local anaesthesia is often difficult to obtain and the incidence of malignancy is higher than with in-hospital treatment.

24.3.2 Size

One should avoid removing large lesions where difficulty in skin closure might be anticipated. In addition, larger lesions tend to have a larger blood supply.

24.3.3 Depth of lesion

The large, diffuse lipoma may extend to a deeper layer than expected. The doctor should be aware of the underlying anatomy, particularly nerves, tendons and arteries.

Similarly, many ganglia need careful dissection down to a joint capsule, through tendons and vessels, in a bloodless operating field. It is better not to start than find oneself in difficulties. (Alternative treatments for ganglia are given in Chapter 4.)

The discharging small ulcer on the face overlying the mandible could be a dental sinus, in which case simple excision will be followed by a recurrence. Examination inside the patient's mouth will reveal the source of the sinus (Fig. 24.4).

24.3.4 Malignant lesions

Excision of a nodular malignant melanoma has no place in minor surgery. Where a thin, small, pigmented lesion is encountered, it may be judicious to excise it and allow a clear margin. Such a judgement depends on the experience and skill of the operator. Basal cell carcinoma and squamous cell carcinoma, particularly if on the face and especially if near the eye, should be referred to a specialist. Small tumours in other sites may be suitable for excision.

Figure 24.2 Basal cell carcinoma near the inner canthus and nasolachrymal duct. This is not suitable for minor surgery and should be referred. (Photograph by courtesy of Dr. R.J. Cairns.)

Figure 24.3 Cellular naevus; tip of the nose. This is a difficult site to obtain a good cosmetic result. This is better referred or not treated. (Photograph by courtesy of Dr. R.J. Cairns.)

Figure 24.4 Beware the small, innocent-looking weeping ulcerated lesion at this site. Excision will be followed by a recurrence. This is a dental sinus. (Photograph by courtesy of Dr. R.J. Cairns.)

24.3.5 Age

The general practitioner should avoid operating on young children who either cannot co-operate, keep still or endure a local anaesthetic.

Finally, if it pulsates, it must not be touched!

24.4 LESIONS THAT DO NOT REQUIRE TREATMENT

Strawberry naevi resolve spontaneously, as do most warts, molluscum contagiosum and even keratoacanthomata.

Small intradermal naevi are often better left alone in case the resulting scar is more unsightly than the original lesion, and histiocytomata are often better left untreated as they extend through the full skin thickness and therefore require excision.

24.5 LESIONS WHERE THERE IS DOUBT ABOUT THE DIAGNOSIS

Not every lesion is readily identifiable, and where there is any significant doubt, it is worth considering referring to a consultant colleague. As a general guide, most skin rashes do not need a biopsy; indeed, histology reports are often very unhelpful in establishing a diagnosis in such cases. A consultant dermatologist is often able to give an immediate clinical diagnosis and decide whether any form of surgical treatment is appropriate.

Skin lesions

25

Naevi materni are those marks which frequently appear on the bodies of children at birth and which originate from impressions made on the mind of the mother during pregnancy.

Encyclopaedia Britannica, 1797

Almost all dermal lesions can be removed in the surgery by a general practitioner (GP), the two exceptions being any lesion which is too large to permit skin closure and the malignant melanoma. Facilities for histological examination are essential and it is good practice to send every specimen excised for histological examination; not only does this improve the doctor's diagnostic acumen, it avoids the pitfall of inadvertently removing an amelanotic malignant melanoma, and provides a permanent record of the tissues and pathology removed. Most of the lesions to be described can be removed leaving a neat inconspicuous scar; where the doctor anticipates otherwise the patient should be advised in advance.

One instrument set will be suitable for all lesions described and the technique with slight variations is applicable to each.

The following instruments are required:

- scalpel handle size 3
- scalpel blade size 10
- Volkmann double-ended sharp-spoon curette
- Kilner needle holder $5\frac{1}{4}$ in. (13.3 cm)
- pair standard stitch scissors, 5 in. (12.7 cm), pointed
- pair toothed dissecting forceps 5 in. (12.7 cm)
- pair Halstead mosquito artery forceps, curved, 5 in. (12.7 cm)
- povidone–iodine in spirit (Betadine alcoholic solution)
- 10 ml syringe
- 25 swg × 5/8 in. (0.5 × 16 mm) needle
- 23 swg × 1 in. (0.6 × 25 mm) needle
- 21 swg × $1\frac{1}{2}$ in. (0.8 × 40 mm) needle
- ampoule 10 ml 1% lignocaine with or without added adrenaline 1:200 000
- skin-closure strips (Steri-strips) 6 × 75 mm (Ref. 3M GP41)
- sterile monofilament Nylon suture 4/0 Ethilon (Ref. W319) (Ethicon) 19 mm curved cutting needle
- electrocautery with platinum-tip burner or equivalent
- unipolar diathermy for coagulation.

25.1 GENERAL TECHNIQUE FOR EXCISION

The first consideration with any dermal lesion is a provisional diagnosis; secondly, does it need to be removed? Lesions such as the infant's strawberry naevus should be left alone as it always resolves completely (Fig. 25.1a–c). Similarly, many warts and molluscum contagiosum may well regress spontaneously and be better left to nature (Fig. 25.2a, b). The third consideration, once it has been decided to remove any dermal lesion, is to decide the line of the final scar, bearing in mind that scars in the line of skin creases and wrinkles are much neater, as are transverse scars across joints, and scars which lie at right-angles to the direction of pull of underlying muscles (Chapter 10). Picking up the skin and squeezing the lesion between finger and thumb will demonstrate skin creases and also help to assess whether excision will result in too much skin tension. The fourth consideration is the method of removal: is this lesion better excised, curetted and cauterized, desiccated, fulgurized, or treated with the diathermy, cryoprobe or radiosurgery, or is the diagnosis such that a preliminary skin biopsy should be taken?

Assuming excision is the method of choice, the lesion and surrounding skin is liberally painted with povidone–iodine in spirit

Figure 25.1 (a) The strawberry naevus, which will disappear completely without any treatment. It should never be excised or cauterized. (b) Large strawberry naevus (superficial angioma) on the forearm. (c) Strawberry naevus showing spontaneous resolution.

Figure 25.2 (a) Many viral warts disappear spontaneously without leaving a scar. (b) Solitary molluscum contagiosum. Many will clear spontaneously.

(Betadine alcoholic solution) and the area anaesthetized using infiltration of local anaesthetic.

For small lesions, a skin bleb of lignocaine is raised at either end of the proposed scar using either a 30 swg needle and dental syringe or a 25 swg × 5/8 in. (0.5 × 16 mm) needle (Fig. 25.3a). The needle is then changed for a larger one, either 23 swg (0.6 mm) or 21 swg (0.8 mm) and inserted through the skin bleb, infiltrating the underlying skin in a fan-shaped distribution from either end. A sterile 'lithotomy type' drape is put over the skin, leaving only the lesion exposed. The hands are washed and scrubbed thoroughly with chlorhexidine in detergent (Hibiscrub), then dried and a pair of sterile surgical gloves is applied.

Figure 25.3 (a) Method of infiltrating the skin with local anaesthetic for excision of intra-dermal lesion, and skin closure with interrupted sutures. (b) Method of skin closure to avoid inversion of the skin edges (vertical mattress suture).

From now on a completely aseptic technique must be used, preferably no-touch, with the minimum of tissue trauma and handling. The wearing of a face-mask is optional; provided the operator does not cough, sneeze or talk continuously over the wound, it is probably not essential. However, wearing a mask protects the patient from droplet infection and enables the doctor to hold a conversation with the patient, explaining the procedure. Similarly, if the patient has any upper respiratory infection, or is liable to cough, sneeze or talk, he or she should likewise wear a mask, as should any assistant.

The lesion is now excised using an elliptical incision through the skin and subcutaneous tissues, attempting to excise a triangular wedge of tissue rather than leaving a flat base. Any small bleeding points can be controlled with pressure alone using a sterile gauze swab. The excised wedge or ellipse of tissue is placed immediately in a histology container and covered with 10% formol-saline as fixative. This container should be promptly labelled with the patient's name, date and nature of specimen and if appropriate, which side or digit. The resulting wound is generally much bigger than expected due to retraction of the skin edges. Bleeding vessels usually stop spontaneously and any brisk bleeding can be controlled by artery forceps.

It is a good idea at this stage to ascertain whether the skin edges will approximate without undue tension. If they can be brought together easily, the wound may be stitched forthwith; if tension is present, it is worth undercutting the edges with a scalpel so that the skin will slide over the subcutaneous tissues, and then suturing the wound.

The two reasons for poor healing are dead spaces and undue skin tension. Dead spaces fill with blood and serum and produce a subcutaneous haematoma which can become infected, while undue tension on skin edges produces ischaemia, non-union and necrosis.

Both dead spaces and skin tension can be dealt with by the judicious use of absorbable subcutaneous sutures such as catgut or coated Vicryl, but only the minimum number necessary should be used as too many act as foreign bodies and increase the risks of infection.

In general, the wound is best closed using interrupted monofilament Nylon sutures, spaced closely together, supported if necessary by the application of self-adhesive skin closure strips (Steri-strips). When inserting sutures, the aim should be to evert the skin edges slightly; this can be achieved by taking slightly more of the subcutaneous tissue in the bite of the needle than skin. If the edges still tend to invert despite this manoeuvre, the suture should be passed through the skin 1 mm from each edge (vertical mattress) (Fig. 25.3b). This is an excellent stitch, but can be difficult to remove. Depending on the site of the scar, the sutures may be removed after 5–10 days, leaving the Steri-strips to give additional external support.

All that remains is the application of a dry, sterile dressing and the instructions to the patient to leave the dressing completely undisturbed until the sutures are removed, unless there is a specific reason to inspect the wound earlier. It is also helpful to rest the limb or part of the body containing the scar for at least 48 h to initiate healing. Thereafter, gentle activity is beneficial.

Figure 25.4 (a) Simple intradermal naevus, suitable for removal with curette. (b) Infiltrating the base with local anaesthetic. (c) Intradermal naevus. Removal with Volkmann sharp-spoon curette (see also Chapter 42).

25.2 CURETTE AND CAUTERY

As an alternative to surgical excision, many lesions may successfully be removed with a sharp-spoon Volkmann curette, then cauterizing the base with the electrocautery to control bleeding. The technique is exactly as described under the section on warts and verrucae (Chapter 27). As with warts, it is important to find the correct plane of cleavage when using the curette; it is also helpful to have a selection of curettes of various sizes corresponding to the size of the lesion (Fig. 25.4a–c).

25.3 INTRADERMAL NAEVI AND PIGMENTED NAEVI

Pigmented naevi are lesions characterized by a proliferation of epidermal melanocytes, later migrating downwards into the dermis. They can be divided into flat lesions, slightly raised lesions, verrucous lesions, dome-shaped lesions and pigmented hairy lesions. The main indication for removal of a naevus is any suspicion that it may be turning malignant, as suggested by sudden enlargement, alteration in the pigment, ulceration or bleeding. Most patients request removal for cosmetic reasons, or because the lesion is catching on clothing or razors when shaving. Surgical excision or radiosurgery is the treatment of choice for all pigmented naevi (Fig. 25.5).

Figure 25.5 (a) Pigmented intradermal naevus which bled regularly after shaving. (b) Excised; closure with fine, interrupted sutures. (Blanching of surrounding skin is from adrenaline in the local anaesthetic.)

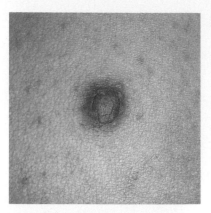

Figure 25.6 Typical fibrous histiocytoma (dermatofibroma). Either no treatment, or excision is the treatment of choice.

25.4 HISTIOCYTOMA (DERMATOFIBROMA)

These are fairly common tumours found frequently on the legs. The cause is unknown, but may be related to trauma. They occur in the dermis and present as a smooth, firm nodule. They are benign and commonly multiple, and the treatment is surgical excision (Fig. 25.6).

25.5 CYLINDROMA (TURBAN TUMOUR)

This is a rare tumour, also benign, occurring commonly on the scalp. Initially it may be mistaken for a sebaceous cyst until excision is attempted, when a firm, granular, adherent lesion is found. Treatment is surgical excision.

25.6 SOLAR KERATOSIS

As the name implies, these lesions are found in areas of skin exposed to light; they are discrete and raised with a crumbling surface. As they are purely epidermal, they may be treated with radiosurgery, curettage and electrocautery or cryotherapy, using a nitrous oxide or liquid nitrogen cryoprobe, or simply shaved off with a scalpel blade and the base cauterized (Figs 25.7–25.11). Where they are extensive, an alternative non-surgical treatment is the application of 5% fluoro-uracil cream (Efudix) twice daily for up to 6 weeks. This causes considerable redness with a risk of infection, so a topical antibiotic cream may be applied during the healing phase. However, the results are good.

25.7 SEBORRHOEIC WARTS

These are due to a benign proliferation of epidermal cells and they become more common with increasing age. They present as multiple, raised, brown or black lesions, often looking as if they had been stuck on the skin. Curettage and cautery, radiosurgery or shaving and cautery is the treatment of choice (Figs 25.8–25.13).

Figure 25.7 (a) Solar keratosis. (b) Multiple solar keratoses, back of hand.

Figure 25.8 Seborrhoeic wart on the back: the base is infilrated with local anaesthetic.

Figure 25.9 Holding the scalpel blade parallel to the skin, the doctor cuts through the base of the wart.

Figure 25.10 Bleeding vessels in the base.

Figure 25.11 Bleeding vessels cauterized with electrocautery.

Figure 25.12 Seborrhoeic wart on the abdomen; easily removed by curette, or shaving with scalpel, followed by cautery to the base.

Figure 25.13 Larger seborrhoeic wart (basal cell papilloma), equally suitable for removal.

25.8 KERATOACANTHOMA

These are not uncommon lesions, which can be mistaken for basal and squamous cell carcinomata; they present as a small papule which grows rapidly in size over a period of 2 or 3 months. The edges are rolled over with a central depression and a thickened keratin

Figure 25.14 Typical keratoacanthoma inside the ear; present for 3 months and enlarging rapidly.

Figure 25.15 Keratoacanthoma; easily curetted with a sharp-spoon curette.

Figure 25.16 The base of the lesion is cauterized with the electrocautery.

Figure 25.17 An atypical, early keratoacanthoma; this could have been mistaken for a basal cell carcinoma.

Figure 25.18 A typical keratoacanthoma, easily curetted and the base cauterized.

plug. Interestingly, they gradually involute over a period of 6 months. The cause is still unknown. Histologically they have an identical appearance to squamous-cell carcinoma.

Treatment is by curettage and cautery or complete excision biopsy (Figs 25.14–25.18).

25.9 GRANULOMA PYOGENICUM (ERUPTIVE ANGIOMA)

This is a type of haemangioma, so called because it was originally thought to be due to infection by *Staphylococcus*. It presents

Figure 25.19 Granuloma pyogenicum on the palmar surface of the hand; treatment by curette and cautery or unipolar diathermy.

Figure 25.20 (a) Granuloma pyogenicum on the lower lip. (b) After removal with a curette and cauterization or the base under infiltration with local anaesthesia.

Figure 25.21 Granuloma pyogenicum on the tongue; treatment by either curette and cautery, or radiosurgical excision with wire-loop. Bleeding, which can be brisk, is controlled by pressure and a coagulation electrode.

as a solitary raised swelling, bright red in colour, and bleeds profusely. The most effective treatment is curettage and cautery under local anaesthesia (Figs 25.19–25.21) or liquid nitrogen cryosurgery.

25.10 SPIDER NAEVI

These are common vascular lesions typified by a very small central red arteriole from which radiate fine, superficial blood vessels. The most effective treatment is radiosurgery or electrocautery to the central arteriole without anaesthetic, or inserting the needle electrode of the Hyfrecator into the arteriole, also without anaesthetic (Figs 25.22–25.25).

Figure 25.22 Typical spider naevus on the face.

Figure 25.23 Pressure applied with a micro-scope slide demonstrates the feeding arteriole.

Figure 25.24 Using the cold-point electro-cautery burner or needle diathermy electrode, the arteriole is coagulated.

Figure 25.25 The appearance immediately following cautery.

Figure 25.26 Single lesion of molluscum contagiosum. Easily treated, but difficult to anaesthetize in young children.

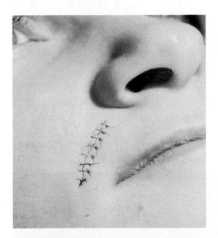

Figure 25.27 Suture line following excision of a dark pigmented naevus. Note the line of the scar to coincide with a skin crease and numerous fine interrupted 6/0 Prolene sutures.

Figure 25.28 Tincture Benzoin Co. being applied to the fine sutures to prevent knots 'slipping'. These sutures will be removed after 4 days and the wound supported with Steri-strips.

25.11 HAEMANGIOMA

Various vascular tumours and lesions are seen on the skin. Cavernous haemangiomata frequently occur on the lower lip and face. The problem with excision is that of haemorrhage, but good cosmetic results may be obtained by desiccation or coagulation using the unipolar diathermy. Treatment consists of inserting either the single-needle electrode or a pair of bipolar electrodes into the centre of the lesion and passing a high-frequency current through the haemangioma. Coagulation occurs rapidly, the procedure is virtually bloodless and healing occurs rapidly over the ensuing 3 weeks. Larger vascular lesions may require more than one treatment.

25.12 MOLLUSCUM CONTAGIOSUM

This is a viral tumour of the skin, commonly seen in children. It has a typically pearly appearance with an umbilicated centre. Treatment is either pricking each lesion with a pointed stick soaked in phenol, or destruction using the electrocautery or diathermy, following anaesthesia with EMLA cream or local infiltration (Fig. 25.26). Good results have also been reported using a fine liquid nitrogen cryoprobe.

25.13 REMOVAL OF TATTOOS

Many patients request the removal of tattoos which have been self-inflicted or professionally performed. Small tattoos are excised exactly as any intradermal lesion, while larger tattoos are better referred to a plastic surgeon or treated with the laser.

25.14 JUVENILE MELANOMA

This is a lightly or non-pigmented naevus which appears in childhood and grows rapidly. Histologically, juvenile melanomata may resemble malignant melanomata, but they are always benign. (Pigmented naevi rarely undergo malignant change before puberty.) Treatment, therefore, is surgical excision (Figs 25.27 and 25.28).

25.15 MALIGNANT MELANOMA

This is a tumour of epidermal melanocytes and the incidence throughout the world is rapidly rising. The exact cause is not fully understood, but appears to be related to increasing exposure to sunlight, particularly short, sharp bursts resulting in burning of the skin.

In the UK the female:male ratio for melanoma is 2:1, and in women 50% occur on the legs, while in males, the trunk is the most common site.

Figure 25.29 (a) Superficial spreading malignant melanoma. (b) Lentigo maligna melanoma. (c) The dreaded malignant melanoma. This is never a minor surgical procedure and must always be referred to hospital urgently.

The following three common varieties are seen in general practice.

- Superficial spreading melanoma is the most common lesion, presenting as irregular, brown/black/bluish lesions with intermingled reddened areas (Fig. 25.29a).
- Lentigo maligna melanoma usually occurs on sun-exposed skin, commonly on the face in the elderly (Fig. 25.29b).
- Nodular melanoma is the most rapidly growing and most malignant. It can occur anywhere on the body, often does not have much melanin, is often very vascular and ultimately ulcerates (Fig. 25.29c).

Figure 25.30 Malignant melanoma, 6 months after Fig. 25.29c. Despite wide excision in hospital and chemotherapy, metastatic spread ensued and the patient died 3 months later.

Figure 25.31 (a) Another malignant melanoma on the leg. This was widely excised and the patient is still alive 20 years later. (b) Close-up of the same malignant melanoma: prognosis unpredictable.

Figure 25.32 Superficial nodular amelanotic malignant melanoma; often very difficult to diagnose. (Photograph by courtesy of Dr. R.J. Cairns.)

Occasionally there may be no pigment – the 'amelanotic malignant melanoma' – which can be extremely difficult to diagnose (Fig. 25.32).

25.15.1 Prognosis of malignant melanoma

Our understanding of the natural history of malignant melanoma has changed in the last 10 years, and it is now recognized that it is the histological depth of the lesion that determines survival or otherwise. This measurement, in millimetres, from the overlying granular layer of the epidermis to the deepest identifiable tumour cells is known as the tumour thickness or Breslow thickness. An alternative classification is the Clarke grading I–IV which is also related to tumour thickness.

If the Breslow thickness is less than 1 mm, there is a 90% 5-year survival rate, whereas lesions measuring 3–3.5 mm or more carry a 40% 5-year survival rate. This knowledge now means that it is not always necessary to excise widely and skin graft all malignant melanomas, but that a more selective approach may be adopted.

If the patient presents with a thick, nodular malignant melanoma, the prognosis is already bad and the chance of metastases is very high (Figs 25.30 and 25.31). In these patients, wide excision, skin grafting and chemotherapy should be tried, with or without lymph-node dissection, and treatment offered in a centre specializing in malignant melanomata.

If, however, the patient presents with a shallow, small melanoma, excision with a 5 mm border is all that is probably required for cure.

Furthermore, if a melanoma is inadvertently excised and the histological report received in less than 10 days, it is safe to reoperate and perform a wider excision without prejudicing the outcome.

Thus, two requests should be made to the histopathologist if a suspected melanoma has been excised.

1. May the histology report be given to you within 10 days.
2. If positive, could you be told the Breslow thickness in millimetres.

As a general guide, malignant melanomas should never be removed by the GP, but referred to a specialist unit.

25.16 BASAL CELL CARCINOMA (RODENT ULCER)

This is the most common malignant tumour of the skin, usually occurring on the face, and appears to be induced by exposure to ultraviolet light. It starts as a small papule which spreads, leaving a central ulcer. The edges are pearl-coloured with fine telangiectasia; left alone they slowly increase in size but practically never metastasize. Treatment is by radiotherapy (95% cure), surgical excision (95% cure) or curettage and cautery (80% cure). Small basal cell carcinomata (BCC) are easily treated by the GP and although curettage and cautery gives a lower cure rate than radiotherapy, it gives a better cosmetic result.

When treating small BCC by curette and cautery, improved results are obtained if the curette/cautery sequence is repeated three times to ensure eradication of the basal layer. Surgical excision is the treatment of choice to give the neatest scar (Figs 25.33–25.35).

Figure 25.33 Basal cell carcinoma (rodent ulcer) on a typical site. The line of the eventual scar is marked with two green dots in the skin creases.

Figure 25.34 Line of excision to coincide with skin creases.

Figure 25.35 (a) Patient with multiple basal cell carcinomata on the face. (b) Unusually large basal-cell carcinoma occurring on the scalp of a patient aged 93 years. Removal was by electrocautery dissection in view of her age. Cure was complete.

Figure 25.36 A large deceptive area of Bowen's disease (carcinoma *in situ*) on the lower leg, present for 18 months, confirmed by biopsy and treated successfully with liquid nitrogen. This could also have been treated with 5% fluoro-uracil ointment.

25.17 SQUAMOUS CELL EPITHELIOMA

This, too, is thought to be due to overexposure to ultraviolet light. It can occur anywhere on the body and can affect the mucous membranes, particularly the lips and tongue. Unlike the basal cell epithelioma, squamous celled carcinomata have the ability to metastasize, but nevertheless if treated early the prognosis is excellent. Treatment is by surgical excision, radiotherapy or both.

25.18 CARCINOMA *IN SITU* (BOWEN'S DISEASE)

This is a form of intraepithelial carcinoma *in situ* which can occasionally metastasize and/or progress to an invasive squamous cell carcinoma. Originally, many Bowen's lesions were thought to be due to arsenic.

It presents as an isolated, scaling, erythematous plaque, not dissimilar to psoriasis. Surgical excision is the treatment of choice, but in carefully selected cases liquid nitrogen cryosurgery is successful (Fig. 25.36). Topical 5% fluoro-uracil cream (Efudix) may also be applied twice daily for up to 6 weeks. This causes considerable reaction, redness and superficial ulceration and usually requires the application of an antibiotic cream during the healing phase to minimize infection, but the results can be very good.

25.19 KELOIDS

Despite meticulous care in skin closure, certain patients develop hypertrophic or keloid scars. These occur more frequently in dark-skinned individuals and in certain sites of the body, particularly in front of the sternum.

If a patient gives a history of developing hypertrophic or keloid scars in previous surgery, serious consideration should be given as to the advisability of performing surgery, as the likelihood of another keloid scar is high. Similarly, a request from a patient to excise a keloid scar should be resisted, as an even larger keloid scar is likely to be the end result.

Faced with a keloid scar, intralesional steroids, e.g. triamcinolone, should be tried monthly, and often give good results. When operating on a patient with a tendency to keloid scar formation, it may be helpful to apply a strong steroid cream during the postoperative healing phase, in an attempt to prevent the hypertrophic reaction. For medicolegal reasons it would be prudent to advise the patient about the risks of hypertrophic scarring and to record this advice in the patient's notes.

25.20 SKIN BIOPSY (see Chapter 31)

One of the advantages of GP minor surgery is the ability to establish a rapid diagnosis of any suspect skin lesion by a simple biopsy. The technique is not difficult and, where histological facilities exist, a firm diagnosis is possible in a matter of days. The object is to choose a representative lesion, including the margin, together with a piece of adjacent healthy skin, and to remove a narrow ellipse, closing the wound with one or two fine interrupted Prolene sutures. Neater results may be obtained by the use of a skin punch-biopsy instrument (Downs Surgical). These are manufactured in different sizes and consist of a sharpened steel tube mounted on a handle. They may be either disposable (Stiefel Laboratories) or reusable (Downs Surgical and Chas Thackray Ltd) (Figs 25.37a–c and 25.38).

After choosing a representative area, which is then anaesthetized, the skin is stretched taut and the punch pressed firmly against the skin. By rotating the handle a core of skin and subcutaneous tissue is obtained. Closure is usually achieved with just one stitch.

Figure 25.37 (a) Skin biopsy; the Hayes Martin skin punch biopsy instrument with three interchangeable heads. Closure is usually with just one stitch. (b) The Hayes Martin skin punch biopsy instrument. (c) Incision and closure for skin biopsy using a scalpel.

Figure 25.38 Disposable, sterile skin biopsy punch (Stiefel Laboratories Ltd).

26 Skin tags and papillomata

It is surprising how many patients have lived with their assorted skin tags and squamous papillomata, feeling that they were too trivial a condition to seek medical advice, even though they have caused much anxiety and embarrassment. The majority are easily removed in a matter of minutes, the diagnosis confirmed histologically and the patient's anxiety allayed.

The following instruments are required:

- 5 ml syringe
- 25 swg × 5/8 in. (0.5 × 16 mm) needle
- ampoule 1% lignocaine with adrenaline 1:200 000
- pair toothed dissecting forceps 5 in. (12.7 cm)
- electrocautery with pointed platinum-tip burner
- Opsite spray or equivalent dressing
- small adhesive plaster dressings
- histology container with 10% formol-saline.

Very small tags may be picked up with the toothed dissecting forceps and separated at the base using the electrocautery. No bleeding occurs, the procedure takes 1 second, a small adhesive dressing is applied, the specimen can be sent for histology and healing takes a matter of days.

Figure 26.1 Typical squamous papilloma; easily removed with the electrocautery.

Figure 26.2 Numerous small skin tags in the axilla; easily removed with the electrocautery.

Figure 26.3 Large fleshy fibrolipoma, on the base of the back; narrow base and easily removed with the electrocautery.

Figure 26.4 Fibrolipoma; Base infiltrated with local anaesthetic and removed with the electrocautery.

Figure 26.5 Squamous papilloma on the posterior pillar of the fauces.

Figure 26.6 Squamous papilloma on the tongue; curetted and base cauterized after local inflitration of anaesthetic.

Figure 26.7 Small cutaneous 'horn'; easily curetted and base cauterized.

Figure 26.8 After removal, base cauterized with electrocautery; rapid healing.

Figure 26.9 Small, warty papilloma on the upper eyelid removed with a small curette and the base cauterized.

Figure 26.10 Multiple skin tags on eyelids; easily removed with electrocautery 'cutting' burner. Anaesthesia by infiltration using 30 swg needle and 1% lignocaine.

Figure 26.11 Following removal with electrocautery. Healing occurs rapidly and no dressing is required.

Figure 26.12 Numerous filiform 'warts' on the neck; Very common. They can be easily picked up with forceps and removed using just the electrocautery, or snipped off with fine scissors and any bleeding vessels touched with the cautery.

Figure 26.13 Picking up skin tags with fine toothed forceps and dividing with electrocautery.

Figure 26.14 Any bleeding points or shallow skin tags may be touched with the ball-ended electrocautery burner.

Larger skin tags or papillomata can still be removed with the electrocautery but it is better to infiltrate the base with local anaesthetic first (Figs 26.1–26.4). Where the base of the lesion is very broad, and particularly where a neat cosmetic result is desired, it is preferable to excise the papilloma under local anaesthesia, using an elliptical incision, and suturing the skin edges.

As an alternative method, if the practitioner does not possess an electrocautery, most small skin tags and papillomata may be tied off using a fine thread and allowed to drop off. This is perfectly acceptable but separation can take 1 or 2 weeks. They may also be snipped off using a pair of fine scissors and the base cauterized with aluminium chloride.

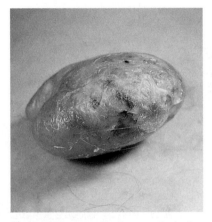

Figure 26.15 Large fibrolipoma at the back of the leg; narrow base, so suitable for division with just the electrocautery.

Figure 26.16 Infiltrating the base with lignocaine 1%.

Figure 26.17 Separating the fibrolipoma from the leg using just electrocautery.

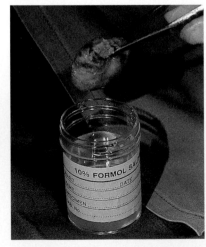

Figure 26.18 Specimen sent for histological examination.

27 Warts and verrucae

> Regardless of this, small morbid swellings arise in the skin such as myrmicia (flat warts) achrocordones, psydraces, and epinytides (herpes zoster) ... All of these are well-known diseases.
>
> *Galen of Pergamum, AD 129–199*

Warts and verrucae are extremely common; they affect children and young adults primarily, are caused by the wart virus and are therefore infectious. They may be single or multiple, painless or painful, slowly growing or rapidly growing, disappear spontaneously after a few weeks, or remain stubbornly resistant to all treatments for years. The multiplicity of treatments and so-called 'cures' give an indication of how ineffective most are. They can cause despair in doctor and patient alike. Fortunately, practically all warts and verrucae eventually disappear spontaneously, never to return, but as this may take several years, most patients seek treatment in an attempt to cure them in a shorter time. Some treatments are undoubtedly harmless and worth trying, whereas others definitely carry certain well-recognized risks and may leave permanent scarring. In a self-limiting condition, therefore, the practitioner must not let his or her surgical enthusiasm inflict a treatment which is worse than the original condition; neither should the treatment be painful, as the majority of sufferers will be young children unlikely to forget or forgive.

Treatments for warts and verrucae fall into two categories: medical and surgical. No apology is made for including a selection of medical treatments before considering surgical approaches.

27.1 MEDICAL TREATMENTS

27.1.1 Psychological therapy

Although warts are known to be caused by a viral infective agent, they can be made to disappear by psychological treatments. This fact was known for centuries by the 'wart charmers' and in recent years by hypnotherapists. If a patient believes that their warts are going to disappear as a result of any treatment, a significant proportion does in fact regress and disappear!

Figure 27.1 Solitary warts may be effectively treated with a saturated solution of monochloroacetic acid, pricked in with a wooden applicator until no more is absorbed.

Figure 27.2 Monochloroacetic acid being applied to a solitary wart on the wrist.

27.1.2 Monochloroacetic acid

Solitary warts or verrucae respond well to a saturated solution of monochloroacetic acid pricked into the wart using a sharp-pointed wooden applicator (Figs 27.1 and 27.2).

One drop of acid is placed on the surface of the wart, and with a wooden applicator is pricked through the horny outer layer. Often the acid appears to soak into the wart very much like soaking into absorbent paper. Further drops of acid are applied and pricked into the wart until no more will soak in. It is most important not to allow any acid on the surrounding skin or a painful burn will result. Should any spread from the wart, it should be immediately removed with a soft paper tissue. Following the application of monochloroacetic acid, there is normally a reddening of the skin over the next 4 or 5 days and signs of healing after 8 days. One application is often successful and the treatment may be repeated if necessary. Ointments containing podophyllin and/or salicylic acid are equally effective.

27.1.3 Podophyllin and/or salicylic acid

The risk in using podophyllin is overenthusiastic treatment in a desperate attempt to cure the verruca. This results in painful burns to the surrounding skin; often the verruca is cured, but at the expense of considerable discomfort (Fig. 27.3). If using podophyllin and salicylic acid ointment (Posalfilin) only enough to cover a pin-head should be used; this should be placed in the centre of the verruca, covered with a plaster dressing and repeated daily until cured. A simple way by which the patient can tell whether the verruca is cured is by

Figure 27.3 Overenthusiastic treatment of verrucae with podophllin and salicylic acid.

Figure 27.4 A simple method to determine whether a wart or a verruca is cured; if there is no pain on lateral compression between the finger and thumb, then it is – cured.

compressing the skin on either side of the verruca: if painful it is still present, if painless it is cured (Fig. 27.4). Plasters with 40% salicylic acid are an effective means of dealing with multiple plantar warts; they macerate the top layers of skin, including the wart.

27.1.4 Aqueous formalin or glutaraldehyde solution

Multiple verrucae may also be treated by soaking the whole foot in 20% aqueous formalin solution for 10 min each day (Fig. 27.5). The skin becomes hard, leathery and liable to crack, particularly between the toes if the solution is not washed off. Using a similar principle, glutaraldehyde solution may be applied just to the wart or verruca daily until it is cured.

27.1.5 Genital warts

Genital warts (condylomata acuminate) are more susceptible to treatment than the ordinary hard wart; in this case the treatment of choice is podophyllin in spirit or tinct. benz. co. applied very carefully to each wart. Traditionally, 25% podophyllin was recommended, but unfortunately this often burned the surrounding skin, and a trial using 0.5% podophyllin resin in 70% ethanol [27] applied twice daily for 3 days gave equally good results. Liquid nitrogen cryosurgery also gives excellent results with less scarring.

Figure 27.5 Multiple verrucae; best treated medically with salicylic acid or formalin.

27.2 SURGICAL TREATMENTS

There are as many surgical as there are medical treatments for warts and verrucae, indicating again that no one treatment offers more than a reasonable chance of cure. Treatments involve burning, freezing, curetting and excision. Various instruments will destroy warts or verrucae by heat. The simplest is the standard electrocautery, by which a platinum electrode is heated to red heat by the passage of an electric current. It is first necessary to infiltrate the base of the wart with local anaesthetic (lignocaine 1% with or without adrenaline, depending on the site) and the wart may then be destroyed using the electrocautery.

Another method of producing heat within tissue is by passing an electric current through it; this is used regularly for coagulating bleeding vessels in the operating theatre. A large pad is strapped to the patient's thigh and connected to one side of the output of the machine, while the other output lead is connected to a small pointed instrument such as a pair of artery forceps. This is a bipolar diathermy apparatus. Similar portable diathermy machines are now available which use just one electrode and these are the unipolar diathermy machines, or Hyfrecators. In use, the needle electrode is inserted into the centre of the wart and the electric current switched on. The heat generated within the wart destroys it; normally a local anaesthetic is used to infiltrate the base of the wart before applying the electrode. No further treatment is required apart from a sterile, dry dressing.

27.2.1 Curetting and cautery

Most solitary warts and verrucae can be removed with a curette and either this or radiosurgery is probably the treatment of choice (Chapter 42).

The following instruments are required (Figs 27.6–27.12):

■ dental syringe and 30 swg needle (0.3 mm)
■ cartridge of 2% lignocaine with 1:80 000 adrenaline

Figure 27.6 Solitary wart on the thumb; present for 1 year and painful. Curette and cautery offer a high chance of permanent cure.

Figure 27.7 Wart being curetted out. A tourniquet and ring-block prevent bleeding at this stage.

Figure 27.8 The base of the wart is now cauterized with the electrocautery.

Figure 27.9 Verruca on the sole of the foot; anaesthesia by posterior tibial nerve block.

Figure 27.10 Technique of using a curette to remove a verruca; firm pressure and a rotating action.

Figure 27.11 After removing the verruca, the base is cauterized with the electrocautery.

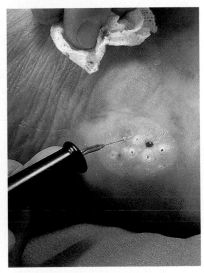

Figure 27.12 A cluster of stubborn verrucae being individually treated with the Hyfrecator needle after preliminary paring of any hard skin.

- 2 ml syringe
- 25 swg × 5/8 in. (0.5 mm × 16 mm) needle
- ampoule 1% lignocaine with adrenaline 1:200 000
- Volkmann double-ended sharp-spoon curette
- electrocautery and pointed burner or unipolar diathermy
- histology container
- dry dressing
- povidone–iodine (Betadine **aqueous** solution).

The wart and adjacent skin is painted with povidone–iodine (Betadine aqueous solution). Using the dental syringe and 30 swg needle or the 2 ml syringe with 25 swg (0.5 mm) needle the base of the wart is infiltrated with local anaesthetic. It is now possible to curette the wart easily from the skin. This is best achieved by holding the handle of the curette firmly, perpendicular to the skin, pressing the curette firmly against the edge of the wart, and then shelling out the wart with a rotating action. When the correct tissue plane is reached the wart or verruca will readily separate, leaving a neat circular hole which bleeds easily despite the adrenaline in the local anaesthetic mixture. To control this bleeding the vessels are coagulated using the electro-cautery, which additionally destroys any remaining fragments of wart. A dry dressing is applied and healing is usually complete in 3 weeks with freedom from pain after 2 days.

27.2.2 Excision of warts

Excision of warts is appropriate in certain sites such as the face where a neat scar is desirable, but as the majority of warts will disappear spontaneously without leaving a scar, excision should only be considered as a last resort.

The following instruments are required:

- dental syringe and 30 swg needle (0.3 mm)
- cartridge of 2% lignocaine with adrenaline 1:80 000
- 10 ml syringe
- 25 swg × 5/8 in. (0.5 mm × 16 mm) needle
- 21 swg × 1½ in. (0.8 × 40 mm) needle
- scalpel handle size 3
- scalpel blade size 10
- pair toothed dissecting forceps
- pair stitch scissors
- Kilner needle holder
- Prolene suture; gauge depending on site, e.g. 6/0 if on face
- 10 ml ampoule 1% lignocaine with adrenaline 1:200 000 dressings
- povidone–iodine in spirit (Betadine alcoholic solution).

The wart and surrounding skin is painted with povidone–iodine in spirit and the base anaesthetized. An ellipse of skin is removed with the wart in the centre; this is sent for confirmatory histology and the wound closed using fine, interrupted Prolene sutures. These are removed between 5 and 10 days, depending on the site of the original lesion.

27.2.3 Cryosurgery for warts and verrucae

As well as destruction by heat, tissues can be destroyed by freezing, and in many situations this method offers a better treatment, relatively free from pain, with an excellent cosmetic result. The different equipment and modes of use are described in Chapter 18 but there are three different machines, using carbon dioxide, nitrous oxide and liquid nitrogen, in ascending order of efficiency. Liquid nitrogen gives the lowest temperature and has the highest success, carbon dioxide has only limited uses, while the nitrous oxide cryoprobe is valuable for superficial lesions. The technique is as follows.

The wart or verruca is pared down and moistened with water-soluble jelly or glycerine, and the cryoprobe applied. As freezing progresses, the probe becomes frozen to the wart, which may now be lifted a few millimetres from subcutaneous tissues by gentle traction on the probe. When the wart is frozen solid, the probe is warmed and detached, and the wart allowed to thaw. The procedure is repeated as this second freeze appears to give improved results. Alternatively, liquid nitrogen may be sprayed on the wart to achieve freezing.

Immediately following freezing little can be seen and the wart appears exactly as before treatment; slight throbbing is experienced during the next few hours, to be followed over the ensuing days by painless necrosis and healing. The relative absence of pain and the very acceptable end result make cryosurgery attractive.

Condylomata acuminate are easily treated with a nitrous oxide cryoprobe. Larger warts are better treated with liquid nitrogen using a spray applicator (Chapter 18; Figs 27.13–27.15), taking care to avoid damage to the underlying tendons, nerves and joints (Figs 27.16 and 27.17).

Figure 27.13 Solitary wart on the forehead; suitable for cryosurgery.

Figure 27.14 Multiple warts on the toes; treatment with either formalin soaks or cryosurgery.

Figure 27.15 Treatment of warts on the hand by liquid nitrogen cryospray.

Figure 27.16 Warts in certain situations require extra care. This wart overlies the joint capsule and extensor tendons. Overzealous treatment could result in damage to these structures.

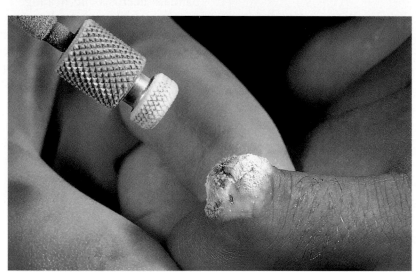

Figure 27.17 Treatment with liquid nitrogen cryospray; several short treatments would be safer than one long freeze.

27.2.4 Radiosurgical treatment of warts (see also Chapter 42)

Solitary warts and verrucae can also be removed using a radiosurgical instrument and wire loop. Treatment is very quick and simple, and causes less tissue damage than electrocautery or diathermy. Local infiltration is still needed. Any bleeding may also be controlled with the radiosurgical unit.

CHAPTER 28

Sebaceous cysts

I made an incision in the scalp, and upon the side on which I stood, which was about three-fourths of its size, I with difficulty detached it from the skin ... The edges of the wound were brought together and lint and plaster applied. The King bore the operation well.

Account by Sir Astley Cooper of the removal of a sebaceous cyst from the scalp of King George IV, 1820

True sebaceous cysts are very rare; however, epidermal and tricholemmal cysts are very common and usually referred to as sebaceous cysts.

Epidermal cysts occur following implantation of epidermis, or from the epidermal lining of pilosebaceous follicles, and are filled with macerated keratin; they can occur anywhere on the body, commonly fingers, from implantation.

The cysts commonly seen on the scalp are tricholemmal (pilar) cysts which are derived from the hair follicle; they occur in families, being inherited as an autosomal dominant gene, and are often multiple. Both types of cyst are ideal for removal in the doctor's treatment room under local anaesthetic. For the remainder of the chapter the term 'sebaceous cyst' will be used as it is better known for both epidermal and tricholemmal cysts.

The following instruments are required:

- dental syringe and 30 swg needle (0.3 mm)
- cartridge of 2% lignocaine with adrenaline 1:80 000
- scalpel handle size 3
- scalpel blade size 15
- pair stitch scissors 5 in. (12.7 cm)
- pair McIndoe curved scissors 7 in. (17.8 cm)
- pair toothed dissecting forceps
- pair Halstead mosquito forceps 5 in. (12.7 cm) curved
- Kilner needle holder $5\frac{1}{4}$ in. (13.3 cm)
- surgical sutures, braided silk, metric gauge 2 (3/0) on curved cutting needle (Ref. Ethicon W533) or equivalent monofilament Nylon or Prolene
- 1% lignocaine with adrenaline 1:200 000
- syringes and 25 swg × 5/8 in. (0.5 mm × 16 mm) needle
- povidone–iodine in spirit (Betadine alcoholic solution).

28.1 TECHNIQUE FOR REMOVAL OF SEBACEOUS CYSTS ON THE SCALP (FIGS 28.1–28.6)

The patient should preferably be lying down rather than sitting in a chair; even the most unlikely character is liable to faint, and it is embarrassing to have to complete the excision of a cyst on the floor!

Figure 28.1 Typical sebaceous cyst on the scalp.

Figure 28.2 The overlying skin is infiltrated with local anaesthetic and a small quantity injected into the base of the cyst.

Figure 28.3 An elliptical incision is made over the cyst, exposing the underlying cyst.

Figure 28.4 Using curved mosquito forceps or curved McIndoe scissors, the cyst is dissected free.

Figure 28.5 With a little patience and careful dissection the cyst may be removed complete.

Figure 28.6 Closure is with interrupted 4/0 Prolene sutures.

Any overlying hairs are clipped with scissors (it is not necessary to shave large areas of scalp) and the overlying skin is painted with povidone–iodine in spirit.

With the finger and thumb of the left hand fixing the cyst, local anaesthetic is injected through the skin using a dental syringe with local anaesthetic and 30 swg needle or 25 swg × 5/8 in. (0.5 × 16 mm) needle, with the bevel flat against the skin. Keeping pressure on the syringe plunger, the needle is slowly advanced, until it reaches the tissue plane between skin and cyst. At this stage, there is a loss of resistance in the syringe plunger, and distension of the cyst may be felt with the palpating finger and thumb of the left hand. Further pressure on the syringe plunger spreads the lignocaine and adrenaline around the cyst, causing the overlying skin to blanch (Fig. 28.2).

Done carefully, this technique separates the tissue planes and makes subsequent excision easier. One additional injection of local anaesthetic is made underneath the cyst before the needle is finally removed. Occasionally, the pressure of the local anaesthetic infiltration causes the cyst to eject some of its contents through the blocked punctum, or rarely may cause the cyst to rupture.

28.1.1 Incision

Very small cysts can be removed merely by a single incision and digital pressure, when the cyst will pop out (Figs 28.7 and 28.8). Closure with one stitch is all that is required. Larger cysts require dissection and the excision of an ellipse of redundant skin. The ellipse of skin should be chosen to include the central punctum; it may be excised, exposing the underlying cyst. Using the blades of a curved McIndoe's scissors, the cyst is freed by gently inserting the closed blades and opening

Figure 28.7   Small inclusion or epidermal cyst in the finger; easily removed under ring block and tourniquet.

Figure 28.8   The same cyst as in Fig. 28.7 being expressed by the application of finger pressure on either side.

Figure 28.9 Method of preventing the skin edges inverting when suturing; vertical mattress suture.

them. Any adhesions can be separated either by this method or by cutting, using the same scissors (Fig. 28.4). At this stage the cyst may be grasped with the toothed dissecting forceps, traction applied and the remaining adhesions divided. Bleeding is not usually a problem, except perhaps with cysts at the back of the neck; it can normally be controlled with firm pressure and usually stops when the edges of the wound are sutured. The aim should be to remove the cyst complete, although this is not always possible, particularly with thin-walled cysts where the centre has become infected. Where there is evidence of infection, the cyst should still be removed, but before closure, a small quantity of fucidic acid gel (Fucidin gel) should be instilled into the cavity and the skin then sutured in the usual way.

28.1.2 Closure

Interrupted Prolene sutures should be used, which may be removed on the 8th–10th postoperative day. Where there is redundant skin which tends to invert on skin closure, the edges should be picked up in the stitch, as shown in Fig. 28.9.

28.2 ALTERNATIVE METHOD FOR REMOVAL OF SEBACEOUS CYSTS

Some practitioners prefer to bisect the cyst, squeeze out the contents with a gauze swab, and then pull out the lining of the cyst with a pair of artery forceps. This is a much quicker procedure than dissection, but is messy and carries a slightly higher infection rate, and the contents of a sebaceous cyst have a slightly unpleasant, persistent odour. Nevertheless, it is a perfectly acceptable method of removal.

28.3 HISTOLOGY

As with all excised specimens, even the humble 'sebaceous cyst' should be sent for histological examination if at all possible; occasionally, an unsuspected squamous cell tumour, cylindroma or other rarity may be discovered.

Figure 28.10 Small earlobe cysts are very common.

Figure 28.11 The application of ring forceps enables the cyst to be held and also controls bleeding.

Figure 28.12 Small epidermal cyst behind the ear, dissected free after infiltration with local anaesthetic.

Figure 28.13 After removal of the cyst, the wound is closed with fine, interrupted 5/0 Prolene sutures.

Figure 28.14 Unusually shaped sebaceous cyst on the neck.

Excision of lipoma

A lipoma is a benign, fatty tumour which can occur anywhere on the body, varying in size from a small marble to larger than a football. On palpation a lipoma feels lobulated and semicystic: smooth in outline and generally painless. Lipomata may be solitary or multiple and the most commonly given reason for requesting removal is cosmetic, although in some sites, pressure effects may cause symptoms. Although appearing to be quite superficial, many lipomata extend deeper than expected and the doctor should be aware of this fact before embarking on excision.

Many lipomata can be enucleated using a gloved finger; others are tethered by fibrous bands which give the lipoma its typical lobulated appearance; these bands need to be dissected free with the curved McIndoe's scissors.

The following instruments are required:

- scalpel handle no. 3
- scalpel blade no. 10
- pair McIndoe's scissors 7 in. (17.8 cm) curved
- pair toothed dissecting forceps
- Kilner needle holder 5¼ in. (13.3 cm)
- Halstead's artery forceps 5 in. (12.7 cm) curved
- povidone–iodine in spirit (Betadine alcoholic solution)
- 10 ml 1% lignocaine with adrenaline 1:200 000
- syringes and needles.

The size, shape and extent of the lipoma are first ascertained, and its relationship to any adjacent structures is noted. The overlying skin is painted with povidone–iodine in spirit and the area infiltrated with 1% lignocaine with adrenaline 1:200 000, remembering to include the deeper part of the lipoma (Fig. 29.1). An incision is made boldly through the skin directly to the lipoma, which will typically bulge into the wound (Fig. 29.2). At this stage a gloved finger can be inserted between skin and lipoma to see whether it will shell out (Fig. 29.3); if not, further blunt dissection is carried out using the McIndoe's curved scissors and an opening action, dividing any fibrous bands tethering the lipoma to deeper tissues. With patience, the complete

Figure 29.1 Lipoma situated in the antecubital fossa; the brachial artery is marked in red.

Figure 29.2 Incising through the skin allows the lipoma to bulge through the wound.

Figure 29.3 Using finger dissection, the lipoma may be removed.

Figure 29.4 Lipoma removed completely; any mild bleeding is controlled with a gauze swab.

Figure 29.5 Wound being closed with sub-cuticular Prolene sutures.

Figure 29.6 Additional support may be given by the use of skin-closure strips.

lipoma can be freed and removed (Fig. 29.4); it is then sent for routine histological examination. Following removal of a large lipoma, a substantial dead space is left which might collect blood and delay healing; in this case it is advisable to close the space with interrupted catgut or Vicryl sutures. In excising larger lipomata, an ellipse of skin should also be removed to enable accurate closure with no redundant skin. Finally, skin closure should be with either interrupted sutures, or a subcuticular Nylon or coated Vicryl suture, the latter probably being more acceptable to the patient who requested removal on cosmetic grounds (Figs 29.5 and 29.6).

CHAPTER 30

Minor operations on the toes

30.1 TREATMENT OF INGROWING TOE-NAILS

Ingrowing toe-nails are extremely common cause much discomfort, and yet can be one of the most rewarding conditions to treat in general practice.

Surgical textbooks abound with scores of treatments, varying from quite minor procedures, often ineffective, to complete removal of the nail, ablation of the nail bed, and even amputation of the terminal phalanx resulting in weeks of painful, messy dressings and much time away from school or work. The cause is still not known; ill-fitting shoes and incorrect cutting of the nails have both been incriminated, and the condition commonly occurs in young males with 'sweaty' feet, but many patients are seen in whom these factors certainly do not apply, and as the condition largely affects the big toenail on either foot and appears to be cured by permanently narrowing the width of the nail, it may be that the width of the nail is an important contributing factor.

Three types of ingrowing toe-nail are seen. The first group is commonly seen in young patients between the ages of 10 and 20 years. Here, the nail is entirely normal in contour but the skin is hypertropied, often with granulations in the nail fold (Figs 30.1–30.3). The second

Figure 30.1 Typical ingrowing toe-nails affecting the big toes on both feet.

Figure 30.2 A severely infected ingrowing toe-nail. Even one as bad as this can easily be cured with matrix phenolization.

Figure 30.3 Ingrowing big toe-nail.

group is more likely to be seen in adults; here the nail has increased its convexity so that its edges press firmly on the shallow nail groove. In the third group, seen in all ages, the nail is incurving and ingrowing so that the nail plate has increased its convexity, particularly at the lateral edges so that the edge of the nail has curved through almost 180° and is digging into the lateral edge of the nail groove.

30.1.1 Medical treatments

Before embarking on surgery, medical treatments may be tried. One of the simplest for mild, early, ingrowing toe-nails is the application of Sofradex drops (dexamethasone 0.05%, framycetin sulphate 0.5% and gramicidin 0.005%) four times daily for 1 week. If by the end of the time there has not been an obvious improvement, surgical treatment is indicated, offering nearly 100% cure.

The operation of choice is one which has been used by chiropodists for many years [28–31], correctly described as nail matrix phenolization, and consists of removing a narrow strip of nail together with nail matrix on the affected side, and the application of liquefied phenol to cauterize the germinal epithelium. It is highly effective and gives rapid, painless healing, with virtually no recurrence [32].

Phenol appears to have a threefold action. First, it destroys the nail matrix and prevents that portion of nail regrowing. Secondly, it destroys the nerve endings, which explains the absence of pain during the healing phase. Thirdly, it destroys all pathogenic organisms, resulting in a sterile, cauterized area.

In the UK pure liquefied phenol containing 80% w/w in water is used; in the USA, liquefied phenol USP containing not less than 89% w/w in water is used. The higher strength used in America is unlikely to make any significant difference to the results, but it should be stored in brown glass bottles, ideally with a glass stopper as the solution changes from colourless to pink or brown when exposed to light, and the phenol can affect plastic caps and washers. Although it appears that phenol which has changed colour is nonetheless effective, it is probably wise to use a relatively fresh and colourless solution.

Wooden applicators with a wisp of cotton wool tightly wound around the tip are the best way of applying the phenol. They must be narrow enough to be easily inserted into the matrix cavity, and only enough phenol to saturate the space should be used, avoiding spilling the solution on adjacent skin.

30.1.2 Nail matrix phenolization

The following instruments are required (Fig. 30.4):

- syringes and needles local anaesthetic **without** adrenaline povidone–iodine in spirit (Betadine alcoholic solution)
- paraffin tulle with 0.5% chlorhexidine (Bactigras)
- Easifix or equivalent bandage 2 in. (5 cm)
- Thwaites nail nipper or sharp-pointed, stitch scissors 5 in. (12.7 cm)
- 25 swg (0.5 mm) needle
- 2 pairs straight artery forceps 5 in. (12.7 cm)
- nail chisel (Nova Instruments)
- wooden applicator sticks
- Volkmann sharp-spoon curette
- rubber-strip tourniquet
- rubber-tube tourniquet
- pure liquefied phenol (BP) (USP)
- 30 swg (0.3 mm) needle

It is helpful to advise the patient to arrange transport home and to bring a large shoe or slipper to accommodate the bandaged toe. Povidone–iodine in spirit is liberally applied to the toe (Fig. 30.5), extending proximally at least 2.5 cm beyond the interdigital clefts. A ring block or digital nerve block is performed using plain lignocaine

Figure 30.4 Instruments required for ingrowing toe-nails; from left to right: nail chisel (Nova) artery forceps, Thwaites nail nipper, artery forceps, wooden applicator, rubber-tube tourniquet.

or prilocaine: under no circumstances should adrenaline or any other vasoconstrictor be added to the local anaesthetic, otherwise ischaemia and possible necrosis could occur (Fig. 30.6).

For greatest comfort, and particularly in children, a 30 swg (0.3 mm) needle should be used with a dental syringe and cartridge. Unfortunately, most dental anaesthetic cartridges contain adrenaline, but prilocaine 4% (Citanest) containing 40 mg/ml is manufactured in 2 ml cartridges (maximum adult dose prilocaine 400 mg). Failing this, a standard 5 ml syringe with a 25 swg × 5/8 in. (0.5 × 16 mm) needle may be used with 1% lignocaine.

The digital nerves to the toe lie on the plantar side of the coronal plane; each should be infiltrated with 0.5 ml local anaesthetic, followed by a 'bridge' of solution across the dorsum of the toe, plus a similar bridge on the plantar surface, producing a complete ring block (Fig. 30.7).

Toes which are very reddened and inflamed are more difficult to anaesthetize, but it is well worth taking additional time and effort to achieve complete anaesthesia before operating.

A sterile gauze swab is now wrapped around the toe (Fig. 30.8) and over this is applied a rubber-strip tourniquet or 1 in. cotton non-stretch

Figure 30.5 The toe-nail and forefoot are liberally painted with povidone–iodine in spirit.

Figure 30.6 The digital nerves are blocked with local anaesthetic (added adrenaline must never be used).

Figure 30.7 A complete ring-block anaesthetic is performed.

Figure 30.8 A sterile gauze swab is wrapped around the toe.

bandage to exsanguinate the toe. (The rubber strip included in the butterfly intravenous cannulae kits makes an ideal tourniquet for fingers and toes.) Next, a fine rubber-tube tourniquet is tied tightly around the base of the toe and fixed with one of the pairs of artery forceps (Figs 30.9 and 30.10). The rubber strip and gauze swab are removed, leaving a bloodless, anaesthetized toe (Fig. 30.11).

More povidone–iodine in spirit is applied and a sterile paper drape is placed over the foot, with the toe protruding through a small hole cut in the paper.

Using the Thwaites nail nipper or pointed stitch scissors, the operator cuts a thin strip of nail adjacent to the granulations, approximately 2–3 mm away from the nail fold and extending to the base of the nail (Fig. 30.12). This cut is then extended to the nail matrix or germinal epithelium, using a special nail chisel which splits the nail, using firm pressure, until resistance is encountered (Fig. 30.13).

Figure 30.9 A rubber-strip tourniquet is wrapped over the gauze swab to exsanguinate the toe.

Figure 30.10 A rubber-tube tourniquet is tied round the base of the toe and secured.

Figure 30.11 The rubber strip and gauze swab are removed, and more povidone–iodine is applied.

Figure 30.12 Using either stitch scissors or Thwaites nail nippers, a strip of nail is cut out as shown.

Figure 30.13 The cut is deepened using the nail chisel, pushing it firmly down to the root of the nail.

The chisel is removed, and the strip of nail is grasped with a pair of straight artery forceps and gently removed using a combination of traction and rotation, making sure not to tear the base of the strip or leave any fragments in the groove (Figs 30.14 and 30.15). Any excess granulations are removed with the curette, and the phenol is applied with the wooden applicator using a massaging action to ensure complete absorption, particularly in the matrix cavity (Fig. 30.16). The phenol is applied for exactly 3 min: if less than this, recurrence is likely. Sufficient is used to cauterize the groove formerly occupied by the strip of nail, but care is taken not to use too much as it might spread over the adjacent skin and delay healing (Figs 30.17 and 30.18). After 3 min, a dry swab is used to mop away any surplus phenol, and an ointment containing an antibiotic, antimycotic and steroid (e.g. Tri-Adcortyl) is applied generously to the nail bed and the area treated with phenol. This appears to accelerate healing. Earlier accounts of the technique described the use of 5% chlorhexidine in spirit to 'neutralize' the phenol, this is now thought not to be necessary.

Figure 30.14   The strip of nail is grasped with artery forceps and removed.

Figure 30.15   The strip of nail which has been removed.

Figure 30.16   Pure phenol is applied, using a wooden applicator and cotton wool.

Figure 30.17   The phenol must be applied for a minimum of 3 min.

Figure 30.18   The appearance of the nail bed after applying the phenol.

A non-adherent dressing of povidone–iodine (Inadine) or paraffin tulle impregnated with 5% chlorhexidine is now applied, covered with one square of sterile absorbent gauze, and the toe bandaged (Figs 30.19 and 30.20).

The tourniquet is released, the dressing checked for any bleeding, and the patient allowed home with instructions to rest the foot for 6 h. If troublesome bleeding occurs after the release of the tourniquet, it can often be controlled by the application of an alginate dressing (Kaltostat or equivalent) under the gauze. Two follow-up dressings are necessary, the first on the third postoperative day and the second 1 week later on the 10th day, and this is usually all that is necessary. Frequently, on the 10th day dressing the toe is found to be moist and messy: this is thought to be due to a delayed 'phenol reaction', is quite common and needs no special treatment. If discharge or granulations persist, an application of povidone–iodine spray powder (Disadine DP) is helpful, covered with a dry dressing.

Incurving, ingrowing nails are treated in an identical manner, removing a narrow strip from either edge of the nail and phenolizing both sides simultaneously.

Figure 30.19 A dressing of Inadine and Tri-adcortyl ointment is applied.

Figure 30.20 This is covered with a gauze swab and cotton bandages and left for 1–3 days.

30.1.3 Cryotherapy for ingrowing toe-nail

Destruction of the granulations of moderately severe ingrowing toe-nails is possible if the doctor possesses a liquid nitrogen cryospray unit.

Technique

Because treatment may be painful, analgesic tablets taken 1 h prior to freezing are advised, and in some patients, infiltration anaesthesia using lignocaine as a ring block will enable the freezing to occur painlessly. The spray is held about 1 cm away from the granulations and liquid nitrogen sprayed on the edge of the nail and toe until ice is seen to extend about 2 mm beyond the edge of the granulations. This normally occurs after 30 s of spraying.

Dermovate-NN cream or similar potent steroid cream is now applied under a dry dressing to minimize the reaction to the liquid nitrogen. Healing is usually complete in 6 weeks.

30.1.4 Wedge excision for ingrowing toe-nail

Many surgeons prefer a simple wedge excision of the granulation tissue to cauterization with phenol. Done carefully, it has the same high cure rate, but demands slightly more surgical skill and experience to judge the amount of tissue to be removed, may require the insertion of one suture and is occasionally accompanied by brisk bleeding when the tourniquet is released. For the doctor starting to treat ingrowing toe-nails, nail matrix phenolization is probably an easier technique to master initially.

Technique

As with nail matrix phenolization, the toe is first liberally painted with povidone–iodine in spirit and a ring block performed using plain lig-nocaine or prilocaine. A rubber tourniquet is next applied to exsan-guinate the toe, and a rubber-tube tourniquet then applied to the base of the toe.

A strip of nail is cut using a no. 15 scalpel blade on a no. 3 handle with the back of the blade adjacent to the nail bed as shown (Fig. 30.21). This cut is extended to the base of the nail to include the germinal epithelium (Fig. 30.22a, b).

A second incision is now made on the lateral side of the toe, down to the first incision, thus removing a wedge of granulation tissue including a thin strip of nail (Fig. 30.23). The nail bed and germinal epithelium are now curetted using a Volkmann sharp-spoon curette. This needs to be done thoroughly to minimize the risks of leaving a small amount of nail matrix behind (Fig. 30.24).

The proximal parts of the wound are brought together with Steri-strips or a single 4/0 Prolene suture (Fig. 30.25), and a non-adherent is Inadine dressing applied, covered by a dry gauze swab and finally bandaged with a cotton conforming bandage (Crinx, Easifix or similar) (Figs 30.26 and 30.27). This dressing is left undisturbed for

Figure 30.21 Wedge excision of an ingrowing toe-nail; initial incision, splitting the nail.

Figure 30.22 (a) Initial incision; a lateral incision would be made if many granulations were present. (b) Wedge resection of nail (redrawn from H.A. Dudley, J.R.T. Eckersley and S. Paterson-Brown, *A Guide to Practical Procedures in Medical Surgery.* By permission of Butterworth-Heinemann Ltd).

Figure 30.23 Granulations being curetted together with any germinal epithelium.

Figure 30.24 Appearance after curetting granulations and nail matrix.

Figure 30.25 (a) Inserting a fine suture. This is not always necessary and the edges may be held together with Steri-strips. (b) Closure after wedge resection (redrawn from H.A. Dudley, J.R.T. Eckersley and S. Paterson-Brown, *A Guide to Practical Procedures in Medical Surgery.* By permission of Butterworth-Heinemann Ltd).

Figure 30.26 One suture, if needed. This is removed on the 7th postoperative day.

Figure 30.27 Non-adherent dressing is applied.

7–10 days, after which time the suture is removed and a smaller dry dressing applied.

Healing usually occurs rapidly, but the immediate postoperative phase may be more uncomfortable than when using phenol, because of the anaesthetic effect of the latter.

30.1.5 Radiosurgical treatment of ingrowing toe-nails (see also Chapter 42)

The germinal epithelium may be destroyed very effectively using the radiosurgical unit and a specially designed nail matrixectomy electrode.

Technique

The preparation of the toe, anaesthesia and removal of the thin strip of nail on the affected side are identical to nail matrix phenolization, but instead of applying a swab soaked in pure liquefied phenol, the special electrode is inserted and a current passed for about 5 seconds (setting 2 on the Ellman Surgitron FFPF, coagulation waveform). The toe is then dressed exactly as with the phenol treatment and reviewed 3 days later.

Healing is quicker than with phenol and there is less reaction. Cure rates in excess of 98% have been reported by Hettinger (see Further reading).

30.1.6 Nail-bed ablation

There are two situations in which total ablation of the nail bed may be the treatment of choice for the patient. The first is when recurrent ingrowing toe-nails fail to respond to either nail matrix phenolization or wedge excision, and the second is the patient with grossly distorted onychogryphotic toe-nails where simply removing the nail will result in the same situation recurring several months later.

Two techniques may be used:

- phenol
- surgical excision.

Technique of phenol ablation of nail bed (see also Onychogryphosis, Fig. 30.28)

The preparation, ring block and application of tourniquet are exactly as described for the treatment of the ingrowing toe-nail. To remove the nail, it is first lifted away from the nail-bed with a McDonald's dissector or special nail elevator and then split in half using the Thwaites nail nipper. Each half may then be grasped with a strong pair of straight artery forceps and pulled off, using a combination of traction and rotation. If nail nippers are unavailable, the nail may be too thickened to be cut with any other instrument; accordingly, it may be removed *in toto* using a strong pair of artery forceps.

Having removed the nail, the nail bed and germinal epithelium are painted with pure phenol, paying particular attention to the groove containing the nail matrix. As with ingrowing toe-nails, the phenol is left in contact for at least 3 min (Fig. 30.29). After 3 min, a dry swab is used to mop away any surplus phenol, and an ointment containing an antibiotic, antimycotic and steroid (e.g. Tri-adcortyl) is applied generously to the nail bed and the area treated with phenol. This appears to accelerate healing. It is then mopped dry and a paraffin-tulle dressing with 0.5% chlorhexidine (Bactigras) applied, covered with a sterile gauze swab and bandage.

Figure 30.28 Incurved, ingrowing, onychogryphotic nail causing much discomfort.

Figure 30.29 After removal of the nail, the nail bed and germinal epithelium are treated with pure, liquefied phenol.

Figure 30.30 Zadik operation. (A) Incisions; (B) block of tissue to be excised (redrawn from H.A. Dudley, J.R.T. Eckersley and S. Paterson-Brown, *A Guide to Practical Procedures in Medical Surgery.* By permission of Butterworth-Heinemann Ltd).

Figure 30.31 Zadik operation; elevation of flap and incision into the nail bed. (redrawn from H.A. Dudley, J.R.T. Eckersley and S. Paterson-Brown, *A Guide to Practical Procedures in Medical Surgery.* By permission of Butterworth-Heinemann Ltd).

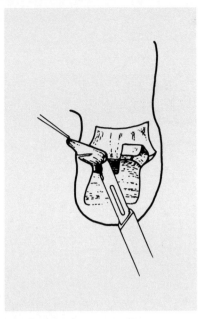

Figure 30.32 Zadik operation; Dissection of the nail bed in two halves (redrawn from H.A. Dudley, J.R.T. Eckersley and S. Paterson-Brown, *A Guide to Practical Procedures in Medical Surgery.* By permission of Butterworth-Heinemann Ltd).

Follow-up dressings are done on the third and 10th days and thereafter as necessary, and any infection is treated with povidone–iodine powder spray. Healing takes 5–7 weeks, leaving a comfortable and cosmetically acceptable toe.

Nail-bed ablation by surgical excision (Zadik)

The toe is prepared exactly as with nail matrix phenolization, a ring block performed and a tourniquet applied.

First, the nail is completely removed. Two incisions 1 cm long are made, diverging proximally and laterally from each nail-fold angle, ensuring that they do not extend as far as the interphalangeal joint (Fig. 30.30). Using skin hooks and a no. 15 scalpel blade, a skin flap overlying the nail germinal epithelium is raised and gently pulled back (Fig. 30.31). The block containing germinal epithelium is now removed in two halves (Fig. 30.32). This leaves a defect, which may now be closed by advancing the flap of skin over it, and closing with 5/0 monofilament (Ethilon) sutures (Ref. W 526). A non-stick Inadine dressing is applied, covered by gauze and bandaged in place.

Any nail regrowth is always due to inadequate excision of the germinal epithelium; thus, it is imperative to make a wide enough incision to see clearly the complete extent of the germinal epithelium.

30.2 ONYCHOGRYPHOSIS

... and his nails were like birds' claws

Daniel, Chapter 4, verse 33 (RSV)

Onychogryphosis, or irregular thickening of the nail, is commonly seen in the elderly; it may follow trauma, or arise secondary to a subungual exostosis or following chronic hyperextension of the hallux. Once it has developed, it tends to be permanent. Removal of the nail alone is followed by a recurrence many months later; softening and burring of the nail likewise only give temporary relief (Figs 30.33 and 30.34). The only permanent cure, therefore, is removal of the nail and total nail-bed ablation.

If the condition is secondary to a subungual exostosis, removal of the nail may predispose to corn formation and further pain; it is therefore important to establish at the outset the possible aetiology of each case. Where total nail-bed ablation is chosen, the method is very similar to that used for ingrowing toe-nails.

A simple, immediate treatment for onychogryphosis is to break off the nail forcibly using thumb and finger (Fig. 30.35). Although such a technique sounds alarming, it is remarkably effective, and can be done under Entonox analgesia, 20 breaths or digital anaesthesia using lignocaine. A loosening onychogryphotic nail may even be snapped off without any anaesthetic at all. As a percentage of such patients may have an impaired peripheral circulation, it causes less risk of trauma to avulse the nail under Entonox or even no anaesthesia than to infiltrate the digit with local anaesthetic.

Having avulsed the nail, a simple, non-stick dressing, e.g. povidone–iodine (Inadine) is applied under a bandage and the wound allowed to heal.

The chance of another onychogryphotic nail recurring is extremely high, and it may be judged preferable to destroy the nail-bed germinal epithelium to prevent any further nail growth (Fig. 30.36–30.39).

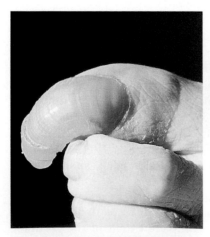

Figure 30.33 Curved, onychogryphotic nail.

Figure 30.34 Another onychogryphotic nail.

Figure 30.35 Onychogryphotic nail removed simply by snapping it off.

Figure 30.36   The nail may either be split and removed in two pieces, or whole with a strong pair of forceps.

Figure 30.37   The nail bed after removal of the onychogryphotic nail.

Figure 30.38   Pure phenol is now applied to the nail bed and nail matrix for 3 min as for ingrowing toe-nails.

Figure 30.39   Appearance of toe following phenol ablation of nail-bed 3 months previously.

30.3 SUBUNGUAL EXOSTOSIS

Occasionally, a patient presents with what at first sight appears to be a typical ingrowing toe-nail, or it may look like a subungual wart, but on closer examination (often after starting the operation) the swelling is found to be bony hard and further dissection reveals a subungual exostosis (Figs 30.40 and 30.41).

It may be necessary to remove half or the whole nail to expose the exostosis. This may then be removed either with a nail chisel or by carefully cutting through with a scalpel blade. A firm, non-stick Inadine dressing is then applied, covered by gauze and a firm bandage. This may then be left undisturbed for 10 days.

Figure 30.40 Subungual exostosis presenting as atypical ingrowing toe-nail.

Figure 30.41 At operation, the bony-hard swelling is seen to arise from the terminal phalanx.

30.4 SOFT CORN

This is a painful condition occurring in the web space between the toes. Initially, it looks like a wart, is very painful and fails to respond to wart cures.

Treatment consists of infiltrating the space with 1% lignocaine and then curetting the 'corn' using a Volkmann sharp-spoon curette, followed by cauterizing the base with the electrocautery or using phenol.

30.5 FUNGAL INFECTION OF THE TOE-NAILS

Established fungal infection of the toe-nails is very hard to eradicate. The best hope of cure consists of removing the toe-nail, sending it for mycological examination and administering oral terbinafine (Lamisil) 250 mg daily while the new nail is growing.

As this may take from 12 to 24 months and entail daily terbinafine for 3–6 months it is very important to establish the diagnosis mycologically beyond doubt.

CHAPTER 31

Biopsy techniques

In many situations it is essential to know the exact histological diagnosis as this will determine the best management for the patient. Lesions such as basal cell carcinoma may be diagnosed with confidence by their naked-eye appearance and may be treated accordingly without the need for a biopsy, but there are occasions when the diagnosis is not immediately obvious and where a biopsy will be helpful, e.g. possible Bowen's disease, an unusual pigmented naevus, suspected mycosis fungoides or granuloma annulare.

As a general guide, biopsy of a skin rash is not usually helpful. Reports such as 'biopsy shows areas of non-specific generalized inflammation' do little to establish a diagnosis and it is better to refer such patients to a consultant dermatologist rather than to perform a biopsy.

In contrast, lesions which may be malignant or premalignant are usually easy to diagnose histologically and a preliminary biopsy will be invaluable.

It is vital when submitting material for histological examination to give the histopathologist as much information as possible, particularly the length of time for which the lesion has been present, its site, method of removal and the clinical diagnosis, where possible (see Chapter 19). Keratoacanthoma and squamous cell carcinoma both have identical histological appearances and only the history will help to differentiate them. If the lesion is 1 cm in diameter and has been present for only 6 weeks, it is very unlikely to be a squamous cell carcinoma but very likely to be a keratoacanthoma. The histopathologist, if faced with such a specimen and no history, will err on the side of reporting 'squamous cell carcinoma', which may result in unnecessary anxiety for both patient and doctor.

When performing any biopsy, it is important that a representative sample is obtained, preferably at the junction of normal and abnormal tissues so that the transformation zone can be examined. In the skin, this is usually as an ellipse including a portion of the lesion, plus healthy skin at the edge. If the lesion can be removed completely, this may be called an excisional biopsy, whereas if only a portion of the lesion is removed, the specimen is labelled an incisional biopsy. It is also helpful to the pathologist to orientate the specimen by marking one end with either an indelible pen or a small suture, indicating that this is the upper, lower, inner or outer margin. This may be important if a malignant lesion has been incompletely excised on one margin and a re-excision needs to be undertaken.

If more than one specimen is taken, they need to be put in separate specimen pots and clearly labelled. This sounds so basic as not to be necessary to mention, but histopathology departments still receive specimen containers with two or more lesions from separate sites; if one is a malignant lesion it will be impossible to identify which came from which site.

31.1 SHAVE BIOPSY (FIGS 31.1–31.7)

This is perhaps the easiest of biopsies to take, particularly when the lesion is raised above the surface of the surrounding skin, but may not always give an exact histological diagnosis. Using a scalpel, razor-blade or special disposable blade the top of the lesion is removed using a sawing action flush with the skin. For all but the smallest lesions, infiltration of the base with local anaesthetic is necessary. Bleeding may either be controlled with firm pressure, or cauterized with the electrocautery or diathermy or radiosurgery unit (see Figs 25.8–25.11).

Figure 31.1 Infiltrating the base of the lesion with local anaesthetic using a dental syringe and 30 swg needle. (Photograph by courtesy of Stiefel Laboratories (UK) Ltd.)

Figure 31.2 By injecting sufficient local anaesthetic, the lesion stands proud of surrounding tissue, making shave-biopsy much easier. (Photograph by courtesy of Stiefel Laboratories (UK) Ltd.)

Figure 31.3 Disposable razor-blades mounted in a rigid plastic handle: rigid.

Figure 31.4 Similar disposable razor-blade mounted in a plastic handle: rigid.

Figure 31.5 Flexible, disposable blade in a plastic handle, held between the finger and thumb.

Figure 31.6 Shave-plane biopsy of lesion.

Figure 31.7 Shave-plane biopsy using a disposable blade.

31.2 PUNCH BIOPSY (FIGS 31.8–31.17)

A punch biopsy is a core of tissue which is removed using a specially designed biopsy instrument (see Figs 25.37b and 25.38). The biopsy punches are made in various sizes from 2 to 8 mm diameter. The base

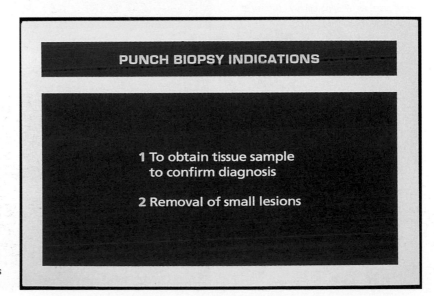

PUNCH BIOPSY INDICATIONS

1 To obtain tissue sample to confirm diagnosis

2 Removal of small lesions

Figure 31.8 Indications for punch biopsy. (Photograph by courtesy of Stiefel Laboratories (UK) Ltd.)

BENEFITS OF PUNCH BIOPSY

- Well established technique in skin surgery

- Rapid and simple procedure

- Wound smaller than elliptical alternative

- May not require suturing

Figure 31.9 Benefits of punch biopsy. (Photograph by courtesy of Stiefel Laboratories (UK) Ltd.)

Figure 31.10 Selection of Stieffel disposable biopsy punches. (Photograph by courtesy of Stiefel Laboratories (UK) Ltd.)

Figure 31.11 A 4 mm biopsy punch.

Figure 31.12 Diagram to show the method of applying traction at right-angles to skin creases to obtain an ellipse giving a better scar. (Photograph by courtesy of Stiefel Laboratories (UK) Ltd.)

Figure 31.13 A representative area is chosen, usually at the edge of the lesion, to include healthy skin.

Figure 31.14 The biopsy punch should be held perpendicular to the skin.

Figure 31.15 Hole left after taking biopsy; closure usually with one or two sutures. (Photograph by courtesy of Stiefel Laboratories (UK) Ltd.)

of the lesion is anaesthetized by infiltration with local anaesthetic, an area chosen to biopsy and the instrument pressed firmly against the skin. The tissue is cut using a rotating action until the instrument is felt to have gone through the full thickness of skin. It is then withdrawn and the core of tissue picked up with fine forceps and the base snipped off with iris scissors or a small scalpel. Closure is with one

Figure 31.16 Using a biopsy punch to remove a small lesion on the face.

Figure 31.17 Closure with just one 6/0 Prolene suture.

or two fine sutures. By applying traction with finger and thumb to the skin at right-angles to the natural skin creases before inserting the biopsy punch, an oval core of tissue is removed rather than a circular one, thus resulting in a neater scar.

31.3 INCISIONAL BIOPSY, INCLUDING CURETTAGE (FIGS 31.18–31.23)

This is the traditional method of taking a biopsy of most skin lesions and consists of removing an ellipse of skin containing both the lesion and healthy skin. In most cases the wound will need to be sutured

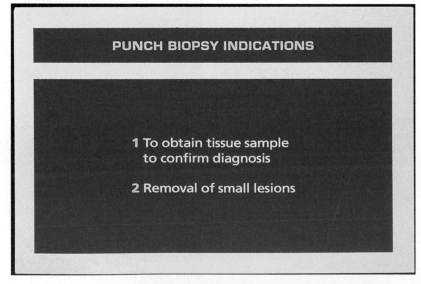

PUNCH BIOPSY INDICATIONS

1 To obtain tissue sample to confirm diagnosis

2 Removal of small lesions

Figure 31.18 Benefits of curettage. (Photograph by courtesy of Stiefel Laboratories (UK) Ltd.)

Figure 31.19 Selection of disposable ring curettes. (Photograph by courtesy of Stiefel Laboratories (UK) Ltd.)

Figure 31.20 Blanching of surrounding skin after the injection of local anaesthetic. (Photograph by courtesy of Stiefel Laboratories (UK) Ltd.)

Figure 31.21 Using a ring curette to obtain a biopsy specimen. (Photograph by courtesy of Stiefel Laboratories (UK) Ltd.)

Figure 31.22 The base is treated with the unipolar diathermy. (Photograph by courtesy of Stiefel Laboratories (UK) Ltd.)

Figure 31.23 A ring-curette attachment for the Ellman radiosurgery unit; this enables biopsies to be taken and blood vessels coagulated with the same instrument.

using fine interrupted Prolene sutures (see Fig. 25.37c). As with any elliptical incision, it is worth ascertaining the Langer's lines or skin creases so that the final scar lies along a crease. If there is a possibility of a malignant melanoma, the specimen should be marked 'urgent' so that a full histological diagnosis is available within 10 days and a wider excision can be offered, or the patient referred to a specialist centre.

31.4 EXCISIONAL BIOPSY

If the suspected lesion is sufficiently small and in a suitable part of the body, it may be possible to remove it entirely at the time of performing the biopsy, thus avoiding the need for a second operation subsequently. The technique is exactly as described for the excision of any skin lesion (Figs 31.24 and 31.25).

Figure 31.24 Excisional biopsy; lines marked out on the skin.

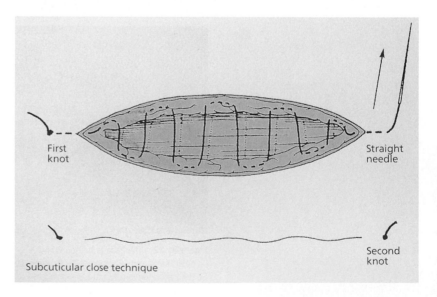

Figure 31.25 Closure may be with subcutaneous Vicryl and intradermal Vicryl or Prolene.

31.5 NEEDLE BIOPSY

Subcutaneous lumps may be diagnosed by fine-needle aspiration rather than total excision. This may give a rapid diagnosis and help to formulate a plan of action for treatment, e.g. lymph nodes or breast lumps. Because the volume of tissue obtained is so small, it is essential to treat it very gently, ensure that it is placed in fixative immediately and, where possible, ensure that the sample is taken from a representative area.

Usually no local anaesthetic is required. A 21 swg needle is attached to a 5 ml syringe. The needle is then inserted into the centre of the lump, moved backwards and forwards a few times, and traction applied to the syringe plunger, creating a vacuum and aspirating cells into the needle and syringe. The syringe and needle are then withdrawn, and the contents 'blown' on to a microscope slide and immediately covered with fixative, exactly as when preparing a cervical smear. The slide is labelled, and the histology form completed with as much information as possible and sent for examination.

31.6 CYTOLOGICAL EXAMINATION OF FLUIDS

Cysts in the breast and thyroid may be aspirated and the contents sent for cytological examination. Similarly, ascitic fluid may be sent for cytological examination and may establish a diagnosis if there is underlying malignancy. Lung cancer may also be diagnosed by cytological examination of the sputum.

CHAPTER 32

Epistaxis

Most nose-bleeds, particularly in children, are self-limiting. Recurrent epistaxes often arise from a small collection of blood vessels in Little's area, just inside the nose on either side of the nasal septum. These can be successfully sealed by a variety of treatments, including the following.

32.1 SILVER NITRATE CAUTERIZATION

This is probably the simplest method. With the patient facing the doctor, and under good illumination, Little's area is inspected on either side. Silver nitrate is now applied, using either a disposable silver nitrate wooden applicator or a pointed silver nitrate pencil stick held in an applicator (Figs 32.1–32.3).

The treated area immediately turns white and some reflex watering of the patient's eyes always occurs. The patient is requested not to blow his or her nose for several hours, and normally only one treatment is necessary. No anaesthetic is required.

Figure 32.1 The majority of nose-bleeds occurs from Little's area just inside the nostril, as shown.

Figure 32.2 Single-use silver nitrate applicators are ideal for cauterizing Little's area.

Figure 32.3 Cauterizing Little's area with silver nitrate.

32.2 ELECTROCAUTERIZATION OF LITTLE'S AREA

More stubborn recurrent epistaxes may be treated with the electro-cautery, but the nose must be anaesthetized. This is achieved by spraying the inside of the nose with Xylocaine pressurized spray (lignocaine metered-dose aerosol 100 µg per dose) or by the application of pledgers of cotton wool soaked in 4% lignocaine or similar topical anaesthetic.

With good illumination, the offending blood vessels are cauterized with the electrocautery. Only dull-red heat is used, and sparingly. Overenthusiastic electrocauterization can lead to perforation of the nasal septum, and only one side should be cauterized at a time.

32.3 DIATHERMY OF LITTLE'S AREA

This may be achieved using the unipolar diathermy or Hyfrecator. As with electrocautery, the preliminary application of local anaesthesia is necessary. The area to be treated may be fulgurized by holding the needle electrode a very short distance away from the tissues and allowing a stream of sparks to play over the area. The current is turned down to minimum to avoid damage to the nasal septum.

32.4 CRYOSURGERY TO LITTLE'S AREA

Effective control may be achieved by freezing; the use of local anaesthesia is desirable but not always necessary. It is important to check that the probe will just cover the area to be frozen without accidentally touching any other part of the nose, otherwise this may become adherent to the probe and result in an additional 'frost-burn'.

32.5 PHOTOCOAGULATION OF LITTLE'S AREA

An infrared photocoagulator with narrow applicator may be used to control recurrent epistaxes. The topical application of local anaesthetic is necessary but the technique is simple and gives good results.

32.6 RADIOSURGICAL COAGULATION

This is a very precise method of coagulationg blood vessels inside the nose. The radiosurgical unit is set to 'coagulation' and a low initial setting, e.g. 2–4. The ball-ended applicator is held over the blood vessel and the current applied. No pressure is needed; in fact, better results are obtained if the electrode is *just* not touching the vessel. The treated area blanches quickly. As with electrocautery, care needs to be taken not to perforate the nasal septum.

32.7 THE ACUTE BLEED

None of the aforementioned treatments is applicable during an acute nosebleed, which must be controlled by either digital pressure or packing the nose with ribbon gauze soaked in 1:1000 adrenaline (plus 4% lignocaine if necessary). Should either of these fail, and particularly if the patient is elderly, in which case the source of bleeding is unlikely to be from Little's area, they should be referred to a hospital.

CHAPTER 33

Use of the proctoscope

The discharge of blood from the rectum is a disease chiefly confined to those advanced in life. It is occasioned by full living, abuse of purgatives, violent passions or habitual melancholy. To this effect, leeches and warm fomentations applied to the anus are the most efficacious remedies.

Encyclopaedia Britannica, 1817

Examination of the anal canal in all patients with rectal symptoms is mandatory, but patients are still seen with inoperable cancers who missed having an early rectal examination.

Rectal bleeding is an extremely common symptom. Fortunately, in the majority it arises from haemorrhoids which can be visualized easily with a proctoscope. Instruments may be disposable or non-disposable, each having its own advantages and disadvantages.

33.1 DISPOSABLE PROCTOSCOPES

These consist of a plastic tube with central obturator; they may be presterilized in individual packs, and if sterilizing facilities are available (Chapter 6) they can be used on more than one occasion. External illumination is necessary for the majority of instruments, although some have provision for internal illumination.

33.2 NON-DISPOSABLE PROCTOSCOPES

These are generally made of stainless steel and consist of an outer tube and handle, together with a central obturator. Illumination can be from an external source, from in-built illumination in the form of a tungsten filament or quartz bulbs, or from an external fibre-optic light source (Fig. 33.1). They can be sterilized by autoclaving, dry-heat oven or immersion (Chapter 6).

33.2.1 Technique

If the patient is lying in the left lateral position, with the knees drawn up, the direction of the anal canal is upwards and forwards. A digital rectal examination is performed and any abnormality in the rectum noted. The muscle tone of the anal sphincter is noted, as is the degree

Figure 33.1 The Naunton Morgan rectal speculum with fibre-light attachment.

Figure 33.2 Anatomy of the anus and rectum (redrawn from G.J. Hill, *Outpatient Surgery*, by permission of W.B. Saunders & Co.).

of discomfort caused by the examination. This may give a clue to the diagnosis of anal fissure, typified by pain and spasm. The examining finger is withdrawn and the glove examined for any signs of blood. Next, the proctoscope is lubricated and very gently inserted into the anal canal; as soon as the instrument is felt to have passed through the sphincter, its direction is changed slightly posteriorly to take account of the direction of the rectum. The instrument is inserted fully to the flange, the obturator withdrawn and the illumination switched on. The normal mucous membrane is pale, but capillaries and tributaries of the superior haemorrhoidal vein are visible. Any pathology is noted and the proctoscope slowly withdrawn, during which the mucous membrane begins to close in. Prolapsing internal haemorrhoids become easily visible at this stage and their positions may be noted for future reference. As the proctoscope is further withdrawn, lesions of the anal canal may be seen, such as proctitis or fissure (Fig. 33.2).

Where the patient gives a history of bleeding on defecation, it is worth reintroducing the proctoscope and asking the patient to strain down as the instrument is slowly withdrawn. In this way, a bleeding haemorrhoid or fissure can be identified. If suspected haemorrhoids are revealed on proctoscopy, it is often convenient to treat them at the time of the initial examination (Chapter 36).

Sigmoidoscopy

34

Signs, forsooth, of ulceration are these: the patient cannot abstain from going to the privy because of aching, and he passes a stinking discharge mixed with watery blood. Ignorant leeches will assure the patient that he has dysentery, when truly it is not. I never saw, nor heard of any man that was cured of cancer of the rectum, but I have known many that died of the aforesaid sickness.

John of Arderne, 1306–1390

Sigmoidoscopy is considerably easier to perform than is generally realized [33, 34]. It is not a difficult technique to learn, and with regular use the practitioner will quickly learn to recognize both the normal and abnormal appearances. The sigmoidoscope can be one of the most valuable instruments in general practice; combined with a pair of biopsy forceps, rapid diagnosis of carcinoma of the rectum, ulcerative colitis, rectal polyp, proctitis and haemorrhoids can be made.

The first sigmoidoscope was invented by Bodenhamer in 1863 and consisted of a flexible tube of reflecting mirrors; unfortunately, it was found to be impractical and it was not until 1895 that Kelly described a sigmoidoscope very similar to those found today. His instrument had the light bulb placed distally, which had the disadvantage of soiling by faeces and bulb failure. In 1912 Yeomans designed an instrument with proximal illumination and air insufflation, and apart from slight modifications today's instruments are very similar.

Improvements in illumination using fibre-optic light sources and cables have enabled better visualization to be obtained, and most recently, flexible fibre-optic sigmoidoscopes have been introduced which will examine more of the rectum and sigmoid colon than the conventional rigid instrument.

34.1 INDICATIONS FOR USE

Sigmoidoscopy forms an integral part of the routine investigation of all patients presenting with rectal bleeding, change in bowel habit and prolonged diarrhoea, and in the follow-up of patients who have had rectal surgery.

The standard adult stainless-steel Lloyd-Davies sigmoidoscope with proximal illumination gives good visualization, and is easy to use, well constructed and virtually indestructible (Fig. 34.1). A smaller diameter instrument is also available, but for the majority of examinations the adult size will be found to be more than adequate. Tungsten filament or quartz halogen bulbs give good illumination, but if a fibre-optic light source can be obtained this is even better and more reliable.

Figure 34.1   The Lloyd-Davies stainless steel adult sigmoidoscope fitted with proximal fibre-light chamber.

Reasonably priced disposable sigmoidoscopes are also available; these have the advantage of not requiring repeated sterilization or cleaning, but will work out more expensive in the long run compared with the stainless-steel models.

A telescope attachment with magnification is a valuable accessory, giving much improved views of the mucosa. Having assembled all of the necessary instruments for sigmoidoscopy it is better to keep them all on a separate 'rectal trolley' ready for immediate use; this may then be taken from one consulting room to another at a moment's notice (Figs 34.2 and 34.3). Biopsy forceps, although expensive, are invaluable and enable the doctor to take an immediate biopsy of any suspicious lesions. In order to take a biopsy, the window or telescope attachment at the operator's end of the sigmoidoscope needs to be removed in order to introduce the forceps, and this occasionally causes slight problems with loss of insufflated air, prolapse of mucosa or poor visibility. Paterson's biopsy forceps (Figs 34.4 and 34.5), Chevalier Jackson's biopsy forceps (Fig. 34.5) and Yeoman's rectal biopsy forceps are all suitable for the taking of biopsies. Other instruments which may be kept on a 'rectal trolley' include a proctoscope, haemorrhoid injection syringe and needles, ampoules of 5% oily phenol, specimen containers with 10% formol-saline for histology, K-Y jelly, swabs, haemorrhoid ligator, grasping forceps and neoprene bands, plus swab holder and swabs.

Figure 34.2   It is a good idea to keep all instruments and accessories for sigmoidoscopy on one trolley for immediate use.

Figure 34.3   Instruments ready for sigmoidoscopy.

Figure 34.4 Paterson biopsy forceps.

Figure 34.5 Chevalier Jackson biopsy forceps.

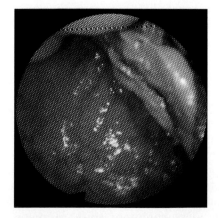

Figure 34.6 View through a sigmoidoscope on entering the rectum. A small quantity of faeces is seen, which is negotiable.

34.2 PREPARATION OF THE PATIENT

Normally no preliminary bowel preparation is necessary or desirable, as the instrument can usually be manoeuvred past any faeces (Fig. 34.6). Enemas or bowel washouts, as well as inflaming the mucosa, will wash away tell-tale bloodstreaks or secretions. If the bowel is completely occluded with faeces, it is better to abandon the examination and attempt it on another occasion after defecation.

34.3 TECHNIQUE OF SIGMOIDOSCOPY

The actual sigmoidoscopic examination only takes a few minutes; thus, if the instruments are always ready assembled for immediate use, it may be included in the initial consultation. The left lateral position is both comfortable and adequate for most sigmoidoscopies. The patient should be positioned with the buttocks at the edge of the couch, and knees and feet at the opposite edge, curled up.

A careful explanation of what will be done should always be given to the patient. In particular, they may feel embarrassed in case they lose faeces or blood and soil the examination couch; reassurance that the patient and doctor are protected by a glass window will allay much anxiety. The sigmoidoscope is assembled, the light checked and the distal end lubricated with water-soluble K-Y jelly. Specimen containers and biopsy forceps are placed in an accessible position for the operator and a digital rectal examination is performed. This will reveal any low-lying masses, as well as lubricating the anal canal. The doctor holds the sigmoidoscope with the palm of the hand covering the obturator to prevent it being extruded, and the instrument is gently inserted into the anal canal, in the direction of the umbilicus. It helps at this stage to ask the patient to breathe quietly in and out of his or her mouth. As soon as the sigmoidoscope has entered the rectum, the obturator is removed, and the inspection window or telescope attached, together with the bellows; a little air is introduced and from now on the instrument is advanced under direct vision. The lower valve of Houston is seen on the left, then the middle valve on the right. The apex of the rectum often appears to be a blind end, but by gently withdrawing the sigmoidoscope and pointing it towards the left and slightly forwards, the entrance to the sigmoid can be seen. This is usually the most difficult part of the examination, but with gentleness and patience, it can usually be negotiated. The instrument may now be passed to 20–25 cm, provided the patient does not complain of pain. Any lesions or blood-stained discharges are noted and the sigmoidoscope is gradually withdrawn.

A better examination of the rectum is obtained as the instrument is being withdrawn than when it is being introduced. Any suspicious lesions can be biopsied and their exact distance from the anus measured on the scale printed on the side of the sigmoidoscope.

If blood or a blood-stained discharge is seen coming from further inside the bowel, a colonoscopy and/or barium enema should be arranged. Similarly, if any infective lesion is suspected, rectal swabs can be taken for culture.

During the examination, air should be gently blown in with the bellows to keep the bowel lumen opened out. Forcible air distension should be avoided as it may cause pain and spasm.

An analysis of sigmoidoscopies performed in one general practice showed that the presenting symptom of bleeding occurred in 49%, of which 14% were found to have rectal cancer; 70% of these could not be felt on digital examination but could all be seen with the sigmoidoscope. Thus, although the most common cause of rectal bleeding is still haemorrhoids, nevertheless one in seven (14%) was found to have a carcinoma [35].

CHAPTER 35

Thrombosed external haemorrhoids

> But wit thou, ... that an abscess breeding near the anus should not be left to burst by itself ... be it boldly opened with a very sharp lancette so that ... the corrupt blood may go out.
>
> *John of Arderne, 1306–1390*

More correctly described as perianal haematoma, the 'thrombosed external haemorrhoid' is a common condition, occurring spontaneously in young adults, sometimes associated with straining at defecation, but often not. They are painful and can vary in size from a small pea to a large walnut; left untreated, they gradually absorb, leaving a small skin tag (Fig. 35.1). Surgical treatment offers a quick and effective cure, takes only a few minutes and gives immediate relief of symptoms.

The following instruments are required:

- 2 ml syringe
- 25 swg × 5/8 in. (0.5 × 16 mm) needle
- 1% lignocaine with adrenaline 1:200 000
- pair toothed dissecting forceps 5 in. (12.7 cm)
- pair iris scissors, straight 4½ in. (11.4 cm).

With the patient lying on his or her left side and the knees drawn up, the base of the haematoma is infiltrated with local anaesthetic. If

Figure 35.1 Typical thrombosed external haemorrhoid.

Figure 35.2 Immediately after incising a thrombosed external haemorrhoid.

an assistant is available, he or she should be asked to pull the upper buttock upwards to expose the thrombosed haemorrhoid; if an assistant is not available, the patient may do this. An ellipse of skin is cut out using the iris scissors and dissecting forceps; this immediately reveals the typical black blood-clot inside the haemorrhoid, which may either be expressed by pressure or lifted out with the forceps. The wound is checked to make sure that there is only one haematoma; occasionally, two or three loculated clots are found and each should be removed. In general, there is only a little bleeding (Fig. 35.2), which can be controlled by the application of a sterile gamgee dressing. The patient is advised to have twice-daily salt baths until healing is complete.

A small perianal haematoma may conveniently be left to absorb spontaneously, but if surgery is contemplated, just a radial incision and expression of the clot may suffice.

Treatment of internal haemorrhoids

When there are chronic haemorrhoids in the anus, sear the patient with three cauterisations over the lower dorsal vertebra.

Albucasis, eleventh century

It is a wise rule to suspect all haemorrhoids as being due to carcinoma of the rectum until proved otherwise. For this reason, it is essential to examine every patient complaining of rectal bleeding with the proctoscope, and if possible the sigmoidoscope as well.

Three types of internal haemorrhoid can be recognized.

36.1 TYPES OF HAEMORRHOID

36.1.1 First-degree haemorroids

The haemorrhoids are small, bleed freely, especially after defecation and, although not palpable with the examining finger, are visible when examined through the proctoscope. This type is eminently suitable for treatment in general practice by injection, photocoagulation or cryotherapy.

36.1.2 Second-degree haemorroids

These haemorrhoids are larger and tend to protrude after defecation, but will generally reduce themselves. Bleeding may be less marked because fibrosis is developing in the pile. Treatment by injection, photocoagulation and cryotherapy is still possible, as is neoprene band ligation, but the results are not consistently as good as first-degree haemorrhoids.

36.1.3 Third-degree or prolapsing haemorrhoids

In this type, prolapse is severe, requiring digital replacement by the patient or doctor, and strangulation is a common complication. Such haemorrhoids are not generally suitable for general practitioner treatment and should be referred to a general surgeon. Most uncomplicated haemorrhoids are painless; the presence of pain indicates inflammation, strangulation, thrombosis or anal fissure.

36.2 TREATMENT OF INTERNAL HAEMORRHOIDS BY INJECTION OF SCLEROSING FLUID

This is still the method favoured by the majority of surgeons in the UK. The solutions used and the technique employed have changed little over the last 100 years and still give excellent results [36, 37].

The following instruments are required:

- proctoscope with illumination
- sigmoidoscope with illumination
- haemorrhoid injection syringe and needle
- 5 ml ampoules of 5% oily phenol BPC.

With the patient lying in the left lateral position a digital rectal examination is performed to exclude any low-lying tumours, followed by a sigmoidoscopy. If there is any suspicion of blood coming from higher in the large bowel, from either the history or examination, colonoscopy and/or barium enema examination should be arranged.

A well-lubricated proctoscope is now inserted to its full length and the obturator removed. On gently withdrawing the instrument, any haemorrhoids will become easily visible; these are commonly situated at the 3 o'clock, 7 o'clock and 11 o'clock positions, corresponding to the termination of the branches of the superior haemorrhoidal artery.

It may be necessary at this stage to reinsert the proctoscope gently so that the base of each haemorrhoid can be seen. A submucosal injection of 5% phenol in almond oil is now given. This must be done at the upper end of the haemorrhoid and above the anorectal ring. Injections given below the anorectal ring are extremely painful. The bevel of the needle should be directed towards the mucosa rather than the lumen of the rectum and the phenol injected slowly, until blanching is seen. The amount injected varies from 1 to 5 ml, or occasionally even more if the mucosa is very lax (Fig. 36.1).

All three primary haemorrhoids may be treated simultaneously, or if one is larger (commonly the right anterior) this may be given two injections, followed by subsequent treatments at a later visit.

The patient is given advice about avoiding constipation, put on a high-roughage diet and allowed home. Follow-up examinations and injections can be at the discretion and preference of the doctor: weekly if other injections are anticipated or after 6 weeks if routine follow-up is desired.

36.3 CRYOSURGICAL TREATMENT OF INTERNAL HAEMORRHOIDS

Where a cryoprobe is available, satisfactory treatment of first- and second-degree haemorrhoids can be obtained, and if the patient is judged to be unfit for haemorrhoidectomy, even third-degree haemorrhoids can be treated [38]. The cryoprobe is applied to the haemorrhoid and a 2 min freeze given.

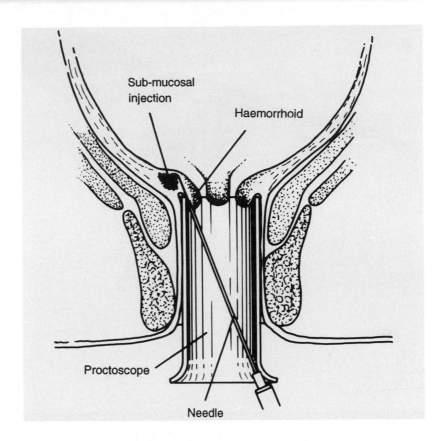

Figure 36.1 Submucosal injection of a haemorrhoid using 5% oily phenol.

The nitrous oxide cryoprobe has the added advantage that it adheres to the tissue, so that gentle traction may be applied to prevent freezing of deeper tissues. The probe must then be rewarmed before it can be separated from the pile. Treatment is well tolerated, although some patients experience a dull ache during and immediately after freezing. The patient should be warned to expect a profuse watery, blood-stained discharge for many weeks following treatment.

36.4 INFRARED PHOTOCOAGULATION OF INTERNAL HAEMORRHOIDS

A relatively new and simple instrument for the treatment of internal haemorrhoids is the infrared photocoagulator. This consists of a low-voltage quartz-halogen bulb with gold-plated reflector and a solid quartz rod which transmits infrared radiation to a Teflon-coated tip (Figs 36.2–36.4). A 1.5 s pulse of infrared radiation produces an accurately defined necrosis 3 mm deep and 3 mm in diameter. The probe may be used through the proctoscope in the same way as injection therapy and is applied at exactly the same sites, i.e. above the base of each haemorrhoid. Three separate areas of coagulation are required at the base of each haemorrhoid for optimum results. Of all treatments currently available for internal haemorrhoids, photocoagulation is one of the simplest, safest and quickest, and can be rapidly learned by any doctor [39].

Figure 36.2 (a) The infrared coagulator; simple to use. Three burns are required at the base of each haemorrhoid (Chilworth Medicals Ltd). (b) The infrared coagulator on base with timer and transformer. (c) Selection of quartz glass light guides: 2, 6 and 10 mm.

Figure 36.3 How the photocoagulator works (Chilworth Medicals Ltd).

Figure 36.4 Placement of photocoagulator within the proctoscope (Chilworth Medicals Ltd).

36.5 NEOPRENE BAND LIGATION OF INTERNAL HAEMORRHOIDS

Rubber-band ligation has been used successfully for the treatment of haemorrhoids, but the technique requires more skill and practice than injection or photocoagulation [40–42]. It is suitable only for haemorrhoids with bases more than 2 cm above the anorectal ring; if bands are applied below this level, severe pain is caused and the removal of any constricting band is extremely difficult. An assistant is required to hold the proctoscope; the haemorrhoids are visualized and the rubber-band ligator, loaded with one band is passed through the proctoscope.

Using a pair of haemorrhoid-grasping forceps, the doctor pulls the mucosa above the base of the haemorrhoid through the ring of the applicator, and the band is slipped over the base by pressing the handle on the instrument (Figs 36.5–36.7). Secondary haemorrhage occurs in 1% of patients and can be severe.

Figure 36.5 The McGivney neoprene band ligator with St George's haemorrhoid-grasping forceps.

Figure 36.6 Close-up of band applicator and neoprene bands.

36.6 MANUAL DILATATION OF THE ANUS

This treatment for haemorrhoids was known in ancient Greece, practised in the Middle Ages and recently revived by Peter Lord [43]. It is normally done under a general anaesthetic, but can be performed under local infiltration or caudal anaesthesia. Young patients with much anal spasm and haemorrhoids associated with anal fissure seem to achieve most relief from this procedure. The elderly and those with a lax anal canal are contraindicated, as they fare particularly badly, with a risk of permanent incontinence of faeces.

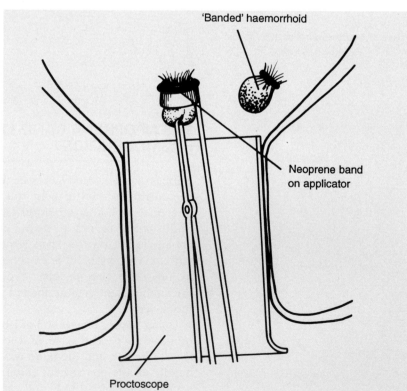

Figure 36.7 Diagrammatic view of the McGivney neoprane band ligator and siting of banding (Redrawn from G.J. Hill, *Outpatient Surgery*, by permission of W.B. Saunders & Co.).

CHAPTER 37

Varicose veins

> Marius, Roman Consul, having both his legs full of great tumours, and disliking the deformity, determined to put himself in the hands of an operator. When, after enduring a most excessive torment in the cutting, never flinching or complaining, the surgeon went to the other, he declined to have it done saying 'I see the cure is not worth the pain'.
>
> *Plutarch's Lives, 186–55 BC*

Varicose veins are one of the most common problems encountered in general practice and it has been estimated that one person in five in the population either has, or will develop varicose veins of the legs. Women are affected more than men, and the most frequent reasons for seeking advice and treatment are discomfort, fear of ulceration and appearance.

As far as minor surgery is concerned, there are three successful treatments: sclerotherapy, stab avulsions and multiple ligations. However, not all varicose veins are suitable for treatment; indeed, in some, treatment might even be contraindicated or give very poor results.

37.1 ANATOMY

There are two sets of veins in the leg, deep and superficial. They are separated from each other by the fascia and connected to each other by perforating veins. The perforating veins have valves which allow blood to pass from the superficial veins to the deep veins, but not the reverse.

The long saphenous vein is the longest vein in the body: it starts at the medial dorsal end of the venous arch on the dorsum of the foot, lying 2 cm in front of the medial malleolus, and passing up the leg to join the femoral vein about 3 cm below the inguinal ligament.

The short saphenous vein starts behind the lateral malleolus as an extension of the dorsal venous arch and passes up the back of the calf in the midline, to join the popliteal veins (Fig. 37.1). Valves are frequent throughout the course of the superficial veins, most notably at the junction of the long saphenous and femoral vein, and it is incompetence of these valves which results in varicosities.

By the action of the calf muscles, blood is actively pumped from the feet to the abdomen; and during exercise, pressures up to 250 mmHg have been recorded in these veins. If valvular breakdown occurs in the

Figure 37.1 Type I varicose veins with competent valves.

perforating veins, blood at this pressure is forced outwards into the superficial veins, causing varicosities and eventual ulceration secondary to capillary stasis.

Varicose veins may conveniently be classified into three categories.

37.1.1 Type I varicose veins (Fig. 37.1)

These veins are dilated, but have competent valves. There is no oedema, but the patient may be troubled with attacks of superficial thrombophlebitis. They are common in men.

Figure 37.2 Type II varicose veins; dilated veins, valves in the superficial veins are incompetent, but valves in the deep and perforating veins are intact. These are ideal for injections.

Figure 37.3 Type III varicose veins. The deep vein is occluded, usually from a previous deep vein thrombosis; all the valves are destroyed; there is considerable oedema and a high incidence of ulceration, and injections or ligations are contraindicated.

37.1.2 Type II varicose veins (Fig. 37.2)

These veins are dilated. The valves in the superficial veins are incompetent, but the valves in the deep and perforating veins are still intact. These veins are therefore ideal for treatment.

37.1.3 Type III varicose veins (Fig. 37.3)

In type III varicose veins, the deep vein is occluded, usually from a previous deep-vein thrombosis. All of the valves are destroyed, and there is considerable oedema, distension of the superficial veins and a high incidence of venous ulceration. As the limb is now relying on the superficial veins to maintain a venous circulation, treatment by ligation or sclerotherapy is contraindicated and will make the situation worse. In many instances, the patient only seeks help when varicose ulceration has occurred; this is still not too late to commence treatment of the veins, as by reducing the superficial venous pressure, healing of the ulcer will be facilitated.

37.2 SELECTION OF PATIENTS

A simple selective procedure will improve results and avoid unnecessary treatment for unsuitable cases.

1. A careful history should be obtained to exclude any serious systemic disease.
2. A past history of deep-vein thrombosis in the affected leg is an absolute contraindication to sclerotherapy.
3. Veins which are confined to below the knee are most suitable for sclerotherapy. Those above the knee are difficult to bandage effectively and are better ligated.

Figure 37.4 Varicose veins affecting the short saphenous vein below the knee; ideal for sclerotherapy.

4. Current medication is noted; patients taking the combined contraceptive pill or oestrogens for any other reasons should be asked to stop medication for 1 month before treatment if this is practicable.
5. If ulceration is present, the arterial system should be checked and the urine tested for sugar.
6. A test of saphenofemoral incompetence is made as follows. The patient lies down and the leg is raised to 30° to empty the superficial veins. A narrow tube is applied as a tourniquet around the upper thigh, the leg is lowered and the patient asked to stand up. If just the saphenofemoral valve is incompetent, the superficial veins will fill slowly over 30 s from below upwards. If the perforating veins at a lower level are leaking, the superficial veins will fill rapidly, in which case other tourniquets may be applied progressively at lower levels until the site of leakage is identified. A second simple test is to apply a tourniquet around the leg at the level of the tibial tubercle and ask the patient to walk around for 1 min. If the perforating vein valves are competent, the superficial veins empty.
7. As the recommended treatment involves daily periods of walking by the patient, it is not advisable to offer injections if for any reason the patient cannot walk at least 3 miles each day.
8. Patients with obese legs should be advised to lose weight before being offered a course of injections.
9. Any known allergic reaction to sodium tetradecyl sulphate (STD) is a contraindication to sclerotherapy.

37.3 SCLEROTHERAPY

The object of sclerotherapy is to obliterate the lumen of the vein by injecting an irritant solution directly inside it and compressing the inflamed surfaces together. Current interest in the technique was revived by Professor Fegan in Dublin [44–46] and, provided suitable patients are selected carefully, i.e. type I or II veins below the knee, the results of treatment are very good.

The following instruments are required (Fig. 37.5):

- 6×1 ml sterile syringes
- 6×25 swg $\times 5/8$ in. (0.5×16 mm) needles
- vial 5 ml of 3% STD solution (Fibrovein) or ampoules of ethanolamine oleate
- elastic web bandage 3 in. (7.6 cm) $\times$ 5 m
- tubular elastic stockinette (Tubigrip)
    size E 8.75 cm $\times$ 1 m or
    size F 10 cm $\times$ 1 m
- Sorbo rubber pads or large cotton dental rolls
- adhesive tape (Micropore) 1 in. (2.5 cm).

Good illumination is essential. The number of injections likely to be given is noted, and the same number of syringes filled with 3% STD or ethanolamine oleate solution; usually 0.7 ml per syringe is sufficient. One strip of adhesive tape, 1×4 in. (2.5 $\times$ 10 cm) per syringe is stuck to the top of the instrument trolley in readiness, and a second strip,

Figure 37.5   Syringes with 3% STD adhesive tapes and cotton-wool rolls in readiness for sclerotherapy.

1 × 4 in., with a large cotton dental roll, per syringe, also attached to the shelf.

With the patient standing on a low stool the veins to be injected are identified using a felt-tip marker (Fig. 37.6). Still with the patient standing and the doctor kneeling, the needle of the preloaded syringe is inserted in the vein and the plunger very slightly withdrawn (Fig. 37.7). Dark blood enters the syringe, confirming that the needle is in the correct place.

Without moving the syringe or needle at all, the doctor carefully tapes them in position using the first strip of adhesive (Micropore) tape. The second injection is performed in exactly the same way, taping the syringe in place as before. Several injections may be given at one session (Fig. 37.8), but the total volume of sclerosant should not exceed 4 ml.

Figure 37.6   The veins to be injected are first marked with a felt-tip pen, with the patient standing.

Figure 37.7   With the patient standing, the first syringe is taped in position with the needle inside the vein.

Figure 37.8   Other syringes are now taped in position after placing the needle inside the vein.

With all syringes taped in position, the operator carefully helps the patient to lie down on the couch or operating table and elevates the leg to about 30° above the horizontal. With an assistant holding the leg, the doctor now applies a finger and thumb over the segment of vein to be injected, thus isolating this short strip of vein. Using the other hand the contents of the syringe are injected into this segment and a compression pad is applied before the needle is removed (Figs 37.9, 37.10). It is important to keep the sclerosant in the empty and isolated segment for at least 30 s. If possible, an assistant maintains pressure over the injected site while the operator proceeds to inject the remaining sites.

When all sites have been injected, an elastic web bandage is applied from the toes to the knee and this is then covered with an elasticated tubular bandage (Tubigrip E or F) doubled back on itself to produce two layers of compression (Figs 37.11 and 37.12). The patient is given an instruction sheet and advised to walk at least 3 miles every day for the next 3 weeks, after which the bandages and pads are removed. It is wise to warn the patient that they may experience severe pain in the leg during the first 48 h, but that this will subside. They may reapply the bandages themselves if they are too tight, but should not disturb the compression pads.

37.3.1 Complications of sclerotherapy

Pain is a common accompaniment of injection treatment and this generally settles in a few days. Occasionally, extravasation of the STD solution results in severe pain, followed by an area of necrosis that may

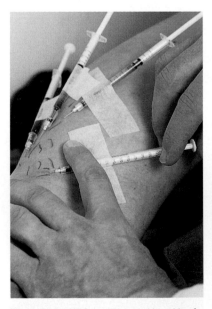

Figure 37.9 With pressure on either side of the injection site, 0.5 ml of 3% STD or ethanolamine oleate is injected into the isolated segment of the vein (gloves should be worn).

Figure 37.10 Cotton-wool rolls or sorbo-rubber pads are placed over each injection site.

Figure 37.11 An elastic web bandage (30) is applied from the toes to the knee.

Figure 37.12 An elasticated tubular bandage (Tubigrip) is applied over the bandage, folding back to give two layers.

slough and produce an ulcer. A dry dressing is all that is required, and healing may take very many months, leaving a permanent depressed scar and a depressed patient. Under these circumstances it may be prudent to excise the ulcer and close the wound by primary suture.

Accidental intra-arterial injection would result in immediate, severe, burning pain over the distal distribution. Should this occur, the needle should be left in the artery and heparin and lignocaine slowly injected; this is the most potentially serious complication in a technique which is otherwise remarkably free of complications.

37.4 STAB AVULSION FOR VARICOSE VEINS (FOR FULL DETAILS SEE CHAPTER 47)

As an alternative to sclerotherapy, or as an adjunct therapy, stab avulsion offers a good treatment for many superficial varicosities.

37.4.1 Technique

Stab incisions of not more than 3 mm are made over the sites of previously marked varicosities. The underlying vein may then be picked up with a single skin-hook, and by grasping with mosquito forceps, as much of the vein gradually teased out and then avulsed. Closure is with skin closure strips, covered with a compression bandage for 3 days followed by graduated compression stockings (class II) for the next 3 weeks (Fig. 37.13).

Figure 37.13 Stab avulsion for varicose veins.

CHAPTER 38

Minor surgical procedures in gynaecology

> If thou examinest a woman suffering in her abdomen so that the menstrual discharge cannot come away from her ... apply Frankincense and incense between her two loins and cause the smoke thereof to enter her flesh.
>
> *Edwin Smith, Surgical Papyrus, 3000–2500 BC*

As well as the usual intradermal lesions that can affect the skin over the perineum and vulva, several lesions of the cervix, vagina and labia can be effectively treated with the minimum of instruments and equipment. The chapter also includes cervical cytology and the insertion of intrauterine contraceptive devices (IUCDs), together with repair of episiotomy following delivery.

38.1 CERVICAL CYTOLOGY

During the last decade most general practitioners (GPs) have learned to take routine cervical smears for cytology. The procedure is quite straightforward. Using a vaginal speculum (preferably not lubricated with jelly) the cervix is visualized. Good illumination is essential, whether external spotlight, integral fibreoptic illumination or tungsten-filament bulbs. The cervix is first inspected, and any unusual features such as excessive discharge, bleeding, erosions or polypi are noted. The purpose-designed wooden cervical spatula is placed at the entrance to the external cervical os and rotated through 360°, thus obtaining cells from the whole area. These are then transferred to a microscope slide by wiping the spatula on the glass in one direction only, followed by immediate fixation with suitable preservative. The slide is then labelled with the patient's name and the appropriate request form completed. Bacterial and viral swabs may also be taken at the same time if necessary (Fig. 38.1).

Figure 38.1 All that is needed to take a cervical smear.

38.2 ENDOMETRIAL CELL SAMPLERS

Using these samplers, the secretions inside the uterine cavity can be aspirated by gentle suction and sent for cytological examination. This will often obviate the need for a transvaginal colour Doppler ultrasound examination, hysteroscopy or dilatation and curettage (D & C).

Figure 38.2 Cervical smear spatula and cytobrush.

38.3 BRUSH CYTOLOGY

As a means of obtaining endometrial cells for cytological examination, small brushes similar to a 'bottle brush' are available. By visualizing the cervical os, the brush is gently inserted as far as possible without causing pain, rotated once and withdrawn. The microscope slide is then prepared in the same way as when using a spatula (Fig. 38.2).

38.4 CAUTERIZATION OF CERVICAL EROSIONS

The popularity of cauterizing every cervical 'erosion' has waned in recent years with the realization that many so-called erosions were not causing any symptoms and were not a sign of disease. Where an erosion is giving symptoms such as a heavy discharge, repeated infections and discomfort, it may be effectively treated with any one of these methods of cautery: silver nitrate, cryotherapy, electrocautery and diathermy. Silver nitrate is still the simplest, cheapest and quickest means of treating a moderate erosion and disposable applicators with a silver nitrate bead are readily available (Chapter 15).

38.4.1 Technique of silver nitrate application

The cervix is visualized and any cervical smears or bacterial swabs are taken. The silver nitrate is applied to the cervix, including the external cervical os, and the area treated immediately turns white. The patient should be warned to expect an increased watery, sometimes blood-stained discharge for several weeks. A topical antiseptic or antibiotic cream may be given during this time to reduce the risks of secondary infection.

38.5 CRYOSURGERY FOR CERVICAL EROSIONS

A nitrous oxide or liquid nitrogen cryoprobe is ideal for cauterizing troublesome cervical erosions. Treatment is quick and simple to apply, and has a high success rate and patient acceptability (Chapter 18).

38.5.1 Technique

Good visualization of the cervix is essential; one hazard of using the cryoprobe is that it can adhere to adjacent vaginal walls if they accidentally touch the probe tip or side and result in a small 'burn'. The cone-shaped applicator is placed on the cervix before starting to freeze and this enables it to be accurately positioned. Once in position the nitrous oxide or liquid nitrogen is switched on and freezing commences. The probe will become adherent to the cervix at this stage, generally 1–2 min is sufficient treatment time, and the probe is allowed either to thaw out spontaneously or to be 'defrosted' with the built-in defroster attachment. One treatment is normally all that is required, but a greater depth of penetration is obtained by giving a second freeze immediately following thawing if this is felt necessary. Follow-up is exactly as for silver nitrate.

38.6 ELECTROCAUTERY OF CERVICAL EROSIONS

As the cervical nerve endings are not sensitive to heat, any erosion may be cauterized using the electrocautery. Care must be taken if cauterizing the cervical os or cervical canal not to cause fibrosis, scarring and stenosis; likewise, during treatment, if steam is produced which passes inside the uterus, pain is caused. To avoid the risk of stenosis, linear radial cauterization should be employed, using the standard V-shaped platinum wire electrode.

38.7 DIATHERMY OF CERVICAL EROSIONS

The use of standard bipolar diathermy requires a general anaesthetic, whereas unipolar high-frequency diathermy may be used successfully without any anaesthetic. The Hyfrecator electrode is held a short distance away from the cervix, the current switched on, and a stream of sparks drawn from the electrode to the cervix (Chapter 17). This fulgurization effectively cauterizes the cervix. As with all other methods of cautery, the patient should be warned to expect an increased watery, blood-stained discharge for several weeks following treatment. An antiseptic or antibiotic cream may be applied during this time to reduce secondary infection.

38.8 VAGINAL VAULT GRANULATIONS FOLLOWING HYSTERECTOMY

Granulations in the vault of the vagina are relatively common following hysterectomy. They may cause a blood-stained discharge or even frank bleeding, both of which can cause anxiety to the patient.

Examination with a vaginal speculum reveals typical messy granulations, which are easily friable and bleed on the slightest touch. Treatment is simple, using silver nitrate to each granulation. Normally one application is sufficient to cure the condition.

38.9 GENITAL WARTS

These warts tend to develop in large clusters, affecting the penile and vulvar skin as well as mucous membranes, and the perianal skin. Examination with the electron microscope clearly shows the human wart virus to be the causative agent.

Genital warts can be confused with condylomata of late syphilis, and as both conditions are sexually transmitted they could coexist; it is therefore essential to examine the sexual partner as well and screen both serologically for venereal diseases.

Treatment can be difficult and requires much patience. Vaginal and rectal examinations should be performed using a speculum to identify the extent of visible lesions.

Cryotherapy is probably the treatment of choice, applied once or twice weekly until effecting a cure. Alternatively, podophyllin 25% in soft paraffin applied daily for 3 days is effective but more uncomfortable. Podophyllotoxin 0.5% solution applied twice daily for 3 days is effective for penile warts. Podophyllin in pregnancy should not be used because of possible teratogenic effects.

The immunosuppressed patient and also some pregnant patients develop warts at an alarming rate, ending up with huge fungating cauliflower-like lesions. The earlier treatment can be offered the better.

38.10 REPAIR OF EPISIOTOMY

A good repair of an episiotomy or second-degree tear following delivery can occasionally be quite difficult; however, time taken identifying each layer is well spent, makes the repair easier and results in better, more comfortable healing. As with any surgical procedure, good illumination is paramount. The patient should be supported in the lithotomy position and a small swab on a cord inserted to the top of the vagina; this helps to control oozing from the uterus as well as helping to identify the extent of the laceration in the posterior vaginal wall. The top of this laceration must be identified and the first suture inserted in the posterior vaginal wall just above the laceration. Chromic catgut 2/0 (metric 3.5) is suitable for this stitch (Ref. Ethicon W 565). Using a continuous stitch, the posterior vaginal wall is closed. Next, one or two interrupted catgut sutures are placed in the muscle layer between the posterior vaginal wall and skin. Finally, the perineal skin is approximated using either interrupted braided silk suture Ethicon W 667 (metric 3, 2/0) on a curved reverse cutting needle, interrupted chromic catgut stitches, or a subcuticular catgut or Vicryl suture, depending on the preference of the operator (Figs 38.3 and 38.4).

38.11 BARTHOLIN'S CYSTS AND ABSCESSES

These can be extremely painful. Some rupture spontaneously; those that do not may be treated either by aspiration, aspiration and injection of fucidic acid gel, or marsupialization.

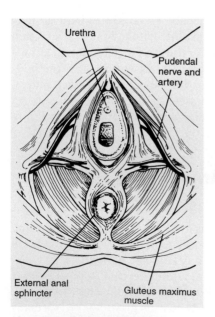

Urethra

Pudendal nerve and artery

External anal sphincter

Gluteus maximus muscle

Figure 38.3 Episiotomy; surgical anatomy.

Figure 38.4 (a) Episiotomy or second-degree tear. (b) Posterior vaginal wall sutured with continuous 2/0 catgut suture. (c) Interrupted catgut sutures to skin and perineal muscles with buried knots. (d) Final result.

38.11.1 Aspiration

Although one would not expect aspiration alone to cure an abscess, nevertheless, it is found that many Bartholin's abscesses respond to a single aspiration using a wide-bore needle and syringe. As an added safeguard, injection of fucidic acid gel following aspiration seems to give improved results.

38.11.2 Marsupialization

Recurrent Bartholin's abscesses are best treated by marsupialization. This consists of creating a permanent sinus by incision, followed by suturing the lining of the cyst to the outside skin; it is very effective and normally results in a permanent cure (Fig. 38.5).

38.12 URETHRAL CARUNCLE

This is a relatively common condition, particularly in postmenopausal women, resulting in prolapse of the urethral mucosa which then causes bleeding, frequency and dysuria. Mild cases may be treated with topical oestrogen-containing creams, possibly supplemented with systemic hormone replacement therapy (HRT). Where this fails, the mucosa

Figure 38.5 Marsupialization of Bartholin's abscess. (a) Abscess. (b) Incised. (c) Inside capsule sutured to outside skin creating a permanent sinus.

may be treated with the diathermy or electrocautery, or cryocautery under local anaesthesia, inserting an indwelling Foley catheter afterwards until the oedema has subsided.

38.13 INSERTION OF INTRAUTERINE CONTRACEPTIVE DEVICES

As a method of contraception, intrauterine devices have become popular in the last 30 years. There are now many different sizes, shapes and materials to choose from, and the practitioner will need to refer to the instruction leaflets provided with each device to determine the method of insertion.

38.13.1 Counselling

The patient and her partner should discuss with the doctor the pros and cons of this method of contraception; they should realize that no coil is 100% effective, that the periods following insertion may be much heavier and longer than previously, that occasionally the coil is expelled spontaneously, and that she should report for regular check-ups and cervical cytology. Although it has been shown to be a far safer procedure than was originally forecast, nevertheless, resuscitation facilities should be available for the unexpected vasovagal attacks. Similarly, the risks of introducing infection are very much less than was anticipated; however, a rigid no-touch technique should be used throughout.

38.13.2 Technique

Whether the patient is lying on her left side or on her back depends on the preference of the doctor; whichever position is used, it is essential to visualize the cervix clearly. Using vulsellum forceps, the anterior lip of the cervix is grasped and downward traction applied; this has the effect of straightening the longitudinal axis of the uterus and makes insertion easier. A uterine sound may be used to ascertain the dimensions and shape of the uterus; however, it is not always necessary as the coil and introducer may serve as a sound during insertion and give just as much information (Figs 38.6 and 38.7).

Figure 38.6 Instruments required for IUCD imsertion.

The coil is loaded into the introducer, which may be given a very slight bend at the tip using the fingers and thumb of the left gloved hand. This simple manoeuvre makes sounding and insertion much easier and is to be recommended. Using gentle pressure, and if necessary slight rotation to 'feel' the direction of the cervical canal, the coil is introduced into the uterine cavity until it is felt to touch the fundus. The introducer is then withdrawn, leaving the coil in position. The threads are cut using McIndoe curved 7 in. (17.8 cm) scissors and the vaginal speculum is removed. The patient is requested to return for a coil check in 4 weeks and, if all is well, annually thereafter. Copper-containing coils have a limited life of 2–5 years and need to

Figure 38.7 IUCD insertion; the cervix is steadied by the application of a pair of vulsellum forceps and slight traction applied. The IUCD is then inserted inside the uterine cavity.

be changed after this interval. In general, the optimum time to insert a coil is at a 6 week postnatal examination or at the end of a menstrual period. Nulliparous patients tend to have more abdominal cramps and side-effects.

38.14 REMOVAL OF THE 'LOST' COIL

Occasionally, the threads of an intrauterine coil are drawn up inside the uterine cavity, so that when the patient reports for a routine check they are not visible. At this point it is not possible to tell whether the coil has been extruded, or the threads are inside the uterus. Ultrasound examination will confirm the presence and situation of the coil, but if subsequently it is necessary to remove the coil, the threads need to be retrieved.

Gentle exploration with an Emmett thread retriever or a very fine single skin hook may bring down the threads, as may the introduction of a cervical cytology brush in the hope of engaging the threads. If all of these measures fail, the patient may need to be referred to a gynaecologist.

38.15 HORMONE IMPLANTS

The discovery that HRT can significantly reduce the incidence of osteoporosis and consequent fractures, as well as reducing the death rate from cardiovascular disease, menopausal symptoms and carcinoma of the ovary, has resulted in renewed interest in the form of therapy.

Earlier attempts at oestrogen replacement alone, whilst abolishing menopausal symptoms, were found to cause endometrial hyperplasia and an increased incidence of carcinoma of the body of the uterus.

By adding progestogens, either cyclically or continuously, the risk of endometrial disease was abolished, but the resumption of menstruation when using cyclical progestogen was not acceptable to many women.

Further research then showed that oestradiol gave better protection against osteoporosis than did synthetic oestrogens [47]. Oestradiol can be given as tablets, injection, vaginal cream or pessary, transdermal patches or subcutaneous implants. Low-dose continuous regimes are now available whereby both oestrogens and progestogens are given continuously. This offers all the advantages of HRT without the withdrawal bleed.

To give adequate protection against osteoporosis it seems necessary to give HRT for at least 5 years following the menopause. In patients who have had a hysterectomy, progestogens, whether cyclical or continuous, need not be given and simple oestrogen therapy is all that is required.

Oestradiol is manufactured as crystalline slow-release pellets in three strengths, 25, 50 and 100 mg. For the average woman 50 mg seems to be adequate and should last for up to 6 months. It is administered as a subcutaneous implant through a trocar and cannula, usually in the abdominal wall.

Figure 38.8 Instruments required for hormone implant.

38.15.1 Technique

The correct size of trocar and cannula should be chosen to match the size of the implant (Fig. 38.8). The point of insertion is chosen: usually this lies on a line 2 in. (5 cm) above the inguinal ligament. A mark is made on the skin, which is then painted with povidone–iodine in spirit.

Using a 30 swg needle and dental syringe (or equivalent) a small quantity of local anaesthetic is infiltrated into the overlying skin and an incision 5 mm long made with a sharp-pointed scalpel blade (size 11) on a no. 3 handle (Figs 38.9 and 38.10).

Whilst this is being done, the assistant opens the sterile tube containing the oestradiol pellet and places it in a sterile gallipot or container. The trocar with obturator is then pushed through the small skin incision into the subcutaneous fat layer (Fig. 38.11) and the obturator removed (Fig. 38.12).

With extreme care the hormone implant is next picked up with sterile forceps and placed in the cannula. It is helpful if the nurse or assistant keeps the sterile gallipot or container under the cannula

Figure 38.9 Local anaesthetic infiltrated at the site of the implant.

Figure 38.10 Small incision using a no. 11 scalpel blade on a no. 3 handle.

Figure 38.11 Trocar and cannula pushed through the incision.

Figure 38.12 Obturator withdrawn.

whilst placing it in position, to avoid dropping it on the floor (Fig. 38.13).

Using the blunt, longer obturator, the implant is pushed through the cannula to lie in the subcutaneous fatty layer (Figs 38.14 and 38.15). The cannula is removed and at the same time firm pressure is applied over the track of the cannula to reduce any bleeding (Fig. 38.16). Closure is by means of one single suture or Steri-strips (Figs 38.17 and 38.18).

Normally, most patients feel the benefits within a few days and can usually tell when it is wearing off. An interesting phenomenon of tachyphylaxis has been observed, where the patient is sure that the implant needs replacing at steadily shorter intervals, whereas if serum oestradiol levels are measured, more than adequate levels are still circulating. Thus, requests for further implants at closer intervals should be resisted, and where possible a 6 monthly schedule adhered to.

Where there is a loss of libido, a simultaneous implant of testosterone 100 mg together with oestradiol 50 mg seems to be helpful.

Figure 38.13 Pellet of oestradiol inserted in the cannula.

Figure 38.14   Obturator ready to insert the pellet through the cannula.

Figure 38.15   Pellet inserted subcutaneously.

Figure 38.16   Trocar and cannula removed. Pressure is applied to reduce any bleeding.

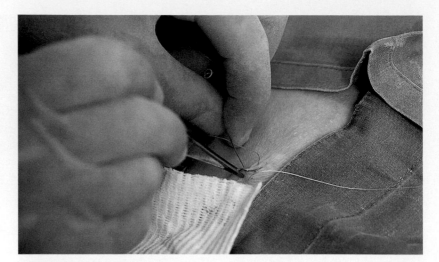

Figure 38.17   One stitch or skin-closure strips to close the incision.

Figure 38.18   The stitch may be absorbable or not, depending on preference.

38.16 REMOVAL OF ENDOCERVICAL POLYPI

Patients presenting with a blood-stained vaginal discharge, often worse after intercourse and occurring throughout the menstrual cycle, may be found to have an endocervical polyp on speculum examination. Many of these are eminently suitable for treatment in general practice. The easiest method of removal is to use a pair of small sponge forceps, grasp the polyp and 'twist' it off. Bleeding is generally slight. The base of the polyp may then be treated with a silver nitrate applicator and the polyp sent for routine histological examination. The patient should be warned to expect a slight increase in the discharge following cauterization with silver nitrate. Some doctors advise the use of an antiseptic vaginal cream for 1 week after removal (e.g. 'Sultrin', triple sulphonamide cream containing Sulphathiazole, sulphacetamide and sulphabenzamide). Because endocervical polypi may coexist with polypi within the uterine cavity, it is good practice to follow up with a transvaginal colour Doppler ultrasound examination of the uterine cavity.

CHAPTER 39

Vasectomy

> But amongst other causes of barreness in men, this also is one that maketh them barren ... the incision, or cutting of their veins behind their ears.
>
> *De Morbis Foemineis, 1686*

Vasectomy as a method of contraception has become increasingly popular during the 1990s. The operation can be performed by the general practitioner surgeon under local anaesthesia, but because of the medicolegal implications, extra attention must be given to counselling, record-keeping, technique, histology and follow-up. It involves resecting a small portion of the vas deferens on either side of the scrotum. Although the operation should be considered irreversible, owing to increasing divorce rates, patients may change their minds, so a technique of vasectomy which will allow reversal should be performed if possible [48].

39.1 PREOPERATIVE COUNSELLING

Where there is a stable relationship, it is preferable to see both patient and wife or partner together although the consent of the spouse is not legally necessary.

The details of the operation need to be carefully explained to the patient, together with the possible risks of failure and the difficulty of reversal should the patient subsequently change his mind. The importance of follow-up is explained and the patient is warned not to relax any contraception until at least two negative sperm tests have been performed.

A consent form (Fig. 39.1) needs to be signed by the patient. The Department of Health has produced a recommended form, HC(90) – Appendix A(2), which can be used for vasectomy.

The following instruments are required:

- warm, aqueous povidone–iodine (Betadine solution)
- 10 ml syringe
- two 25 swg × 5/8 in. (0.5 × 16 mm) needles
- scalpel handle size 3
- scalpel blade size 15
- pair fine-pointed, straight iris scissors $4^1/_2$ in. (11.4 cm)
- pair toothed dissecting forceps 5 in. (12.7 cm)
- two pairs fine, curved Halstead mosquito artery forceps
- pair 'vasectomy' forceps or fine Allis forceps

CONSENT FORM
For sterilisation or vasectomy

Health Authority . . . .   Patient's Surname . . . .

Hospital . . . .   Other Names . . . .

Unit Number . . . .   Date of Birth . . . .

Sex: *(please tick)*   Male ☐   Female ☐

DOCTORS (This part to be completed by doctor. See notes on the reverse)

TYPE OF OPERATION: STERILISATION OR VASECTOMY

Complete this part of the form
I confirm that I have explained the procedure and any anaesthetic (general/regional) required, to the patient in terms which in my judgement are suited to his/her understanding.

Signature . . . .   Date . . . .

Name of doctor . . . .

PATIENT

1   Please read this form very carefully.

2   It there is anything that you don't understand about the explanation, or if you want more information, you should ask the doctor.

3   Please check that all the information on the form is correct. If it is, and you understand the explanation, then sign the form.

I am the patient

I agree	■ to have this operation, which has been explained to me by the doctor named on this form.
	■ to have the type of anaesthetic that I have been told about.
I understand	■ that the operation may not be done by the doctor who has been treating me so far.
	■ that the aim of the operation is to stop me having any children and it might not be possible to reverse the effects of the operation.
	■ that sterilisation/vasectomy can sometimes fail, and that there is a very small chance that I may become fertile again after some time.
	■ that any procedure in addition to the investigation or treatment described on this form will only be carried out if it is necessary and in my best interests and can be justified for medical reasons.
I have told	■ the doctor about any additional procedures I would **not** wish to be carried out straightaway without my having the opportunity to consider them first.
For vasectomy I understand	■ that I may remain fertile or become fertile again after some time.
	■ that I will have to use some other contraceptive method until 2 tests in a row show that I am not producing sperm, if I do not want to father any children.

Signature . . . .

Figure 39.1   Form of consent for vasectomy.

- Kilner needle holder
- Hyfrecator (optional)
- surgical sutures: catgut metric gauge 2 (4/0) curved cutting needle, Ref. Ethicon W 480 (chromic) or W 470 (plain)
- braided polyester (Mersilene) metric gauge 1.5 (4/0) curved cutting needle, Ref. Ethicon W 316

39.2 TECHNIQUE (Figs 39.2–39.24)

All instruments should be sterilized by autoclaving or using a hot-air oven, and an absolutely aseptic technique employed throughout; an infected postoperative scrotal haematoma is disastrous. The patient should shave the scrotal skin on both sides and follow this with a bath.

A right-handed surgeon should stand on the left of the patient; this allows gentle traction to be applied to each vas with the left hand. Each

Figure 39.2 The vas is always isolated lateral to the cord and held between the finger and thumb of the left hand. After raising a small intradermal weal with lignocaine, a 1 cm incision is made through it down to the outer surface of the sheath of the vas (Figs 39.2–39.24 by permission of the late Mr W. Keith Yeates' widow).

Figure 39.3 After another very small amount of lignocaine has been injected in each side of the vas and into its sheath; the sheath is delineated by introducing and opening the blades of fine-pointed iris scissors.

Figure 39.4 The vas in its sheath is picked up with a fine pair of Allis forceps.

Figure 39.5 A blunted towel-clip is applied around the vas in its sheath; the latter is then opened with fine-pointed iris scissors, exposing the bare vas.

Figure 39.6 The exposed vas is held with toothed dissecting forceps while the towel clip is opened and then reapplied inside the sheath under the vas itself. The lower part of the sheath of the vas is then picked up with small-toothed dissecting forceps, and the fine adhesions between it and the vas are divided with the scissors.

Figure 39.7 The lower edge of the pocket created is held with haemostatic forceps, which are then left on.

Figure 39.8 A short section of vas is picked up with the toothed dissecting forceps and isolated from the posterior part of its sheath.

Figure 39.9 A pair of haemostatic forceps is applied at each end of the isolated vas.

Figure 39.10 The vas is divided.

Figure 39.11 A portion of the vas is excised and sent for histological examination.

Figure 39.12   The 'mesentery' attached to the upper end of the vas is held with haemostatic forceps, which are used to strip off the mesentery from the upper end for about 1 cm.

Figure 39.13   Proximal end of vas freed from the mesentery.

vas is identified by careful palpation and the presence of any abnormality such as a varicocele excluded.

The skin is painted with warmed povidone–iodine aqueous solution (Betadine), and the vas identified and isolated to the lateral side of the cord. A small intradermal weal of lignocaine is raised and a 1 cm incision made in the skin, down to the outer sheath of the vas, which is then further anaesthetized with a second injection of lignocaine into the sheath surrounding the vas. Using special vasectomy forceps or fine Allis forceps, the vas in its sheath is picked up and the sheath separated using fine-pointed iris scissors. The vasectomy forceps are now reapplied, this time around the vas inside the sheath, and a short section of vas is freed from its sheath posteriorly. The sheath is mobilized from the front of the vas distally for about 1 cm

Figure 39.14   The mesentery is ligated with 4/0 catgut.

Figure 39.15 The upper end of the vas is ligated with 4/0 catgut.

Figure 39.16 The lower end is ligated with non-absorbable material (silk or braided Nylon).

Figure 39.17 The ligatures around each end of the vas are left long and held in haemostatic forceps, which keeps the field in full view throughout the procedure. Diathermy is applied to both cut ends.

Figure 39.18 The lower end is buried in the pocket in the sheath previously prepared. The closing suture of non-absorbable material is first tied around a haemostat, which picks up the site of ligation of the mesentery.

to prepare a pocket for burying the vas later. It is now possible to apply a pair of fine Halstead mosquito artery forceps at either end of the isolated portion of vas and excise the middle piece, which is sent for histology. A 1 cm portion of 'mesentery' is separated from the proximal portion of vas and then ligated with 4/0 (metric gauge 2) catgut, as is the vas itself.

The distal end of the vas is ligated with non-absorbable braided polyester 4/0 (metric gauge 1.5). Each end of the divided vas is now coagulated with the unipolar diathermy (Hyfrecator). To prevent any chances of reanastamosis, the proximal and distal ends of the vas are enclosed in different fascial planes as follows: the lower end is buried in the pocket of the previously prepared sheath, while the upper end of the vas is secured outside the sheath.

Skin closure is achieved by inserting one blade of a small pair of Allis forceps inside the incision deep to the dartos muscle and the other in the skin, and suturing through both with 4/0 (metric gauge 2) plain catgut. The same procedure is then performed on the opposite side and both skin incisions are painted with Whitehead's varnish, Opsite or collodion.

A scrotal support or close-fitting pants are applied and the patient is allowed to return home after 15 min rest.

It is essential to warn the patient that he will continue to produce viable spermatozoa for 3 months or more following vasectomy, and thus must continue with alternative forms of contraception until two consecutive sperm tests are returned showing no motile spermatozoa in fresh (less than 2 h old) specimens. Failure to take notice of this advice has resulted in more than one unplanned pregnancy.

For medicolegal reasons, it is important to record the following in writing:

- that the patient and his wife have had the operation carefully explained to them
- that the exceptionally rare possibility of failure has been explained and is understood
- a histology report confirming that a portion of vas has been excised on either side
- two negative sperm tests following operation.

Figure 39.19 The lower edge of the pocket is opened by traction on the haemostat previously applied.

Figure 39.20 The ligature around the lower end of the sectioned vas is cut.

Figure 39.21 The suture is passed through the margins of the sheath.

Figure 39.22 The sheath is closed over the lower end of the vas.

Figure 39.23 The ends of the catgut ligature round the upper end of the vas are tied round a tented-up piece of loose fascia outside the sheath and then cut short.

Photocopies of duplicate forms of each should be given to the patient, with the originals being kept permanently by the doctor.

39.3 POSTOPERATIVE CARE

The patient may experience discomfort, but not usually pain, which can be controlled with mild analgesics. He should be advised to keep the skin dry for 4 days; no restrictions need be imposed on intercourse, provided contraception is practised until azoospermia is achieved. Mild bruising is common and of no significance; very rarely, a large haematoma occurs, which can look alarming, but which normally settles on conservative treatment alone. Given careful selection, adequate counselling and the doctor's personal knowledge of the patient, vasectomy is an excellent method of contraception once a couple feels that their family is complete.

Figure 39.24 The skin is closed by inserting the blade of a small pair of Allis forceps inside the incision deep to the dartos, the other end being held in a similar fashion with fine-toothed dissecting forceps. The effect of this is to ensure that the suture of 4/0 plain catgut will include the dartos layer. This is very important for haemostasis. A similar procedure is then performed on the opposite side. At the end of the operation, both incisions are painted with Whitehead's varnish, and the scrotum is powdered to remove the stickiness of the povidone–iodine. A scrotal support is applied.

Lymph-gland biopsy

> A Scrofula is an indurated gland, mostly forming in the neck, armpits and groins ... When the base of the scrofulous tumour runs out into a narrow point, we may cut it away readily.
>
> *Paul of Aegina, seventh century* AD

Excision of an enlarged lymph node for histological examination may give valuable information and help to establish a definite diagnosis, but it can be a difficult operation and the doctor should be aware of certain possible problems.

- Many lymph nodes give the appearance of being quite superficial, but are found at operation to be situated much deeper than anticipated.
- Bleeding may be more brisk than with other excision procedures.
- The lymph nodes need very careful handling to preserve their histology, as they tend to be somewhat friable.
- The inguinal area and axilla should be avoided if possible because of the risk to underlying structures.

Given these constraints, however, excision biopsy of suitably accessible lymph glands is a useful procedure which on occasions gives important information in establishing a diagnosis.

40.1 SELECTION OF PATIENTS

Certain preliminary investigations will help to establish a diagnosis and may make the need for lymph-node biopsy unnecessary. These include a full blood count, haemoglobin, differential white cell count and platelets, erythrocyte sedimentation rate (ESR), or plasma viscosity, serum proteins and electrophoresis, liver function tests, Lupas Erythematosus (LE) cells, autoantibody screening, chest X-ray, and possibly blood culture, if pyrexial, and bone marrow.

These tests, together with a careful clinical examination, will establish a diagnosis in the majority of patients; those remaining will be helped by excision of a gland for histological examination. Before embarking on surgery, a representative gland should be chosen and excision should be undertaken.

40.2 TECHNIQUE FOR EXCISION OF GLAND

The following instruments are required:

- scalpel size 3 scalpel blade size 10
- toothed dissecting forceps 5 in. (12.7 cm)
- McIndoe's scissors, curved 7 in. (17.8 cm)
- Kilner needle holder 5¼ in. (13.3 cm)
- two pairs Halstead mosquito artery forceps curved 5 in. (12.7 cm)
- surgical suture 4/0 (1.5 metric) monofilament Ethilon (Ref. Ethicon W 319) with curved, reverse cutting needle
- povidone–iodine in spirit (Betadine alcoholic solution)
- 10 ml 1% lignocaine with adrenaline 1:200 000
- syringes and needles.

The overlying skin is painted with povidone–iodine in spirit and the area anaesthetized by infiltration using 1% lignocaine and adrenaline 1:200 000. An incision is made down to the gland, which may be dissected free using the curved McIndoe's scissors and scalpel, holding the gland with the toothed dissecting forceps. Bleeding can be troublesome, but normally responds to firm pressure; should any small bleeding points not be controlled by pressure, they may be clipped and ligated (Figs 40.1 and 40.2).

Closure is by interrupted 4/0 sutures to the skin, with coated Vicryl sutures to the deeper layers if a dead space has been left. The excised gland should be placed in 10% formol saline, immediately labelled and sent for histological examination.

Figure 40.1 Lymph-gland biopsy; technique similar to removal of sebaceous cyst.

Figure 40.2 Lymph-gland biopsy; closure with interrupted braided silk or Prolene sutures.

Treatment of ganglia

Ganglia are extremely common. They are cystic swellings surrounded by a fibrous tissue wall, occurring in the vicinity of joint capsules and tendon sheaths. Most have crystal clear gelatinous contents, apart from some in which bleeding has occurred. The cause is not fully understood, but may be a degenerative process in the mesoblastic tissues surrounding the joint [49]. The most common site is the dorsum of the wrist (Fig. 41.1) (60–80%), followed by the flexor aspect of the wrist adjacent to the radial artery (15–20%). Smaller ganglia occur in the flexor sheaths of the fingers, dorsum of foot, ankle and head of fibula.

Untreated, many ganglia disappear spontaneously, and many others appear not to trouble the patient and may be left alone. Treatment is indicated if the patient is complaining of unacceptable symptoms, usually pain or limitation of function. Many treatments have been advocated, but all carry a recurrence rate and the patient should be advised of this accordingly.

41.1 INDICATIONS FOR TREATMENT

Many ganglia give no symptoms and do not worry the patient. If the diagnosis is certain, such ganglia may be left alone and a high percentage will rupture spontaneously during the next 3 years.

Figure 41.1 Typical ganglion on dorsum of the wrist.

The following are indications for treatment:

■ pain
■ interference with function
■ uncertainty about diagnosis
■ cosmetic reasons.

41.1.1 Pain

Many patients complain that their ganglion is painful, particularly those on the dorsum of the wrist and those adjacent to the radial artery on the palmar surface of the wrist. Often the capsule is tense and the ganglion has recently increased in size.

41.1.2 Interference with function

Very small, pea-sized ganglia adjacent to the flexor tender sheaths in the palm of the hand may interfere with flexion of the fingers. Treatment is justified in such circumstances to restore normal function.

41.1.3 Uncertainty about diagnosis

A small, tense ganglion may feel bony hard and be mistaken for an exostosis. Usually, X-ray examination will confirm or exclude the diagnosis. If, however, doubt still exists, and the patient or doctor is worried, aspiration or exploration should be undertaken.

41.1.4 Cosmetic

As aspiration and sclerosing injection leaves virtually no scar, it may be offered to those patients who are very concerned about the appearance of their ganglion.

Excision always leaves a scar and often a depressed area, so if the patient is worried about the appearance of the ganglion, excision is not an appropriate treatment unless the patient is fully prepared to accept the scar.

41.2 CHOICE OF TREATMENTS FOR GANGLIA

41.2.1 Simple rupture

Traditionally, the treatment of a ganglion was to hit it firmly with the family Bible! This was marginally successful, but the recurrence rate was high and not all patients volunteered to have the treatment repeated.

41.2.2 Incision with tenotomy knife

This is done under a local anaesthetic. As with rupture of the ganglion, recurrence rates are high, but the treatment is quick and simple, and generally leaves no scar (Figs 41.2 and 41.3).

Figure 41.2 Ganglion on dorsum of the wrist; incision with a tenotomy knife.

Figure 41.3 Incision with a tenotomy knife; contents are expressed by pressure. Recurrence is likely.

41.2.3 Catgut suture transfixing the ganglion

Described in the eighteenth century, the treatment consisted of drawing a thread through the ganglion. This may most conveniently be done by inserting a chromic catgut suture through the skin and through the ganglion. The action of the suture is to pierce the wall of the ganglion, allowing the contents to leak away under the skin, and secondly to produce an irritant inflammatory reaction within the ganglion in the hope of causing fibrosis and cure.

41.2.4 Aspiration and sclerosant injection

In recent years good results have been obtained by aspirating the gelatinous contents and reinjecting a sclerosing solution. This simple treatment offers an 80% cure rate, the same as excision, but does not leave a scar, and is considerably quicker and easier to perform.

41.2.5 Excision

If all other treatments fail excision under a bloodless field may be performed, but even this treatment has a failure rate, and it is wise to warn the patient of this possibility at the initial consultation. It is a time-consuming operation which needs to be done meticulously, and if general anaesthesia is unavailable, an intravenous regional block needs to be performed, which demands a qualified assistant [50].

41.3 TECHNIQUE FOR ASPIRATION AND SCLEROSANT INJECTION

The following instruments are required:

- 2 2 ml syringes, 19 swg needle (white) and 25 swg needle (orange)
- 3% sodium tetradecyl sulphate (STD) injection or 6% aqueous phenol injection
- 2 dental rolls
- micropore tape
- 1 in. Elastocrepe bandage 3 in.
- povidone–iodine in spirit (Betadine alcoholic solution)
- 2% lignocaine

The skin overlying the ganglion is liberally painted with povidone–iodine in spirit (Fig. 41.4).

Lignocaine 2% is now infiltrated from a point on the skin, through to the ganglion itself, injecting 0.5–1 ml local anaesthetic into the cyst. This has the effect of thinning the gelatinous contents, which will make aspiration easier as well as anaesthetizing the area (Fig. 41.5).

One millilitre of 3% STD or 6% aqueous phenol is drawn up in a 2 ml syringe and the needle discarded. Using the 19 swg needle attached to an empty sterile 2 ml syringe the ganglion is entered and the contents are aspirated. This may be assisted by simultaneous pressure over the ganglion with the thumb or finger of the opposite hand (Figs 41.6 and 41.7).

With patience, all the gelatinous contents of the ganglion can be aspirated through the 19 swg needle. When the ganglion has been emptied, the syringe is disconnected from the needle, which is left inside the empty ganglion sac, the volume of aspirate noted and STD, exactly half the volume aspirated, is now injected through the needle (Fig. 41.8).

Figure 41.4 The skin overlying the ganglion is painted with povidone–iodine.

Figure 41.5 Lignocaine 1% is infiltrated into the overlying skin and into the ganglion.

Figure 41.6 Using a 19 swg needle the contents of the ganglion are aspirated.

Figure 41.7 Pressure applied whilst aspirating helps to empty the cyst.

Figure 41.8 Sclerosant is injected into the emptied cyst.

Figure 41.9 A dental roll or cotton-wool ball is applied over the site of the ganglion.

Pressure is applied over the ganglion with a gauze swab while the needle and syringe are withdrawn. A dental roll is taped over the site of the ganglion and covered by a firm elastocrepe bandage (Figs 41.9 and 41.10). This is left undisturbed for 2 weeks, after which time it is removed. No further follow-up is needed. This simple treatment offers an 80% cure rate, similar to that for excision, and is now the treatment of choice for ganglion.

Three per cent STD is known to cause marked inflammation when injected in leg veins; it is interesting to note that such reactions are rare when the sclerosant is injected into ganglia, but the reason for this is not fully understood.

41.4 THE MUCOUS CYST (GANGLION) ON THE FINGER

Mucous cysts are commonly seen over the terminal interphalangeal joints of the fingers. They frequently occur over the lateral edge and interfere with writing and knitting. Some disappear spontaneously but

Figure 41.10 A firm bandage is applied over the dental roll and left for 2 weeks, keeping the pressure applied during that time.

many recur. They may be excised, sclerosed, cauterized chemically or electrically, or treated with cryotherapy or radiosurgery, but a very simple treatment which patients can undertake themselves once shown is to prick with a sterile needle, express the clear jelly and apply a firm tape dressing daily for 6 weeks. Micropore tape ($\frac{1}{2}$ in.) is ideal. It should be applied around three-quarters of the finger and replaced whenever it becomes loose. If the patient is given a supply of sterile needles they can be instructed to repeat the procedure should the cyst recur (Figs 41.11–41.13).

Figure 41.11   A typical synovial or mucus cyst overlying the terminal interphalangeal joint.

Figure 41.12   After pricking with a sterile needle, jelly may be expressed and the cyst emptied.

Figure 41.13   The finger should then be taped daily for 6 weeks to prevent recurrence.

CHAPTER 42

Radiosurgery

Radiosurgery now has an established place throughout the world in dermatology, gynaecology, facial and cosmetic surgery, vascular and podiatric practice. Its use in minor surgery is increasing rapidly and it can now achieve far more superior results than other more conventional surgical techniques.

Radiosurgery is a procedure in which tissue is removed or destroyed by electrical energy. This energy is converted to heat as a result of tissue resistance but, unlike electrocautery, the heat is generated in the tissues themselves and the actual electrode remains cold.

42.1 BACKGROUND

The control of bleeding by the application of heat was probably first used by the Ancient Egyptians and there are numerous accounts of heated metal instruments being used to destroy tissues and control haemorrhage.

Electric current has been used in medical equipment for over a century. The traditional electrocautery consisted of a platinum wire which could be heated to red heat by the application of an electric current; and this had the ability to both cut and coagulate tissues.

Later, with the advent of alternating current and transformer circuitry, high-frequency electric currents were used in medicine to coagulate, cut and destroy tissues, and today diathermy equipment is found in every operating theatre in the world.

In standard diathermy, a high-frequency electric current is passed through the patient. Two electrodes are used: a large plate electrode which is moistened and strapped to the patient's leg, and an 'active' electrode which is used to touch tissues. The heating effect is dependent on the electrical 'density', i.e. where the current is spread over a large surface area there is minimal generation of heat, but where it is concentrated at a small point, enough heat is generated to cut, coagulate or destroy tissue (Fig. 42.1).

Low-frequency alternating current caused muscle contractions (the Faradic effect as used in physiotherapy), whereas high-frequency (>10 000 Hz) currents did not have this effect, but resulted mainly in heating of the tissues.

Figure 42.1 Diagrammatic illustration of radiosurgery showing the distribution of energy.

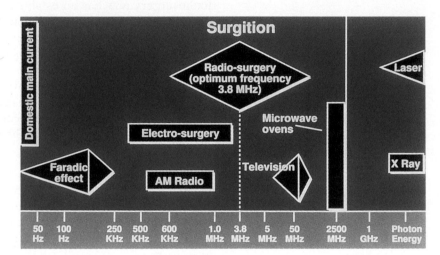

Figure 42.2 Comparison of different electrical frequencies and their respective uses.

The invention of the vacuum tube, as used in radios and televisions, allowed the production of amplified electric currents which would cut tissues, and in 1978 Maness showed that 3.8 million cycles per second (3.8 MHz) was the optimal frequency for cutting soft tissues. This frequency is still used in modern radiosurgery units (Fig. 42.2).

Furthermore, in modern radiosurgical instruments several different waveforms can be generated, each having different characteristic effects on tissues, namely incision, excision and coagulation (Fig. 42.3).

Radiosurgery is an atraumatic method of cutting and coagulating soft tissues. No pressure is needed and the cells are vapourized in the path of the radiowaves, causing them to split apart much like a hot wire through polystyrene. This results in less trauma to the cells, less fibrous scarring and less postoperative discomfort; the other advantage is that the electrodes are also self-sterilizing in use.

	Waveform	Use	Oscilloscope configuration
I	Fully filtered and fully rectified	Cutting	
II	Fully rectified	Cut and coagulate	
III	Partially rectified	Hemostasis	
IV	Markedly damped (spark gap)	Fulguration and electra desiccation	

Figure 42.3 Different waveforms and modes of action.

42.2 DIFFERENT WAVEFORMS

The five different waveforms commonly used are as follows.

1. A pure filtered waveform (pure microsmooth cutting) (Fig. 42.4) is used for skin incisions and wire loop excisions where haemostasis is not expected to be a problem. This waveform gives the least lateral heat, and therefore the least tissue damage.
2. A fully rectified waveform (blended cutting and coagulation) (Fig. 42.5) is used for skin tags, papillomata, keloids, keratoses and removal of naevi where slight bleeding might be expected. It cuts as well as coagulates small blood vessels and gives slight lateral heat to the tissues.
3. A partially rectified waveform (hospital-type control of bleeders) (Fig. 42.6) is primarily for haemostasis; it cannot be used for cutting but is excellent for coagulation, telangectasia and spider veins.

Figure 42.4 Fully filtered waveform (cutting).

Figure 42.5 Fully rectified waveform (cutting and coagulation).

Figure 42.6 Partially rectified waveform (coagulation).

Figure 42.7 Marked damped (spark-gap) waveform (fulguration).

4. A fulgurating current (spark-gap tissue destruction) (Fig. 42.7) is very similar to the unipolar diathermy (Hyfrecator) and causes superficial tissue damage by holding the needle electrode close to the tissue and allowing a stream of sparks to burn the tissues. It is suitable for superficial haemostasis and destruction of small basal cell carcinomata and cysts.

5. Bipolar coagulation (Fig. 42.8): very precise haemostasis may be obtained by using bipolar forceps. Each blade is connected to the radiosurgical unit so that the current passes between the points of the forceps. It is very useful for picking off individual bleeding vessels in microsurgery. The heat generated in the tissues as the electrode passes through them is described as lateral heat and can be calculated from the formula:

$$H = T \times I \times W \times S \times F$$

where T = time during which the electrode is in contact with the tissues, I = power intensity, W = waveform (pure filtered gives

Figure 42.8 Finger-switch and bipolar forceps.

least lateral heat and partially rectified gives the most lateral heat), S = surface area of the electrode in contact with the tissues (the smaller, the less heat), and F = frequency of application (one must allow time between successive treatments for the tissues to cool).

The more lateral heat produced, the more is the tissue damaged, so it follows that for the best results, the needle electrode should be of the finest diameter, the power setting should be the lowest compatible with smooth cutting, the appropriate waveform should be selected and no pressure should be used.

There are several radiosurgical units on the market (Fig. 42.9a–e), each with different characteristics, waveforms and power outputs. The author uses an Ellman Surgitron FFPF unit, and all settings and waveforms refer to this machine. Where the doctor possesses an alternative instrument, reference should be made to the maker's handbook for power settings, etc.

Most radiosurgical units will comprise the following:

- an electrical generator connected to the domestic electricity supply which converts the mains voltage (110 V at 60 Hz or 240 V at 50 Hz) to a high-frequency current of 3.8 MHz. It has a switch which will select different waveforms (Figs 42.9 and 42.10)
- a passive electrode or ground plate or dispersive electrode (Fig. 42.9b). This is usually a small plastic covered plate which is placed in close proximity to the patient. It does not need to make electrical contact with the patient (unlike hospital diathermy) and acts like an antenna to concentrate the radiowaves

Figure 42.9 (a) The Ellman Surgitron FFPF radiosurgical unit. (b) The Ellman Dento-surg 90. (c) The Ellman Surgitron IEC unit. (d) The Ellman Surgitron IEC II (dual-frequency unit). This uses 4 MHz for cutting, coagulation and fulguration, and 1.7 MHz for bipolar coagulation. (e) The Ellman Surgitron Radiolase 50 W unit.

Figure 42.10   The Ellman Surgitron on a trolley with the Vapor-vac smoke extraction unit.

Figure 42.11   A selection of needle electrodes (Ellman).

- a treatment handle connected to the generator by a flexible wire. Different shaped electrodes are inserted into this handle and clamped in position. Electrodes, manufactured from surgical quality tungsten, may be single wire for incision or fulguration, loop electrodes for cutting (electrosection) (Figs 42.11–42.13) or ball-ended for haemostasis (Fig. 42.14). Fine, bipolar forceps are also available for precise haemostasis. A handle which holds a standard scalpel blade or ring curettes is also available so that the surgeon can use both conventional cutting as well as radiosection (Fig. 42.15).
- a foot switch or finger-operated switch on the electrode handle (Figs 42.8 and 42.18)
- a smoke evacuator (Figs 42.19–42.21). This is essential where any number of radiosurgical procedures is being performed, particularly in wire loop excision of the cervix in gynaecology. Viral filters and activated charcoal filters can be incorporated in the extraction circuit, making the radiosurgery operation almost odourless. A room ventilator is also a very good idea.

Other necessary equipment includes:

- latex gloves: these should be worn at all times; for the majority of superficial skin lesions they need not be sterile, but for deeper procedures sterile gloves should be worn
- masks: where viral lesions are being removed it is a sensible precaution to wear a surgical mask. There has been documented evidence that the wart virus DNA is liberated during carbon dioxide laser surgery, and it is possible that this can occur with the plume of smoke released during radiosurgery
- appropriate sterile instruments to handle tissues, e.g. fine forceps and skin-hooks
- an autoclave to sterilize the electrodes and instruments.

Figure 42.12   (a) Selection of electrodes for Ellman radiosurgical unit. (b) Selection of flat electrodes for Ellman radiosurgical units.

Figure 42.13 The tungsten-wire loop electrode.

Figure 42.14 The ball-ended 'coagulation' electrode.

Figure 42.15 (a) Conventional scalpel blades may be used with a radiosurgical unit, combining both modes of cutting. (b) Universal handle with size 15 scalpel blade (Ellman). (c) Universal handle with ring-curette attachment (Ellman).

Figure 42.16 Attachment which can take disposable 30 swg needles to use as scalpel.

Figure 42.17 Needle electrode.

Figure 42.18 Hand-piece with finger-switch and switching unit which plugs into the side of the Surgitron FFPF.

Figure 42.19 (a) Considerable smoke is produced with radiosurgery. (b) The Quiet Vac Smoke Evacuation System (Ellman). (c) Using the smoke extraction unit during removal of naevus.

42.3 LEARNING THE TECHNIQUE OF RADIOSURGERY

Radiosurgical instruments are powerful and a totally different technique from that of conventional scalpel surgery has to be learned. Most of the poor results are entirely due to inexperience and faulty technique.

The first major difference is that **no pressure must be used.** This is hard to learn for a surgeon who has been trained to press the scalpel firmly through the tissues. In radiosurgery it is the radiowave which does the cutting.

Secondly, there are no absolute power settings on the machine; these need to be learned by trial and error and experience. For example, a small moist lesion will require much less power to remove than a larger fibrous keratinized lesion.

Thirdly, if repeated incisions are to be made on the same lesion, time should be allowed to let the edges cool between cuts; usually up to 10 seconds.

Figure 42.20 The use of a vacuum extractor unit is strongly recommended for both visibility and patient comfort.

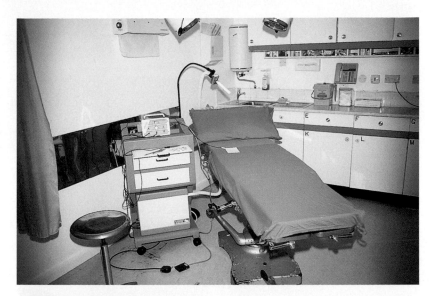

Figure 42.21 Radiosurgery unit and trolley with vacuum exttraction unit alongside treatment couch.

Figure 42.22 Histological appearance of tissue cut with scalpel.

Figure 42.23 Histological appearance of tissue cut with radiosurgery. Note less cellular damage.

Fourthly, rather than removing the whole lesion at the first attempt, better cosmetic results are obtained by first removing a representative sample for histological examination and then gradually 'planing' off the remainder of the lesion until it is flush with the surrounding skin.

One of the simplest teaching aids is a piece of raw steak placed on the passive base electrode. Starting with high power, different techniques of cutting and coagulation may be tried, and then, by reducing the power, the effects of too low or too high current are discovered (Figs 42.24–42.27).

Many videotapes have now been produced demonstrating radiosurgery and these can be highly recommended for teaching. Tuition by a colleague familiar with the technique of radiosurgery is well worth the time and effort, followed by treating several patients under supervision.

Figure 42.24 To practise radiosurgery, a piece of beef-steak is placed over the ground-plate electrode.

Figure 42.25 Demonstrating cutting with needle electrode and beef-steak.

Figure 42.26 Removing a small piece of tissue using the loop electrode.

Figure 42.27 Beef-steak showing areas of coagulation, incisions and 'biopsies'.

42.4 WARNINGS

1. Cardiac pacemakers. No patient with a cardiac pacemaker should be treated with radiosurgery without prior consultation with their cardiologist. Fixed-rate pacemakers are least likely to experience problems, but demand-led pacemakers may well be affected and result in arrhythmias. It is, therefore, essential to ask every patient in advance whether they have a pacemaker.
2. No spirit-based or inflammable skin antiseptic should be used. In fact, it is probably unnecessary to use any form of skin preparation.
3. Any allergic history of the patient to local anaesthetics (very rare), skin preparations and postoperative skin applications and tapes should be noted.
4. Delayed bleeding can occur. This is usually light but can cause alarm to the patient. It can be minimized by not using adrenaline with the local anaesthetic, and by applying a solution of 20% aluminium chloride or Monsell's solution on a cotton-wool applicator at the end of the procedure. It is also helpful to advise the patient about applying finger pressure for 10 min should any oozing occur.

5. Explosion risks exist in the presence of bowel gases and/or oxygen, as they do with diathermy and electrocautery.
6. Electrical shocks and burns can be minimized by not allowing any part of the patient to touch any metal and by the operator wearing rubber gloves.
7. Finally, inexperience can cause problems.

42.5 AVOIDANCE OF COMPLICATIONS

As with all medical and surgical treatments, complications can occur, but the majority are avoidable, and careful preoperative assessment of both patient and equipment will prevent many mishaps.

The following precautions should be taken.

1. All wires should be checked and any which are frayed or where there is a break in the insulation must be replaced.
2. All electrodes must be checked. Broken wires will cause lacerations. Any worn tips should be discarded.
3. Too deep an excision will result in unnecessary scarring.
4. The doctor should watch the foot switch or finger switch. Both the operator and any assistants should be careful not to tread accidentally on the foot switch, as accidental burns can occur to the patient.
5. The hand-piece must be inserted in correct socket.
6. The doctor should check that the power control has not been increased at the end of a previous procedure, e.g. to steam-clean electrodes.
7. Too much tissue destruction makes histology impossible. This may be due to an incorrect power or waveform setting, or a lesion which is too shallow. In this case the top may be cut off with a conventional scalpel and then the base treated with the radio-surgical unit.
8. The doctor must check that the patient does not have a cardiac pacemaker.
9. The patient must not be on aspirin or anticoagulants.
10. One should beware of lower limbs in diabetic patients.

42.6 CLEANING ELECTRODES

All electrodes can be steam sterilized in an autoclave, as can the wires, plugs and antenna baseplate. Furthermore, in use the electrodes are self-sterilizing. However, during use, carbon particles and debris can become adherent to the tungsten wire, reducing the efficiency and causing 'drag'. A very simple way of removing this and also for sterilizing the electrode is steam-cleaning. (Fig. 42.28), as follows.

1. Gloves should be worn.
2. The unit is set to cutting waveform (pure filtered).
3. The power dial is set to 5 (or equivalent).
4. Two gauze pads are placed together and folded in half.
5. They are saturated with water.

Care of electrodes

Preventing electrode breakage

Electrodes are made of surgical grade tungsten wire and will eventually volatize and break. If misused, they will carbonize and rapidly wear out. To increase their efficiency and prolong their life follow these recommendations.

1. Plug handpiece into the correct terminal.

2. The correct waveform should be used. **Never** try to cut on partially rectified.

3. The antenna plate should be in close proximity to the operative site. (i.e. in face surgery, place behind the head). The antenna may be placed behind cloth or under a pad. **It does not need** to have skin contact.

4. Have your assistants handle the electrodes by the **insulated shafts only**. The wires are surgical grade tungsten with very thin diameters.

5. If using bendable electrodes, **only bend** the electrodes at their insulated shaft.

6. Tissue should be moist.

7. Always activate the unit **before** making contact with the tissue.

8. **Never apply pressure**. Always remember that the radiowaves are doing the cutting.

9. If there is resistance, drag, or tissue sticking to the electrode, the power setting is **too low**. This will cause bending and breakage. Adjust accordingly by raising power gradually.

10. If there is sparking (which causes carbonization), the power is **too high**. Adjust accordingly by lowering power gradually.

11. Electrode loops need slightly **higher power** than straight wires (adjust up gradually) and are more fragile.

12. If you get stuck in the tissue, **do not force** the electrode. De-activate the unit and carefully remove the electrode from the tissue.

Cleaning electrodes during surgery

1. Set radiosurgical instrument at cut or cut/coag waveform.

2. Set power dial between 3 and 5.

3. Place two gauze pads together and fold in half.

4. Saturate the gauze with tap water.

5. With electrode in the handpiece, place it between the folds of the gauze.

6. Activate unit for 1–2 seconds while moving electrode back and forth within the gauze with little or no finger pressure. Repeat procedure (you should hear a 'sizzling' sound). This volatizes the water molecules and 'steam cleans' your electrodes.

**Note: OSHA requires that gloves be worn during all clinical procedures and during cleaning, disinfecting, and sterilizing of instruments including electrodes.

Care and cleaning of electrodes after use

1. **Do not scrub** electrodes with a brush or an abrasive.

2. To remove blood or tissue, place the electrode in hydrogen peroxide or in an ultrasonic cleaner for 3–5 minutes.

3. Place electrodes in an autoclave bag, being sure that electrodes lay side by side and **not** on top of each other.

4. Place electrode autoclave bag on top of other surgical instrument bags to prevent breakage.

Important: A periodic visual inspection of your electrodes is strongly recommended. If the tungsten wire is broken or if the insulated coating is 'nicked', torn, cracked, or damaged in any way, replace the electrode.

Figure 42.28 Care of electrodes.

6. With the electrode in the hand-piece, it is placed between the folds of the gauze.
7. The electrode is activated for 2 s while moving back and forth within the gauze, with almost no finger pressure. This is repeated. A sizzling sound can be heard as steam is generated. One must be careful not to burn the fingers holding the swab.

Certain electrodes are bendable to make for easier access, but the tungsten wire should always be treated with great respect as it is very fragile.

42.7 GENERAL GUIDELINES FOR RADIOSURGERY

1. The correct waveform must be selected.
2. One must never try to cut on partially rectified waveform (coagulation).
3. The antenna plate should be as near as possible to the operative site, but it does not need to have skin contact with the patient.
4. Tissues should be moist.
5. The unit must be activated before making contact with the tissues.
6. The doctor must never apply pressure, but instead let the radiowave do the cutting.
7. If there is resistance or 'drag', or tissue sticking to the electrode, the power setting is too low.
8. If there is sparking the power setting is too high.

42.8 CARE OF ELECTRODES AFTER USE

1. Electrodes must not be scrubbed with a brush or abrasive.
2. Blood and secretions may be removed by soaking in a solution of hydrogen peroxide, or by using an ultrasonic bath for 5 min.
3. Electrodes must be autoclaved in a separate container to avoid damage from other larger instruments.

42.9 PREPARATION OF THE PATIENT

1. It is essential to explain to the patient in advance the technique of radiosurgery, and what to expect both during the procedure and during the postoperative management.
2. Where a vacuum extractor unit is used it is helpful to explain to the patient that most of the noise will be coming from that, and that the operative electrode and unit is silent.
3. Any rings and jewellery must be removed, particularly if situated near the operation site.
4. The patient is made comfortable, and asked not to make any jerky or unexpected movements if at all possible.
5. The patient should be warned about the smell of burning and also to expect to see some smoke, even if the vacuum extractor is used.
6. Preprinted preoperative and postoperative information sheets are invaluable and usually answer most of the patient's questions.

42.10 ANAESTHESIA

With few exceptions, local infiltration anaesthesia is required, exactly as with conventional surgery or electrocautery. This should be with plain lignocaine rather than with added adrenaline as there is a slightly increased risk of postoperative oozing where adrenaline has been used. The finest gauge needle should be used to administer the anaesthetic (30 swg or finer).

Because infiltration of the tissues might distort the size and shape of skin lesions, it is helpful to mark the boundaries of the 'mole' or 'naevus' with a skin-marking pen before injecting the local anaesthetic.

42.11 APPLICATIONS OF RADIOSURGERY

A chart showing the applications of radiosurgery, lesions which may be treated, choice of waveform and which electrode to use is shown in Fig. 42.29.

Radiosurgery may be used in the following conditions and applications:

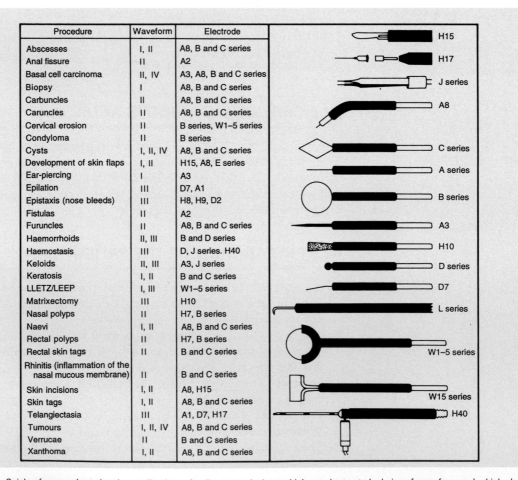

Procedure	Waveform	Electrode
Abscesses	I, II	A8, B and C series
Anal fissure	II	A2
Basal cell carcinoma	II, IV	A3, A8, B and C series
Biopsy	I	A8, B and C series
Carbuncles	II	A8, B and C series
Caruncles	II	A8, B and C series
Cervical erosion	II	B series, W1–5 series
Condyloma	II	B series
Cysts	I, II, IV	A8, B and C series
Development of skin flaps	I, II	H15, A8, E series
Ear-piercing	I	A3
Epilation	III	D7, A1
Epistaxis (nose bleeds)	III	H8, H9, D2
Fistulas	II	A2
Furuncles	II	A8, B and C series
Haemorrhoids	II, III	B and D series
Haemostasis	III	D, J series. H40
Keloids	II, III	A3, J series
Keratosis	I, II	B and C series
LLETZ/LEEP	I, III	W1–5 series
Matrixectomy	III	H10
Nasal polyps	II	H7, B series
Naevi	I, II	A8, B and C series
Rectal polyps	II	H7, B series
Rectal skin tags	II	B and C series
Rhinitis (inflammation of the nasal mucous membrane)	II	B and C series
Skin incisions	I, II	A8, H15
Skin tags	I, II	A8, B and C series
Telangiectasia	III	A1, D7, H17
Tumours	I, II, IV	A8, B and C series
Verrucae	II	B and C series
Xanthoma	I, II	A8, B and C series

Figure 42.29 Quick reference chart showing applications of radiosurgery, lesions which may be treated, choice of waveform and which electrode to use (Ellman International Inc.).

- actinic keratoses
- basal cell carcinoma
- blepharoplasty
- Bowen's disease
- cauterization of bleeding vessels
- cervical biopsies
- cervical conization (LLETZ)
- chalazion
- condylomata accuminata
- cosmetic surgery
- epilation
- excision of skin lesions
- fibroepithelial polyps
- hair transplants
- haemorrhoids
- ingrowing toe-nails
- keloids
- mucosal lesions inside the mouth
- naevi
- palato-uvuloplasty
- pyogenic granuloma
- rhinophyma
- sebaceous cysts
- seborrhoeic warts
- skin tags
- syringoma
- tattoo removal
- telangectasia
- xanthelasmata.

Some of these procedures are beyond the scope of this book, but those which can be considered minor surgical procedures are included under the following headings:

- removal of skin lesions (Figs 42.30–42.61)

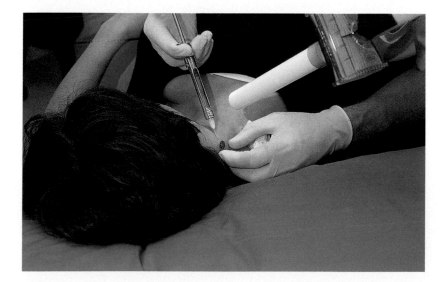

Figure 42.30 Removal of pigmented naevus on neck. Stage 1: injection of the base with local anaesthetic.

Figure 42.31 Removal of pigmented naevus on neck. Stage 2: moistening the lesion with water or saline.

Figure 42.32 Removal of pigmented naevus on neck. Stage 3: removing the lesion using a wire-loop and forceps.

Figure 42.33 Removal of pigmented naevus on neck. Stage 4: planing down the base flush with surrounding skin.

Figure 42.34 Removal of pigmented naevus on neck. Stage 5: specimen ready to put in histology pot.

Figure 42.35 Removal of intradermal naevus with the tungsten wire-loop electrode.

Figure 42.36 Patient with multiple pigmented intradermal melanocytic naevi on the face.

Figure 42.37 Each naevus is marked with a skin pen.

Figure 42.38 Immediately after removal with the wire-loop electrode.

Figure 42.39 The same patient as in Fig. 42.38, 6 weeks later.

Figure 42.40 Patient with fibroepithelial polyp on the chin and two intradermal naevi on the face.

Figure 42.41 The same patient as in Fig. 42.40, 6 weeks later.

Figure 42.42 A common site for intradermal naevus (photograph by courtesy of Dr Sheldon Pollack).

Figure 42.43 Removal with the wire-loop electrode (photograph by courtesy of Dr Sheldon Pollack).

Figure 42.44 The same patient as in Fig. 42.43, 3 months later (photograph by courtesy of Dr Sheldon Pollack).

Figure 42.45 Pigmented melanocytic naevus on the upper lip (photograph by courtesy of Dr Randolph Waldman).

Figure 42.46 The same patient as in Fig. 42.45, 3 months later (photograph by courtesy of Dr Randolph Waldman).

Figure 42.47 Patient with actinic keratosis on the right of the face; marking with a skin pen.

Figure 42.48 The same patient as in Fig. 42.47; infiltrating the base with local anaesthetic.

Figure 42.49 Removal of keratosis with a wire-loop electrode.

Figure 42.50 The same patient as in Fig. 42.49, 4 weeks later.

Figure 42.51 Two darkly pigmented seborrhoeic warts on the abdomen.

Figure 42.52 The same patient immediately after removal of warts with a wire-loop electrode.

Figure 42.53 (a) Possible squamous cell carcinoma; preliminary marking of the margin to be excised. (b) Starting the incision using the vari-tip needle electrode.

Figure 42.54 (a) Excising the lesion using the needle electrode; note the absence of bleeding. (b) Note also the sharp edges to the wound which will simplify subsequent suturing.

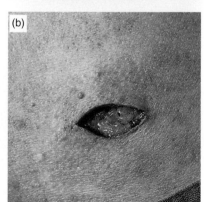

Figure 42.55 Conventional suturing of the wound after excision.

Figure 42.56 Wire-loop excision of seborrhoeic keratosis at back of neck; too much pressure is being applied, resulting in a deep cut.

Figure 42.57 The cut is too deep in this case; these lesions are very superficial and only need 'planing' off.

Figure 42.58 The same patient as in Fig. 42.57, 3 weeks later; the wound will heal eventually and will be acceptable, but better results would have been obtained with a shallower cut.

Figure 42.59 Wire-loop too small and cut too deep.

Figure 42.60 Intradermal naevus on the left cheek.

Figure 42.61 Minor bleeding may be controlled by pressure from a swab soaked in 20% aluminium chloride (Driclor) or Monsell's solution.

■ treatment of ingrowing toe-nails (Figs 42.62–42.67)
■ telangectasia and thread veins (Figs 42.68 and 42.69).

42.12 RADIOSURGERY IN CONJUNCTION WITH CRYOSURGERY

Excellent cosmetic results can be achieved with radiosurgery alone, but even better results may sometimes be obtained if the area treated by radiosurgery is sprayed with liquid nitrogen immediately postoperatively.

The rationale behind this is, first, to blend the edges of the wound and make for a smoother junction between healthy and treated skin and, secondly, when treating lesions such as basal cell carcinoma, squamous cell carcinoma and intraepithelial carcinoma (Bowen's disease) any microscopic spread by neoplastic cells may be destroyed.

In practice, the lesion is marked with a skin pen, removed or destroyed using the radiosurgical electrode, any bleeding vessels are coagulated using the ball-ended electrode, and the base is then frozen using liquid nitrogen cryospray, extending the freezing to 1 or 2 mm beyond the edge of the wound.

Healing will then be a combination of the effects of radio-surgery and freezing.

42.13 INTRADERMAL NAEVI

Some of the most impressive results of radiosurgery are with the removal of intradermal naevi and other similar lesions. Because the amount of thermal damage is so slight, remarkable cosmetic results can be obtained (Figs 42.30–42.61 and 42.73–42.75).

A wire loop electrode is used, and this should be held at right-angles to the skin. A smooth, light action is required with no pressure.

42.13.1 Technique

1. The edges of the naevus are marked with a skin marker pen (Fig. 42.37).
2. Lignocaine is infiltrated beneath and around the base of the naevus using a 30 swg needle and dental syringe.
3. The antenna plate electrode is positioned near the lesion; skin contact is not necessary.
4. The unit is switched on and allowed to warm up.
5. The power setting is turned to 2, on 'cut' or 'cut and coagulate'.
6. The assistant should have a histology pot available, with 10% formol saline in which to preserve the specimen, and also have the vacuum extractor ready for use.
7. The naevus is moistened with a small gauze swab soaked in water.
8. Holding the wire loop electrode at right-angles to the lesion, the doctor makes one or two practice strokes to ensure accuracy and avoidance of shakes or unwanted movements.
9. The power is switched on using the foot switch or fingertip control.
10. The wire loop is passed smoothly through the lesion (Fig. 42.35). If sticking occurs, the power may be increased; if sparking occurs, it should be reduced.
11. The specimen is placed in the histology pot and labelled.
12. The remainder of the lesion is trimmed using small, smooth strokes, wiping any charred debris away from the base of the lesion with a moist gauze swab. Finally, the edges are 'feathered' to blend with adjacent skin.
13. If any bleeding vessels are noticed, they may be sealed with the ball-ended electrode at setting 3 on 'coagulation' (partially rectified).

14. If mild oozing occurs, a cotton bud swab soaked in 20% aluminium chloride in spirit is applied (Fig. 42.61). Since this is inflammable the electrode must not be reapplied.
15. A small 'spot' plaster may be applied, or the lesion left exposed to the air.

42.13.2 Postoperative care

Various regimes have been advocated for the postoperative management of lesions treated with radiosurgery. The aim is to prevent infection and to keep the area relatively moist to accelerate healing. Small lesions are probably best left exposed to the air and frequently washed with warm soapy water using cotton wool, taking care not to rub the surface too vigorously in case it causes bleeding from capillaries. Larger or deeper wounds are probably best covered with non-adherent dressing and antibiotic ointment, changing every other day or more frequently if there is much discharge. Any signs of spreading infection should be promptly treated with systemic antibiotics as well as topical antibiotics. A patient information sheet given at the end of the operation helps to remind the patient how to look after the wound (Chapter 50).

42.14 INGROWING TOE-NAILS (Figs 42.62–42.65)

Excellent results have been reported using radiosurgery to ablate the germinal epithelium, and cure rates in excess of 98% have been reported.

The technique is basically identical to nail matrix phenolization (Chapter 30), but instead of destroying the germinal epithelium with phenol the matrix is destroyed electrically. This is achieved by using a specially designed matrixectomy electrode which is insulated on one side to protect the overlying eponychium (Fig. 42.62).

Figure 42.62 Selection of electrodes for ingrowing toe-nails.

42.14.1 Technique

1. Some doctors prefer to use a tourniquet and a bloodless field, while others prefer not to use a tourniquet. As the radiowave will coagulate any bleeding vessels, a tourniquet is certainly not essential.
2. A ring block of local anaesthetic is performed and the antenna plate is placed under the leg.
3. Using a pair of Thwaites nail nippers, stitch scissors or a scalpel blade, a thin strip of nail including the nail base on the affected side is removed.
4. Any granulations are removed with a sharp-spoon Volkmann curette.
5. The nail matrixectomy electrode is now inserted its full length so that the exposed part lies next to the germinal epithelium and the insulated part lies under the eponychium (Figs 42.63–42.65).
6. The power dial is set at '3' on 'partially rectified' (coagulation).
7. The current is applied for 2–4 s and the electrode is then slowly withdrawn over the next 5 s. Better results are obtained if the metal side of the electrode is raised slightly away from the nail matrix rather than pressing firmly against it.
8. Normally bleeding is not a problem.
9. A dressing of Bactigras or similar non-adherent material is applied, with or without triple antibiotic cream, depending on the degree of preoperative infection.
10. Where there is any significant preoperative infection, it is advisable to give the patient systemic antibiotics as well as topical applications.
11. The first postoperative dressing is done on the third day, and thereafter at approximately weekly intervals until fully healed.
12. The patient is seen again at 3 months to ensure that there has been no regrowth of nail.
13. Where there have been granulations and infection alongside the nail, some doctors spray these with liquid nitrogen followed by a strong steroid and antibiotic ointment and a final dressing.

Figure 42.63   The nail matrixectomy electrode.

Figure 42.64   Diagram showing placement of the electrode with the insulated side uppermost beneath the eponychium and the metal side face downwards, in proximity to but not pressing against the germinal epithelium.

Figure 42.65   The nail matrixectomy electrode in use.

Figure 42.66 Total nail-bed ablation with phenol 3 months previously; note the small spicule of nail regrowing at the edge.

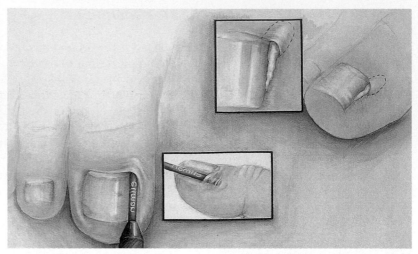

Figure 42.67 Diagram showing the use of the nail spicule electrode.

42.15 RECURRENT 'SPICULES' OF NAIL

1. Occasionally, a small 'spicule' of nail regrows despite what appeared to be a matrixectomy (Fig. 42.66). These can occur whatever the original method of matrix destruction.
2. A specially designed spicule electrode is available to deal with this situation. It comprises a Teflon-insulated shaft and a small, pointed metal electrode at the end (Fig. 42.67). After removal of the spicule under local anaesthesia, the 'spicule' electrode is inserted under the eponychium down to the germinal epithelium, and the offending matrix destroyed using the partially rectified (coagulation) current waveform at setting '2' for 5 s. To be absolutely sure of success, it is helpful to wait 15 s for the tissues to cool and then repeat the treatment.
3. Postoperative dressings are the same as for matrixectomy.

42.16 TELANGIECTASIA AND THREAD VEINS
(Figs 42.68 and 42.69)

Spider naevi and thread veins can be obliterated very successfully using radiosurgery. The technique is quick, simple and easy to learn, and gives excellent results.

42.16.1 Materials and method

1. The radiosurgical unit is set to partially rectified (coagulation).
2. The power setting is between 'low' and '1'.
3. A fine 30 swg needle is attached to the hand-piece and, if necessary, bent to an angle of 45°. Alternatively, the specially designed insulated shaft needles may be used.
4. With the patient in a comfortable position, the foot switch is continuously depressed and each telangectasis is lightly touched or 'tapped' along its course (Fig. 42.69).

Figure 42.68 Telangiectasia on the side of the nose (photograph by courtesy of Dr Lewis Kaminester, Florida).

Figure 42.69 (a) Needle electrode being used to treat telangiectasia (photograph by courtesy of Dr Lewis Kaminester, Florida). (b) Postoperative result (photograph by courtesy of Dr Lewis Kaminester, Florida).

5. Any bleeding points can be treated with a cotton-wool bud soaked in 20% aluminium chloride in spirit (remembering that this is inflammable) or Monsell's solution.
6. More than one treatment session may be required.
7. Thread veins are dealt with in the same manner.
8. In general, facial telangiectasia respond better to radiosurgery than do the thread veins found on the lower limbs.

42.17 EPILATION

Radiosurgery is very effective for epilation. Fine, insulated needle electrodes are best (Fig. 42.70). The needle is inserted to the hair root, parallel to the hair, and the waveform set to the partially rectified (coagulation) lowest setting, 0–1. Gentle traction on the hair will free it.

Figure 42.70 Diagram showing insulated needle electrode for epilation.

Figure 42.71 Patient with rhinophyma suitable for treatment with radiosurgery.

42.18 RHINOPHYMA

This distressing condition (Fig. 42.71) can now be very effectively treated using radiosurgery and the large wire loop electrode. Local infiltration anaesthesia may be employed and successive layers of excess tissue planed off. Any troublesome bleeding vessels can be coagulated using the ball-ended electrode and partially rectified waveform. Following planing and coagulation, the raw area and adjacent margins may be treated with liquid nitrogen cryospray for 15–20 s.

42.19 XANTHELASMATA

These can be treated either by fulguration using a very fine spark, or by coagulation using the ball-ended electrode. Larger lesions can be planed off using the fully rectified (cut and coagulation) waveform and a wire loop. As they are very superficial, only minimal treatment is needed.

42.20 SEBORRHOEIC KERATOSES

These are generally very superficial and only light 'planing' is needed. The wire loop electrode at power setting 2–3 on fully rectified (cut and coagulation) gives very good results. It is important to keep the keratosis moistened during treatment. Some dermatologists also give the base a freeze with liquid nitrogen cryospray immediately after radiosurgery.

Figure 42.72 Diagram showing the use of radiosurgery for vasectomy.

Figure 42.73 Raised intradermal naevus on upper lid margin. Very suitable for radio surgery (photograph by courtesy of Dr Chedly Bououaya, Tunisia).

Figure 42.74 Diagram showing removal of a naevus from the the eyelid using a loop electrode. Note the protective plastic eye-shield to prevent any damage to the cornea (photograph by courtesy of Dr Chedly Bououaya, Tunisia).

Figure 42.75 Postoperative result (photograph by courtesy of Dr Chedly Bououaya, Tunisia).

42.21 CERVICAL DYSPLASIA

For those doctors trained in colposcopy and the treatment of cervical intraepithelial neoplasia, radiosurgery using the specially designed wire loop electrodes offers a very quick and efficient method of removing suspicious areas of cervix, by the LLETZ technique (large loop excision of the transformation zone) or LEEP (loop electrosurgical excision procedure). A good vacuum extraction system is needed. Any troublesome bleeding can be controlled using the ball-ended electrode and partially rectified (coagulation) waveform. For full details of this technique the reader should refer to a textbook of gynaecology.

42.22 VASECTOMY

Radiosurgery can be used for both cutting and coagulation in vasectomy (Fig. 42.72).

42.23 MISCELLANEOUS OTHER USES FOR RADIOSURGERY

Radiosurgery is also widely used in dentistry, plastic and reconstructive surgery, ear, nose and throat and ophthalmology, and is not covered in this book. The reader who wishes to learn these techniques is advised to refer to the relevant papers or textbooks.

CHAPTER 43

Miscellaneous minor surgical procedures

To draw out splinters
Incence, Dough, Sea-salt, Wasp's Dung, Fat, Red-lead and Wax,
Apply thereto: it draws the matter out.

Ebers Papyrus, 1500 BC

43.1 SUBUNGUAL HAEMATOMA

This is extremely painful because of the pressure of trapped blood underneath the nail. Release of the blood results in an immediate relief of pain. One of the simplest methods is to rest the electrocautery V tip against the nail, switch on the current, and allow the wire to burn a small hole through the nail. As the nail itself is devoid of any nerve endings, the procedure is totally painless, provided undue pressure is not applied to the nail by the cautery. Once all the blood is released, the hole may be sealed with collodion or clear nail varnish, and allowed to grow out (Figs 43.1–43.5). An even neater hole may be produced by using the cold-point electrocautery burner.

Figure 43.1 Subungual haematoma.

Figure 43.2 A fine-pointed electrocautery burner is rested against the nail.

Figure 43.3 No anaesthetic is required and the blood is released.

Figure 43.4 The residual hole is allowed to grow out. When dry, it may be sealed with clear nail varnish.

Figure 43.5 . An even neater hole may be made using a cold-point electrocautery burner.

43.2 REMOVAL OF SUBUNGUAL SPLINTERS

These can be extremely painful, as can any attempts at removal. It may help to leave the splinter for 2 days, during which slight suppuration will occur, loosening the splinter and making subsequent removal easier.

Many splinters may be removed under Entonox analgesia. The patient takes 20 deep breaths of the gas and most splinters may then be removed painlessly. Alternatively, the digit may be anaesthetized by performing a digital nerve or ring block with or without a rubber-strip tourniquet. The splinter is then grasped with a pair of splinter forceps or straight Halstead's mosquito forceps and removed. Very deeply embedded splinters may sometimes be removed by using a 21 swg (0.8 mm) needle which has had the point bent backwards to form a hooked barb.

43.3 SMALL SCALP LESIONS

Where a suture is judged inappropriate, small scalp lacerations can be closed by twisting a few hairs on either side of the wound and knotting them together over the centre of the laceration. To prevent the knots slipping undone, they should be sprayed with tinct. benz. co., Whitehead's varnish, collodion or Nobecutane. Thereafter, the knot is left to grow out or is cut out after 10 days. Alternatively, the wound may be closed using a cyanoacrylic tissue adhesive (Histoacryl or Dermabond) (Chapter 11).

43.4 XANTHELASMATA

These may be treated with topical applications of monochloroacetic acid or pure liquefied phenol BPC. Great care is needed to avoid accidental burns to the eye or surrounding skin, and repeated small applications are preferred (Figs 43.6 and 43.7).

Other treatments include cauterization using the unipolar diathermy (Hyfrecator) electrocautery, freezing with the cryoprobe or infrared coagulation with a sapphire interface.

43.5 REMOVAL OF FOREIGN BODIES IN EARS AND NOSES

Young children frequently insert small pieces of rubber, paper, plastic, peas and nuts, etc., into the nostrils and ears. If not noticed at the time, the first symptom may be a unilateral, offensive, blood-stained discharge. Examination of the nose or ear with an auriscope reveals the cause and the offending object may usually be removed with a pair of Tilley's aural forceps. Foreign bodies in ears may be difficult to

Figure 43.6 Typical shallow xanthelasmata, suitable for treatment with monochloroacetic acid.

Figure 43.7 More prominent xanthelasmata, also very near the inner canthus of the eye. Great care is needed if treatment is judged to be necessary.

grasp, and may be more conveniently syringed out using an ear syringe and warm water. Steel ball-bearings may need a powerful ophthalmic electromagnet for removal.

43.6 STONE IN THE SALIVARY DUCT

Obstruction to a salivary gland by a calculus in the duct gives a classical picture of intermittent swelling of the gland whenever the patient attempts to eat. If the calculus can be felt with the examining finger, a small bleb of local anaesthetic is injected and a suture placed deeply behind the stone, which serves to steady the duct and also prevents the stone slipping into the hilum of the gland. An incision in the long axis of the duct is made over the stone, which may then be easily lifted out. The suture is removed and no further treatment is needed.

43.7 EAR-LOBE CYSTS

These are particularly common and troublesome, occurring more frequently in young male patients. Many of the cysts become infected and discharge spontaneously. Treatment consists of either dissecting the cyst free after infiltrating the area with local anaesthetic, or incising the cyst, expressing the contents, and cauterizing the lining of the cyst with a small cotton-wool swab applicator soaked in pure liquefied phenol.

If the doctor possesses a pair of chalazion ring forceps, these are ideal for holding the ear-lobe and fixing the cyst. The introduction of fucidic acid gel into the cavity before closure enables healing by primary intention to occur.

43.8 HAEMANGIOMA OF THE LIP

These lesions are relatively common, and may be readily treated by electrocautery, diathermy, cryotherapy or photocoagulation. After preliminary infiltration with local anaesthetic, the needle of the Hyfrecator or electrocautery is inserted into the centre of the haemangioma; more than one treatment may be necessary to obtain a good cosmetic result (Figs 43.8–43.10).

Figure 43.8 (a) Haemangioma on the lower lip; easily treated with electrocautery or the Hyfrecator. (b) Haemangioma on the upper lip.

Figure 43.9 Needle of the Hyfrecator inserted in the centre of a haemangioma.

Figure 43.10 Appearance immediately following fulguration with the Hyfrecator.

43.9 SKIN GRAFTING

Small skin grafts may be performed in the general practitioner's (GP's) surgery, usually to treat skin loss following accidents. Tips of fingers are the most common site; if only a small piece of skin has been lost, grafting is unnecessary, but if the complete tip of the digit has been removed, a pinch-skin graft may be attempted.

A donor site is chosen, usually the thigh or arm, and after preliminary infiltration, the chosen piece of skin excised. This is then carefully sutured in place over the injured digit, a tulle-gras dressing applied, and a firm, dry sterile gauze dressing applied and left in place for at least a week.

43.10 NASAL POLYPI

These may be removed with a wire snare; often they are multiple and are situated in inaccessible sites, but if the doctor is fortunate enough to see a solitary nasal polyp situated near the entrance, it can be snared off after preliminary topical local anaesthesia. Bleeding can be brisk, but usually stops spontaneously. Good illumination, preferably a spotlight and a head-mirror, is essential.

43.11 CONGENITAL EXTRA DIGITS

Most extra digits are inherited, and may be removed easily at birth either by tying a braided silk suture around the base, or preferably using the electrocautery (Figs 43.11–43.14).

Figure 43.11   Baby with an extra 'thumb'.

Figure 43.12   Thread may be tied around the base, or alternatively the digit may be removed immediately with the electrocautery.

Figure 43.13   After 2 weeks, the extra digit begins to separate.

Figure 43.14   The end-result, 4 weeks later.

43.12 ACCESSORY AURICLES

Accessory auricles or preauricular skin tags or polypi may be removed either by tying a braided silk suture around the base, or by excision and suturing, occasionally using the electrocautery or with radiosurgery (Figs 43.15–43.18).

Figure 43.15   An accessory auricle.

Figure 43.16   Thread may be tied round the base, or alternatively the papilloma may be removed immediately with the electrocautery.

Figure 43.17 Accessor auricle too broad to tie off.

Figure 43.18 Accessor auricle excised under local anaesthetic.

43.13 SUPERNUMERARY NIPPLES

Many patients suffer considerable embarrassment by the presence of supernumerary nipples but feel that their problem is too trivial to consider treatment. Excision is simple, effective and quick, and may be performed under local infiltration anaesthesia (see Intradermal lesions, Chapter 22, and Incisions, Chapter 10), paying particular attention to the direction of the ultimate scar.

43.14 REMOVAL OF PACEMAKER

One prerequisite before cremation can be authorized is the removal of any cardiac pacemakers or implants, and the GP may be asked to do this by the undertaker or relatives (Fig. 43.19). A simple suture pack is all that is required (Chapter 2). An incision is made over the pacemaker, which may be easily removed, together with the flexible wire electrode. The skin is then closed with interrupted sutures or adhesive tape.

Figure 43.19 Typical site for cardiac pacemaker.

43.15 FOREIGN-BODY REMOVAL UTILIZING A BLOODLESS FIELD

The removal of small pieces of glass or metal can be extremely difficult if the operating field is covered with blood. Attempts to locate or remove such objects usually provoke further bleeding. It tends to be forgotten that a bloodless operating area can be obtained in any limb or digit by the use of a rubber tourniquet.

Any injection of local anaesthetic, either infiltration, digital nerve block or ring block, should be given first and the injured site then covered with a dry dressing or small ring pad if fragments of glass are likely to be embedded. A rubber-strip or Esmarch bandage may then be applied to exsanguinate the part, and a tourniquet applied. In the case of digits, this can be a thin rubber tube and artery forceps, while limbs should have a pneumatic tourniquet applied. The absence of bleeding then enables the doctor to locate and remove any fragments of glass or metal more easily.

43.16 CIRCUMCISION

The majority of boys should have fully retractile foreskins by the age of 4 years. Where recurrent attacks of balanitis have occurred, or where there is a marked phimosis or paraphimosis, circumcision may be considered.

General anaesthesia is normally used, but where this is unavailable or contraindicated, local infiltration using 1% plain lignocaine may be used, forming a ring block around the base of the penis.

Under anaesthesia, the foreskin should be retracted fully if possible and the glans cleaned with a moist swab. Using fine, straight mosquito forceps the tip of the foreskin is grasped, and dorsal and ventral midline cuts are made using straight scissors up to within 5 mm of the coronal sulcus. Next, using curved scissors, the foreskin is trimmed parallel to the sulcus, also leaving a margin of 5 mm.

Figure 43.20 Circumcision; dissection method. (a) Dorsal slit. (b)The prepuce is trimmed parallel with the coronal sulcus. (c) All bleeding points are ligated and the deep skin layer is trimmed. (d) Skin closure.

Figure 43.21 The 'three-in-one' fraenal stitch.

Any bleeding points can be secured using 4/0 catgut or Dexon, and the skin edges sutured using interrupted 4/0 Dexon or similar absorbable suture. Finally, the stitch line is sprayed with Nobecutane spray or painted with tinct. benz. co. and a dry gauze swab applied (Fig. 43.20).

It is important not to damage the urethra, and unipolar diathermy is not recommended to control bleeding because of the risk of vascular thrombosis. It is also important to arrange postoperative supervision, to check regularly for any postoperative bleeding. This can arise from the fraenal artery and may be picked up in a special three-in-one stitch (Fig. 43.21).

43.17 REMOVAL OF FISH-HOOKS

During the fishing season, patients may be seen with fish-hooks embedded in various parts of their anatomy. Attempts by the patient to remove the hook usually fail because of the barb. If a pair of strong wirecutters is available, the eye of the hook should be cut off, and then with a needle holder or artery forceps, the hook pushed through the skin and removed (Figs 43.22–43.24).

43.18 PINCH-GRAFTS TO VARICOSE ULCERS

Every doctor and every nurse has one or two 'heart-sink' patients with varicose ulcers which stubbornly fail to heal. Occasionally, in suitable patients, pinch-grafts will heal such ulcers and are well worth trying.

Before attempting grafting, the base of the ulcer should be clean, granulating, free from infection as much as possible, and fairly shallow. To this end, Inadine non-stick dressing applied directly to the ulcer under gauze and pressure bandages, changed frequently if necessary, will ensure optimum grafting conditions.

Figure 43.22 A fish-hook embedded in the cheek, complete with maggot.

Figure 43.23 One end of the hook is cut off with wire-cutters.

Figure 43.24 The hook may now be pushed through and removed.

The donor site is normally the upper outer thigh. An area is chosen and anaesthetized. This may be by infiltration, but a simple method of anaesthetizing the skin is by the use of EMLA cream under waterproof occlusion. This is applied 2 h before the grafting.

Pinch-skin grafts are taken as follows. Using a 21 swg needle, a small piece of skin is picked up and cut off using a scalpel. This is then laid on the ulcer. Similar 'islands' of skin are prepared until the ulcer is covered with small pieces of skin, spaced about 5 mm apart or less (Figs 43.25–43.28).

Figure 43.25 Chronic, painful varicose ulcer defying attempts to heal it.

Figure 43.26 The doctor aims to clean the ulcer and encourage granulations in the base.

Figure 43.27 The ulcer, treated with inadine dressings, ready for pinch-grafting.

Figure 43.28 Islands of skin taken from the thigh are laid evenly over the ulcer.

A dressing of Inadine (povidone–iodine in non-stick base) is carefully placed over the grafted area, taking care not to dislodge the grafts (Fig. 43.29). A layer of sterile gamgee or multiple layers of gauze are then applied, covered by an elastocrepe bandage, which in turn is covered by an elasticated tubular bandage (Tubigrip E or F). The donor site (Fig. 43.30) is covered with a similar dressing.

The grafted area is left undisturbed for up to 2 weeks: the absence of pain is a promising sign that epithelialization is occurring. After 2 weeks the dressing is changed and another applied. When successful, the ulcer is found to be healed after 6 weeks (Fig. 43.31).

Figure 43.29 These are covered with Inadine dressing and bandaged firmly in place.

Figure 43.30 The donor sites on the thigh. These are covered with non-stick dressing.

Figure 43.31 The healed ulcer, 6 weeks later (it remained healed for 2 years, then there was a small recurrence).

43.19 SPIDER NAEVI

These vascular lesions are quite common in children and young adults. They may be solitary or multiple and are due to a cutaneous arteriole feeding a leash of fine blood vessels radiating from the centre.

Treatment consists of sealing the feeding arteriole. This may most conveniently be done using the cold-point electrocautery.

The needle of the cold-point burner is rested against the centre of the spider naevus and gentle pressure applied. If correctly positioned, the naevus will blanch and disappear. By resting the needle against this arteriole and switching on the current, a localized burn in the skin occurs.

No anaesthetic is used, and the procedure takes less than 1 second, and is extremely successful (Fig. 43.32), (see Chapter 16). Radio-surgery ablation of the feeding arteriole is also very successful using a needle electrode and a low setting (Chapter 42).

Figure 43.32   Spider naevus being treated with the cold-point electrocautery burner; no anaesthetic is used and the central arteriole blanches when pressure is gently applied.

In the absence of a cold-point burner, a conventional ∧-shaped platinum wire burner or the needle electrode of the Hyfrecator diathermy may be used; alternatively, the centre may be touched with a sharpened wooden applicator dipped in monochloroacetic acid.

43.20 BIOPSY OF THE TEMPORAL ARTERY (Figs 43.33 and 43.34)

Polymyalgia rheumatica and temporal arteritis are relatively common in the elderly. Untreated, temporal arteritis may be followed by sudden loss of vision, which is permanent and occurs without warning. Systemic steroids give dramatic results and prevent the onset of blindness.

Superficial temporal artery

Figure 43.33   Temporal artery; anatomy.

Figure 43.34   Temporal artery; biopsy.

The diagnosis is usually made on clinical findings plus a markedly raised erythrocyte sedimentation rate (ESR), but occasionally the diagnosis is not straightforward and it may be helpful to biopsy a branch of the superficial temporal artery. As these vessels lie above the deep fascia on the temporalis muscle, they are easily palpated.

43.20.1 The operation

Any overlying hair is shaved, and the area painted with povidone–iodine in spirit and infiltrated with 1% or 2% lignocaine with added adrenaline 1:80 000. An incision is made over the artery, in a skin crease line. If possible the edge of the wound is retracted, either by an assistant or by using a small self-retaining retractor.

By blunt dissection using a pair of curved Halstead's mosquito forceps, the artery is freed, and two ligatures of 3/0 coated Vicryl are applied, spaced 1.5 cm apart. The isolated segment of artery is carefully excised and placed immediately in a histology pot with 10% formol-saline.

The wound is then closed with interrupted 4/0 monofilament Nylon sutures and sprayed with Nobecutane spray. No other dressing is required.

43.21 DIVISION OF TONGUE-TIE

Where a very tight fraenum is preventing the tongue from protruding to its full length, and particularly if it is thought to be interfering with the development of speech, it may be easily divided using the electro-cautery or radiosurgical unit. Any bleeding points can normally be sealed with the cautery or coagulation tip of the radiosurgical electrode, and it is not normally necessary to suture the divided edges.

43.21.1 The operation

Fifteen minutes before the operation, the patient (usually a child) is asked to apply 4% topical lignocaine on a cotton-wool swab to the underneath part of the tongue, and to keep repeating the application to anaesthetize the fraenum. Using a dental syringe and 30 swg needle, a small quantity (1 ml) of lignocaine is infiltrated into the area at either end of the fraenum to supplement the topical anaesthesia. Using a gauze swab, the tongue is held with the operator's left hand and drawn upwards to stretch the fraenum.

With the C28 cordless electrocautery and ring cutter electrode, or radiosurgical unit and diamond wire loop electrode and cutting and coagulation waveform, the fraenum is carefully divided. Any bleeding vessels are sealed using the ball-ended electrode (Figs 43.35 and 43.36).

Postoperatively, the patient is instructed to keep the mouth clean with frequent mouth rinses, and healing occurs rapidly over the next few days.

Figure 43.35 Typical tongue-tie showing tight fraenum.

Figure 43.36 Fraenum divided using either electrocautery or radiowave surgery.

43.22 CHONDRODERMATITIS HELICIS CHRONICUS (Figs 43.37 and 43.38)

This is a common, painful nodule arising on the edge of the ear. The patient finds it is painful to lie on it when in bed.

Intralesional injection of triamcinolone using a dental syringe and a 30 swg needle sometimes effects a cure, as does careful use of liquid nitrogen cryosurgery.

Where these two methods fail, wedge excision and suture is the treatment of choice. Closure is with the finest monofilament Prolene sutures (6/0 or finer), which are removed after 7 days and the edges held together with skin adhesive strips for another 7 days.

Figure 43.37 A typical lesion of chondrodermatitis helicis chronicus.

Figure 43.38 This looks similar to chondrodermatitis helicis chronicus but there are two areas of actinic keratosis, both of which cleared with liquid nitrogen.

CHAPTER 44

Resuscitation

Every hospital and doctor's surgery should have facilities for giving emergency resuscitation for the 'collapsed' patient, and a basic knowledge of first aid and cardiopulmonary resuscitation is essential for members of the staff working in these premises.

The combined manual of first aid produced by the St John Ambulance Association, the St Andrew's Ambulance Association and British Red Cross Society is excellent. A patient who has collapsed at the surgery may be suffering from any of the following:

- a vasovagal attack (faint)
- profound vasovagal attack leading to a convulsion
- epileptic attack
- myocardial infarction
- allergic reaction to drugs administered
- anaphylactic reaction to drugs administered
- pulmonary embolism
- concealed haemorrhage
- cerebrovascular attack (stroke)
- acute psychiatric crisis
- cardiac arrest.

It is helpful to keep all resuscitation equipment together in one place, which is known to all members of the staff. The exact contents of any 'resuscitation kit' will vary depending on the preference of the doctors, but the following will provide a nucleus which can be supplemented with additional equipment if needed:

- a selection of plastic airways
- endotracheal tubes
- laryngoscope
- intravenous cannulae
- giving sets for intravenous fluids
- oxygen cylinders and giving sets
- suction apparatus
- positive-pressure inflator (Ambu)
- sphygmomanometer
- electrocardiogram machine or monitor

- cardiac defibrillator
- large selection of syringes and needles
- emergency drugs, intravenous fluids and plasma expanders.

44.1 THE VASOVAGAL ATTACK

This is undoubtedly the most common cause of collapse seen by the doctor. The patient may complain of not feeling well, and becomes pale, sweaty and anxious, with cold, clammy skin and a slow, imperceptible pulse. The patient is usually sitting or standing at the time, and if left in this position, will lose consciousness owing to cerebral ischaemia secondary to hypotension. It is a common accompaniment to injections or painful or unpleasant experiences and is usually self-limiting as consciousness returns as soon as the patient falls to the ground.

First-aid treatment consists of laying the patient on the floor and elevating the lower limbs to increase the venous return to the heart, watching the airway at the same time. Recovery is normally rapid. Because vasovagal attacks can occur in the most unexpected patients it is a good rule always to insist that the patient lies on the couch or operating-theatre table rather than be seated in a chair for any minor surgical procedure.

44.2 PROFOUND VASOVAGAL ATTACK LEADING TO CONVULSION

In this, the patient appears to faint, but then has a short epileptiform convulsion. Unlike a major epileptic fit, the patient recovers consciousness quickly and is able to resume his or her activities without any impairment. Treatment consists of laying the patient down and placing him or her in the recovery position. If the airway can be guarded, the patient may be placed on his or her back and the lower limbs elevated to hasten recovery of consciousness.

44.3 MAJOR EPILEPTIC CONVULSION

This may arise in a patient known to suffer from epilepsy or may occur without any previous history of attacks. If a solitary fit occurs, the patient should be placed in the recovery position and the airway guarded. Should multiple fits occur (status epilepticus) intravenous diazepam should be given and oxygen administered via a high-concentration mask.

44.4 MYOCARDIAL INFARCTION

A patient may suffer a myocardial infarction while in the doctor's surgery and immediate resuscitation may be life-saving. Nitrites and aspirin given immediately may reduce the severity of the infarction.

Oxygen should be given via a high-concentration face-mask, pain relieved by diamorphine or morphine, nausea by cyclizine and bradycardia by intravenous atropine. The early insertion of an intravenous cannula is valuable as it gives access to the circulation should subsequent collapse occur or should thrombolytic therapy be considered. Arrangements to transfer the patient to hospital should be made, and if possible electrocardiographic monitoring done, with cardiac defibrillation available should cardiac arrest occur.

44.5 ALLERGIC REACTION TO DRUGS ADMINISTERED

It is always wise to enquire from the patient whether he or she has any allergies or drug sensitivities, and beware of any interactions with drugs to be administered. Should a reaction occur, intravenous antihistamines and steroids should be administered, an intravenous cannula inserted, regular blood-pressure checks made and any shock corrected.

44.6 ANAPHYLACTIC REACTION

These are extremely rare, but very frightening when they occur. Sudden circulatory collapse occurs. The patient should be immediately placed on the floor or a couch, the legs elevated and adrenaline administered, together with intravenous steroids, antihistamines and fluid replacement. Oxygen and ventilation may be necessary. The expiry date for adrenaline must be checked regularly.

44.7 PULMONARY EMBOLISM

This may be very difficult to diagnose outside hospital. First-aid treatment consists of maintaining an airway, the administration of oxygen, the introduction of an intravenous cannula and urgent admission to hospital.

44.8 CONCEALED HAEMORRHAGE

This may arise from a bleeding duodenal ulcer or ruptured ectopic pregnancy, or following trauma from a ruptured liver, kidneys or spleen. The patient will be shocked, with a rising, rapid, feeble pulse and falling blood pressure. First-aid treatment aims to restore the blood volume by the insertion of an intravenous cannula and administration of plasma expanders after first taking blood for grouping and cross-matching.

44.9 CEREBROVASCULAR ATTACK

As with a myocardial infarction, any patient may suddenly develop a cerebrovascular attack while attending the doctor. The patient with a cerebral haemorrhage suddenly loses consciousness, may have localizing signs and may die within 48 h. The only first-aid treatment is the maintenance of an adequate airway and oxygen if necessary, with transfer to hospital. Occlusion of a cerebral artery from thrombosis or embolus may respond initially to rebreathing via a polythene bag. In this, a large polythene bag is placed over the nose and mouth and the patient requested to rebreathe until they find it uncomfortable. This allows the carbon dioxide levels in the lung to rise, giving cerebral vasodilatation. In addition, intravenous dexamethasone has been used to reduce intracranial oedema.

44.10 THE ACUTE PSYCHIATRIC CRISIS

This may manifest itself as hypomania, excitability, confusion, delusions or violence. There is usually a preceding history of psychiatric disturbance. First-aid treatment consists of reassurance and, if necessary, intravenous chlorpromazine or diazepam.

44.11 CARDIAC ARREST (Figs 44.1–44.7)

This is the most serious of all collapses. It may arise following a myocardial infarction, following fright or spontaneously with no obvious cause. It is diagnosed by an unconscious patient with absent pulses, and irregular, infrequent respirations which eventually stop. Following this, the pupils become widely dilated and fixed.

Figure 44.1 Cardiac defibrillator.

Figure 44.2 Cardiac defibrillator monitor and ECG machine.

Figure 44.3 CR5 cardiorater monitor.

Figure 44.4 A tripod chest electrode gives immediate tracings.

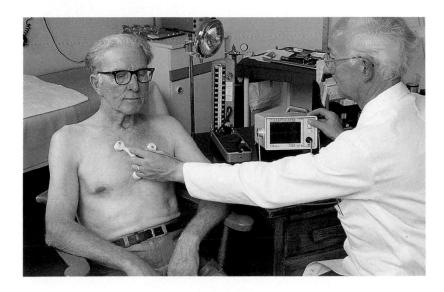

Figure 44.5 The use of the tripod electrode with cardiac monitor.

Figure 44.6 Contents of a simple 'cardiac arrest' box.

Figure 44.7 A comprehensive resuscitation kit which may be kept in the treatment room, or in the boot of the doctor's car for immediate use both at road-traffic accidents and in the patient's home (Laerdal Medical Ltd).

44.11.1 First-aid treatment

If an electrocardiographic monitor is immediately available and the cause is shown to be ventricular fibrillation, immediate cardiac defibrillation should be performed, giving a d.c. shock of up to 400 J and, repeating if necessary. Oxygen and endotracheal intubation should be instituted, together with the insertion of an intravenous cannula. Following successful defibrillation, intravenous lignocaine 100 mg and dexamethasone 5 mg should be given.

ECG

Electromechanical dissociation
QRS without palpable pulse

Ventricular fibrillation (VF)

Apparent asystole
isoelectric ECG

where VF can   where VF cannot
be excluded   be excluded

Adrenaline 1mg IV

Consider specific
therapy
for - hypovolaemia
    - pneumothorax
    - cardiac tamponade
    - pulmonary embolism

Consider calcium
chloride (10ml of 10%)
for - hyperkalaemia
    - hypocalcaemia
    - calcium antagonists

Defibrillate 200J

Defibrillate 200J

Defibrillate 360J

Adrenaline 1mg IV

Defibrillate 360J

Lignocaine 100mg IV

Repeated
defibrillations 360J

Consider - different paddle positions
         - different defibrillator
         - other antiarrhythmic drugs

Defibrillate 200J

Defibrillate 200J

Defibrillate 360J

Adrenaline 1mg IV

Atropine 2mg IV

Consider pacing
If P waves or any other
electrical activity present

**Continue CPR for up to 2 min. after each drug. Do not interrupt CPR
for more than 10 sec., except for defibrillation.
If an IV line cannot be established, consider giving double doses of
adrenaline, lignocaine or atropine via an endotracheal tube.**

PROLONGED RESUSCITATION
Give 1mg adrenaline IV every 5 minutes.
Consider 50mmol sodium bicarbonate (50 ml of 8.4%)
or according to blood gas results.

POST RESUSCITATION CARE
Check - arterial blood gases
      - electrolytes
      - chest X-ray
Observe monitor and treat patient
in an intensive care area.

Figure 44.8 Protocol for resuscitation
produced by the Resuscitation Council of the
UK 1984.

Severe bradycardia should be treated with intravenous atropine
300–600 µg while asystole should be treated with intravenous adrenaline 1 ml of 1:1000 to induce ventricular fibrillation, which can be
converted to sinus rhythm by d.c. defibrillation.

Acidosis is treated by intravenous sodium bicarbonate 8.4%
50–150 ml and cardiac failure by intravenous frusemide 20–40 mg.

Throughout all of these procedures, cardiopulmonary resuscitation
by mouth-to-mouth artificial respiration and external cardiac
compression should be maintained (Fig. 44.8).

Advanced minor surgery

In the following five chapters are described four additional operations – decompression of the carpal tunnel, release of trigger finger, excision of ganglion and stab avulsion of varicose veins – which are well within the capability of the experienced general practitioner surgeon but carry additional risks. These should therefore only be undertaken after the doctor has had personal tuition from a colleague and has done several under supervision before embarking on his or her own.

Chapter 49 concludes with two more complex anaesthetic techniques – caudal epidural and intravenous regional anaesthesia (Bier's block). There are few occasions when the average doctor will use either of these methods of anaesthesia, particularly intravenous regional blocks which carry considerable risks should the cuffs fail. However, if the practitioner is faced with a situation where either would be appropriate, the risks are fully understood, and the necessary backup and resuscitation facilities exist, then it is helpful to know the procedures.

In the first edition of *Minor Surgery* decompression of the carpal tunnel, excision of ganglion and release of trigger finger were all described using intravenous regional anaesthesia (Bier's block) which in itself carries a significant risk, and this was the reason why it was decided not to include these procedures in the second edition. However, it is perfectly possible to produce a bloodless anaesthetic area without resorting to intravenous regional blocks, so it has been decided to reintroduce them in this edition.

Stab avulsion of varicose veins is a relatively new technique which lends itself admirably to minor surgery provided, again, that the doctor has had personal tuition and has performed several under supervision.

All four operations are supplemented with a small intravenous 'premedication' injection of fentanyl and midazolam to reduce the awareness of the orthopaedic tourniquet in operations on the hand, and to reduce awareness of avulsing segments of veins in the leg. It is therefore essential that an assistant is present throughout the whole of the operation and that suitable resuscitation facilities are available, a benzodiazepine reverser is available, and ideally blood-oxygen monitoring should be carried out.

Given all these restraints, these operations are nevertheless some of the more rewarding to do, giving excellent results.

Decompression of the carpal tunnel

> She is woke up nightly by pains in the fingers, hands and up the fore-arms. The hands seem to become stiff and useless, and when she gets up – look, she says, as if they were dead. The pain is severe and prevents sleep. She connects her complaint with the use of water for scrubbing floors – she gave up her place as a servant on this account and her hands improved afterwards.
>
> *J. A. Ormerod, On a peculiar numbness and paresis of the hands, 1883*

Decompression of the median nerve in the carpal tunnel is now one of the most common operations on the hand, yet the first recorded carpal tunnel decompression was only carried out in 1941. The presenting symptoms are paraesthesia affecting the middle three fingers, with pain up the forearm. The patient is commonly a woman and the right hand is affected more than the left. Typically, the pain and 'pins and needles' wake the patient at night, and relief is obtained by shaking the arm and hanging it out of bed.

Confirmation of the diagnosis may be obtained by applying pressure over the carpal tunnel to reproduce the symptoms, by tapping the carpal tunnel or by acutely flexing the wrist for 1 min (Chapter 22).

If early warning symptoms are ignored, wasting of the thenar muscles occurs and, even if the nerve is subsequently decompressed, recovery of wasted muscle seldom recovers occurs (Fig. 45.1). It should

Figure 45.1 Untreated, compression of the median nerve may result in severe wasting of the thenar muscles.

be remembered that cervical nerve root entrapment at C7 level will also give pain in the hand and numbness of the middle finger, so it is important to check the neck at the time of the initial examination.

Non-surgical treatment consisting of splinting, diuretics and steroid injection is worth trying (Chapter 22). If a steroid injection relieves the symptoms which later recur, at least the doctor knows that decompression will work and can thus confidently recommend it.

Surgical decompression is a much simpler operation than is generally realized. A bloodless operating field is essential, so an orthopaedic tourniquet and Esmarch bandage are required. Likewise, complete aseptic operation conditions are mandatory: this means central sterile supplies department (CSSD) packs or autoclaving, gowns, masks and sterile surgical gloves.

45.1 INSTRUMENTS

The following instruments are required:

- Povidone–iodine in spirit (Betadine alcoholic solution)
- 1 dental syringe and 30 swg needle
- 1 cartridge local anaesthetic (without added adrenaline)
- 1 orthopaedic tourniquet
- 1 Esmarch bandage
- sterile pads, bandages and gauze
- 1 scalpel handle size 3
- 1 scalpel blade size 15
- 1 self-retaining retractor (West Weitlander or similar)
- 1 double-ended McDonald's dissector
- 1 stitch scissors
- 1 Kilner needle-holder 5¼ in. (13.3 cm)
- 1 pair fine-toothed Adson's dissecting forceps 4¾ in. (12 cm)
- 1 surgical suture 3/0 monofilament Nylon or Prolene on curved cutting needle
- skin closure strips 3M Ref. R1547 12 × 100 mm (1/2 × 4 in.)

Where the doctor requires a bloodless field and anaesthesia in a limb, a safer alternative to a Bier's block is to infiltrate the area with local anaesthesia and then to apply an orthopaedic tourniquet and Esmarch bandage. This is particularly effective for decompression of the carpal tunnel, release of trigger finger and exploration for foreign bodies.

45.2 TECHNIQUE FOR PRODUCING ANAESTHETIC BLOODLESS FIELD

1. Any rings are removed from fingers on the affected hand.
2. The procedure is explained in detail to the patient.
3. An intravenous 'premedication injection' of fentanyl 100 µg and midazolam 2–4 mg is given slowly over 1–2 min into a vein in the opposite arm. If an intravenous cannula is inserted at this stage

Figure 45.2 Infiltrating the line of the incision with local anaesthetic.

and taped in position, the doctor then has access to the circulation for the remainder of the operation. This would be valuable if the midazolam needed to be reversed.

4. The palmar surface of the hand and wrist is painted with povidone–iodine in spirit.
5. The line of the thenar crease is infiltrated with local anaesthetic (without added adrenaline) using a dental syringe and 30 swg needle (Fig. 45.2).
6. The skin is painted a second time with povidone–iodine in spirit and covered with a sterile pad.
7. The orthopaedic tourniquet is applied over a layer of cotton wool over the upper arm and bandaged in position.
8. The arm is raised, keeping the sterile pad in position over the palm, and the Esmarch bandage applied tightly from the fingertips to the lower edge of the orthopaedic tourniquet.
9. The tourniquet is pumped to above arterial pressure (approx. 300 mmHg)
10. The Esmarch bandage is unwound and the sterile pad removed.

45.3 THE OPERATION

The overlying skin is again painted with povidone–iodine in spirit (Betadine alcoholic solution) and a sterile drape placed over the area. As with excision of ganglion and release of trigger finger, full aseptic technique is employed: this means wearing sterile surgical gown, mask and gloves.

A skin incision is made in the thenar crease (Fig. 45.3); correctly placed it will be exactly between the thenar and hypothenar muscles, exactly over the median nerve. Self-retaining or individual handheld retractors are placed in the wound and opened to expose the underlying fatty tissues and dense fibrous transverse ligament (Fig. 45.4). The incision is cautiously deepened until the glistening median nerve is seen. At this stage, the McDonald's dissector (Fig. 45.5) is gently

Figure 45.3 The incision is made in the proximal palmar crease as shown.

Figure 45.4 A self-retaining retractor makes the operation much easier.

Figure 45.5 The McDonald's dissector is slipped under the retinaculum, in front of the nerve.

introduced below the transverse ligament and in front of the median nerve, and the ligament is divided by cutting down on the blade of the dissector which is protecting the nerve (Fig. 45.6). The median nerve may now be freed both proximally and distally with the aid of the McDonald's dissector, and particular note made of any branches to the thenar muscles or skin, which should be preserved (Figs 45.7 and 45.8).

When the operator is satisfied that the median nerve is no longer compressed within the carpal tunnel, the retractors may be removed

Figure 45.6 The McDonald's dissector is inserted in front of the median nerve to protect it, and the deep transverse ligament is divided using a no. 15 scalpel blade with the back of the blade resting against the McDonald's dissector.

Figure 45.7 With the McDonald's dissector protecting the nerve, the retinaculum is split with a small scalpel blade.

Figure 45.8 The median nerve is exposed; note what a large a structure it is.

Figure 45.9 The retractor may now be removed.

Figure 45.10 Skin closure is with a sub-cuticular monofilament Nylon or Prolene suture.

Figure 45.11 A subcuticular stitch gives a neat scar, and is quick to insert and easy to remove.

Figure 45.12 The scar 6 weeks later.

(Fig. 45.9) and the wound closed. Just the skin is sutured; either with interrupted 3/0 Prolene sutures, or a neater scar may be obtained by using a subcuticular monofilament polyamide 6 3/0 (metric gauge 2) suture, strengthened with adhesive skin closure strips Ref. 3M R1547 1/2 in. × 4 in. (12 × 100 mm) (Figs 45.10 and 45.11). Sterile gauze swabs are now folded in half and taped in position over the incision to act as a mild pressure dressing; these are then covered with cotton wool and a firm elastocrepe bandage. When applying the cotton wool, it is important to place it between all of the fingers.

The arm is now elevated, and the assistant applies pressure over the incision while the doctor releases the tourniquet. Pressure is maintained for at least 5 min; following this the arm is placed in a triangular sling with the palm of the operated hand on the opposite shoulder.

Assuming all is well, the dressing is left undisturbed until the 14th postoperative day when the sutures are removed, leaving the Steri-strips. A sterile dry dressing is reapplied over the strips and lightly bandaged and left in place for a further 4 days, by which time healing is complete (Fig. 45.12).

The patient usually obtains immediate relief of all symptoms. Occasionally, the condition may take several months to recover, and frequently there is a tender area underneath the scar which arises from the exposed nerve and likewise recovers gradually over several months; however, if any significant degree of muscle wasting has occurred, this does not usually recover.

Carpal tunnel syndrome, if diagnosed before irreversible damage to the nerve has occurred, is one of the most satisfactory conditions to treat surgically.

CHAPTER 46

Release of trigger finger

It seemed most likely that it was a thickening of the tendon sheath at a specific point. On March 7th 1894, I excised the common tunnel of extensor pollicis brevis over a length of one centimetre.

Fritz de Quervain, Concerning a Form of Chronic Tenovaginitis, 1868–1940

Trigger finger and trigger thumb (tenovaginitis stenosans and de Quervain's syndrome) are cause by a constriction of the flexor tendon sheath combined with a secondary localized thickening of the tendon. This results in difficulty in extending the joint, which often straightens suddenly with a palpable 'click'. Commonly, the constriction occurs in front of the metacarpophalangeal joint under the annular ligament. Relief may be obtained by injecting corticosteroid (methylprednisolonc acetate) into the sheath but, if the condition recurs, surgery is indicated.

A bloodless operating field is essential, and therefore an orthopaedic tourniquet and Esmarch bandage are required. Likewise, complete aseptic operation conditions are mandatory: this means central sterile supplies department (CSSD) packs or autoclaving, gowns, masks and sterile surgical gloves.

46.1 INSTRUMENTS

The following instruments are required:

- Povidone–iodine in spirit (Betadine alcoholic solution)
- 1 dental syringe and 30 swg needle
- 1 cartridge local anaesthetic (without added adrenaline)
- 1 orthopaedic tourniquet
- 1 Esmarch bandage
- sterile pads, bandages and gauze
- 1 scalpel handle size 3
- 1 scalpel blade size 15
- 1 self-retaining retractor (West Weitlander or similar)
- or 2 Kilner double-ended retractors (cat's paw retractors)
- 2 pair Halstead's mosquito artery forceps, curved 5 in. (12.7 cm)
- 1 double-ended McDonald's dissector
- 1 pair stitch scissors
- 1 Kilner needle-holder $5^{1}/_{4}$ in. (13.3 cm)
- 1 pair fine-toothed Adson's dissecting forceps $4^{3}/_{4}$ in. (12 cm)
- 1 surgical suture 4/0 monofilament Nylon or Prolene on curved cutting needle
- skin closure strips 3M Ref. GP 41, 6 × 75 mm

Where the doctor requires a bloodless field and anaesthesia in a limb, a safer alternative to a Bier's block is to infiltrate the area with local anaesthesia and then to apply an orthopaedic tourniquet and Esmarch bandage. This is particularly effective for decompression of the carpal tunnel, release of trigger finger and exploration for foreign bodies.

46.2 TECHNIQUE FOR PRODUCING ANAESTHETIC BLOODLESS FIELD

1. Any rings are removed from fingers on the affected hand.
2. The procedure is explained in detail to the patient.
3. An intravenous 'premedication injection' of fentanyl 100 µg and midazolam 2–4 mg is given slowly over 1–2 min into a vein in the opposite arm. If an intravenous cannula is inserted at this stage and taped in position for the duration of the operation, the doctor then has access to the circulation. This is valuable should the midazolam need to be reversed.
4. The palmar surface of the hand and wrist is painted with povidone–iodine in spirit.
5. The line of the distal palmar crease is infiltrated with local anaesthetic (without added adrenaline) using a dental syringe and 30 swg needle (Fig. 46.1).
6. The skin is painted a second time with povidone–iodine in spirit and covered with a sterile pad.
7. The orthopaedic tourniquet is applied over a layer of cotton wool over the upper arm, and bandaged in position.
8. The arm is raised, keeping the sterile pad in position over the palm, and the Esmarch bandage applied tightly from the fingertips to the lower edge of the orthopaedic tourniquet.
9. The tourniquet is pumped to above arterial pressure (approx. 300 mmHg).
10. The Esmarch bandage is unwound and the sterile pad removed.

Figure 46.1 The line of the distal palmar crease is infiltrated with local anaesthetic (without added adrenaline) using a dental syringe and 30 swg needle.

46.3 THE OPERATION

The overlying skin is liberally painted with povidone–iodine in spirit (Betadine alcoholic solution), a sterile drape is placed over the area and full aseptic precautions are observed. A surgical gown, mask and gloves should be worn.

A small transverse incision is made in the distal palmar crease for trigger fingers, and the proximal thumb crease for trigger thumb (Fig. 46.2).

The incision is deepened until the flexor sheath is exposed, taking care to avoid the digital nerves and blood vessels on either side. For this stage of the operation it is easier and safer to use curved fine artery forceps for dissection rather than scissors or scalpel (Fig. 46.3).

The proximal part of the annular ligament and tendon sheath is divided, and the patient is asked to move the fingers to demonstrate that any triggering has been released. It is preferable to leave the distal portion of the annular ligament, as troublesome bowing of the tendon can occur if this is divided. It is neither necessary nor desirable to remove any thickening of the tendon itself, for fear of subsequent weakening and spontaneous rupture.

Closure is by one subcuticular monofilament suture or interrupted sutures (Fig. 46.4) supplemented by skin closure strips.

A sterile dressing is applied over the incision, covered with cotton wool and an elastocrepe bandage, and the arm placed in a triangular sling with the affected hand on the opposite shoulder.

The dressing is left completely undisturbed until the suture is removed on the 10th postoperative day. The skin closure strips are left in place and the hand lightly bandaged for two more days, after which no restrictions need be imposed and the patient is encouraged to use the fingers as much as possible.

Figure 46.2 Small transverse incision in the distal palmar crease.

Figure 46.3 The incision is deepened using curved fine artery forceps.

Figure 46.4 Closure of the wound.

CHAPTER 47

Stab-avulsion varicose veins

Anatomy, types of varicose veins and sclerotherapy have been covered in Chapter 37 and, for the majority of veins below the knee, sclerotherapy still gives very good results. However, even better results can be achieved by the multiple stab avulsion technique by the purchase of just one additional instrument, namely, vein forceps (see Fig. 47.5a).

The principle of treatment is to make numerous small stab incisions along the course of the vein, and then to tease out segments of vein through these incisions. By grasping this vein with strong artery forceps it may be forcibly avulsed.

In effect one is 'stripping' the vein, but in small sections. The advantage over stripping is that irregular tributaries may be treated, and both long and short saphenous veins treated.

As with sclerotherapy, if there is any evidence of saphenofemoral incompetence, these patients should be referred for ligation in the groin. Failure to recognize this will result in a high recurrence rate and disappointed patients.

Normally, stab avulsions are done under general anaesthesia, but it is perfectly possible to perform them under local anaesthesia. Because the actual avulsion of the vein can be uncomfortable, an intravenous premedication injection of midazolam and fentanyl is given. This enables the patient to remain relaxed and pain free, and it also has an amnesic effect.

It is important to warn the patient in advance not to drive for at least 24 h following the injection and to arrange transport home.

A scrubbed assistant is needed for this operation.

47.1 INSTRUMENTS

The following instruments are required:

- 1 pair of vein forceps (see Fig. 47.5a)
- 1 pair of strong, straight, artery forceps
- 1 scalpel handle size 3 with size 15 blade

- 1 10 ml syringe with 25 swg needle
- 1 skin marker-pen
- Steri-strips size l/2 in. × 4 in. (12 mm × 100 mm) Ref. 3M R1547
- Micropore tape 1 in.
- Sterile gauze swabs
- Elastocrepe bandages 4 in.
- Tubigrip size F, 2 × 1 m
- Elastic web bandage 3 in. × 5 metres
- ampoules, midazolam and fentanyl
- 5 ml syringe and 23 swg needle
- 10 ml ampoule 1% lignocaine, plain
- 1 aerosol spray skin adhesive (Dow Corning Medical Adhesive 'B' or Opsite Spray).

47.2 OPERATIVE TECHNIQUE (Figs 47.1–47.12)

1. With the patient standing, all varicose veins are marked using the skin marker-pen and the proposed sites of incisions are marked (Fig. 47.1).
2. With the patient lying down an intravenous premedication injection of midazolam (2–4mg) and fentanyl (100 μg) is given slowly. If 'sleep doses' of midazolam are given it is advisable to use a pulse oximeter to monitor oxygen saturation.
3. Sterile drapes are placed under the leg and injections of 1% lignocaine given where marked along the course of the veins (Fig. 47.3).
4. Starting distally, a small stab incision is now made adjacent and parallel to the segment of vein to be removed (Fig. 47.4).
5. Using the vein forceps, the vein is brought out through the incision (Fig. 47.5b) and grasped with artery forceps (Fig. 47.6).
6. Using a twisting action much like a windlass, more vein may be pulled out (Fig. 47.7) until it eventually tears free.
7. The assistant now places a folded gauze swab over the incision and applies firm pressure to prevent bleeding.

Figure 47.1 With the patient standing, the veins are marked out.

Figure 47.2 Marked branches of the long saphenous vein.

Figure 47.3 Lignocaine 1% is injected at the sites along the vein.

Figure 47.4 Using a no. 15 blade, a small stab incision is made alongside the vein.

Figure 47.5 (a) The vein forceps look like a pair of very fine mosquito artery forceps with the tips turned back to form two very small hooks (Caterham Surgical Supplies Ltd). (b) The vein forceps are inserted through the stab incision and the vein is pulled through the skin.

Figure 47.6 Using artery forceps, the vein is gradually 'teased' out of the wound.

Figure 47.7 By twisting the forceps a longer section of vein may be avulsed.

Figure 47.8   Instruments needed, together with typical sections of avulsed vein.

8. The operator moves along the course of the vein and repeats the procedure at the next point which has been marked. If a good segment of vein was obtained it may be possible to miss out a marked spot and move on to the next.

9. It is not always possible to obtain good segments of vein, usually because they are friable and tear easily. This does not seem to make a significant difference to the outcome as there has been an interruption of the vein itself.

10. When all segments of veins have been avulsed, the incisions are closed with Steri-strips. To ensure good adhesion, the skin is sprayed liberally with a medical adhesive prior to the application of each Steri-strip.

11. Folded gauze swabs are now placed over each incision and taped in position with 1 in. micropore tape.

12. A 4 in. Elastocrepe bandage is now applied from the toes to above the topmost incision (Fig. 47.9).

13. This is then covered with two layers of Tubigrip F (Fig. 47.10).

Figure 47.9   The leg is bandaged with 4 in. Elastocrepe from the toes to above the top incision.

Figure 47.10 Two layers of elasticated tubular bandage (Tubigrip size F) are applied.

14. Finally, a 3 in. elastic web bandage is applied firmly over the Tubigrip extending from the toes to above the previous bandages. This is primarily to prevent any bleeding on the way home.
15. The patient then remains on the premises for at least 2 h, during which the effects of the midazolam wears off.
16. Before going home the bandages are checked and a postoperative patient information sheet is given to the patient.
17. The patient is advised to go straight home and straight to bed, and to remain there for the next 12 h.
18. Once the patient is in his or her own bed, the outermost elastic web bandage may be removed after 1 h.

Figure 47.11 Typical varicosities before operation.

Figure 47.12 'Before and after'. The leg on the left was treated 6 months previously. The scars of the stab avulsions can still be seen. The leg on the right has been marked and is ready for treatment.

19. The patient is encouraged to be fully ambulant after the initial 12 h rest and to remove all bandages and dressings after 10 days. This is best done in the bath where they can be soaked off.
20. The Tubigrip bandage is reapplied for the next 4 days when the patient is seen for a check-up.
21. Some bruising is normal, but this disappears quickly over the next few weeks.
22. The patient is seen for a final check at 2 months.

It is helpful to give the patient both a preoperative and a postoperative information sheet.

CHAPTER 48

Excision of ganglia

They are most frequently met with over the tendons upon the back of the wrist: the most certain method of treatment is to make a small puncture into the sac, and to draw a cord through it, or after the puncture is made, to press out the contents and then inject some gently stimulating fluid, as port wine and water heated blood warm.

Encyclopaedia Britannica, 1797

Ganglia are extremely common; they are cystic swellings surrounded by a fibrous tissue wall, occurring in the vicinity of joint capsules and tendon sheaths. Most have crystal-clear gelatinous contents, apart from some in which bleeding has occurred. The cause is not fully understood, but may be a degenerative process in the mesoblastic tissues surrounding the joint. The most common site is the dorsum of the wrist (Fig. 48.1) (60–80%), followed by the flexor aspect of the wrist adjacent to the radial artery (15–20%). Smaller ganglia occur in the flexor sheaths of the fingers, dorsum of foot, ankle and head of fibula.

Untreated, many ganglia disappear spontaneously; many others appear not to trouble the patient and may be left alone. Treatment is indicated if the patient is complaining of unacceptable symptoms, usually pain or limitation of function. Many treatments have been advocated, but all carry a recurrence rate, and the patient should be advised of this accordingly. Simple rupture of the cyst by pressure occasionally succeeds, as does incision with a tenotomy knife, aspiration and injection of sclerosants, but many surgeons recommend excision as offering the best chance of cure [50].

Figure 48.1 Typical ganglion on the dorsum of the wrist.

It is essential to have a bloodless operating field, secured by a pneumatic tourniquet, as the dissection can be quite difficult and the ganglion extend deeper than anticipated. Thus, a general anaesthetic or intravenous regional block or tourniquet and local infiltration is required, the latter being the method chosen for the average general practitioner.

Many patients will assume that excision of a ganglion will be no different from a small sebaceous cyst; it is therefore important to let them know that it is quite a complicated procedure, that they should not drive a car immediately following operation and that, despite a meticulous dissection, recurrence is still possible.

48.1 INSTRUMENTS

The following instruments are required:

- povidone-iodine in spirit (Betadine alcoholic solution)
- 1 dental syringe and 30 swg needle
- 1 cartridge local anaesthetic (without added adrenaline)
- 1 orthopaedic tourniquet
- 1 Esmarch bandage
- sterile pads, bandages and gauze
- 1 scalpel handle size 3
- 1 scalpel blade size 15
- 1 self-retaining retractor (West Weitlander or similar)
- or 2 Kilner double-ended retractors (cat's paw retractors)
- 2 pairs Halstead's mosquito artery forceps, curved 5 in. (12.7 cm)
- 1 stitch scissors
- 1 Kilner needle-holder 5¼ in. (13.3cm)
- 1 pair fine-toothed Adson's dissecting forceps 4¾ in. (12 cm)
- 1 surgical suture 4/0 monofilament Nylon or Prolene on curved cutting needle.
- skin closure strips 3M Ref. GP 41, 6 × 75 mm.

Where the doctor requires a bloodless field and anaesthesia in a limb, a safer alternative to a Bier's block is to infiltrate the area with local anaesthesia and then to apply an orthopaedic tourniquet and Esmarch bandage. This is particularly effective for decompression of the carpal tunnel, release of trigger finger and exploration for foreign bodies.

48.2 TECHNIQUE FOR PRODUCING ANAESTHETIC BLOODLESS FIELD

1. Any rings are removed from fingers on the affected hand.
2. The procedure is explained in detail to the patient.
3. An intravenous premedication injection of fentanyl 100 µg and midazolam 2–4 mg is given slowly over 1–2 min into a vein in the opposite arm. If an intravenous cannula is inserted at this stage and taped in position, the doctor then has access to the circulation for the remainder of the operation. This is valuable should the midazolam need to be reversed.

4. The skin overlying the ganglion is painted with povidone–iodine in spirit.
5. The skin over the ganglion is infiltrated with local anaesthetic (without added adrenaline) using a dental syringe and 30 swg needle.
6. The skin is painted a second time with povidone–iodine in spirit and covered with a sterile pad.
7. The orthopaedic tourniquet is applied over a layer of cotton wool over the upper arm and bandaged in position.
8. The arm is raised, keeping the sterile pad in position, and the Esmarch bandage applied tightly from the fingertips to the lower edge of the orthopaedic tourniquet.
9. The tourniquet is pumped to above arterial pressure (approx. 300 mmHg).
10. The Esmarch bandage is unwound and the sterile pad removed.

48.3 THE OPERATION

The overlying skin is liberally painted with povidone–iodine in spirit (Betadine alcoholic solution), a sterile drape is applied over the area and full aseptic precautions are observed. A surgical gown, mask and gloves should be worn.

The incision should follow a skin crease, normally transverse (Fig. 48.2), about 4 cm long, and any underlying nerves are dissected free. The extensor retinaculum overlying the ganglion is incised and a self-retaining retractor inserted. The bulk of the ganglion is seen superficial to the tendons, but when these are retracted, the deeper part of the ganglion may be seen (Figs 48.3 and 48.4) extending to the wrist joint or intercarpal joint. Gradually, the main part of the ganglion is dissected free using a scalpel, applying traction with toothed dissecting forceps. Usually at this stage, the capsule is incised, liberating the

Figure 48.2 A transverse incision is made over the ganglion in the line of a skin crease.

Figure 48.3 A self-retaining retractor is inserted.

Figure 48.4 If necessary, two 'cat's-paw' retractors may be used as well to improve access.

Figure 48.5 The ganglion has been opened; blood-stained jelly is seen, which indicates possible previous trauma. Normally, the jelly is clear.

Figure 48.6 The capsule of the ganglion has been excised.

typical clear jelly. This is often an advantage and makes the remaining dissection easier. The ganglion is now detached (Fig. 48.6) excising part of the joint capsule as well. It is quite in order to leave adjacent tendons without a synovial covering.

Closure is by one subcuticular prolene or monofilament polyamide suture, strengthened by skin closure strips (Figs 48.7–48.10). A sterile dry gauze dressing is applied covered with cotton wool and an elastocrepe bandage. The assistant now applies direct pressure over the site of the incision and the doctor releases both tourniquets.

If all is well, the dressings are left undisturbed until the 10th postoperative day, when the suture is removed, leaving the Steri-strips in position. A light sterile dressing is reapplied over these for four more days and then removed.

Figure 48.7 A subcuticular monofilament Nylon or Prolene suture gives a neat scar.

Figure 48.8 Skin edges approximated with a subcuticular Nylon suture.

Figure 48.9 Additional support may be given by the application of skin-closure strips.

Figure 48.10 The ends of the Nylon suture are folded over a cotton-wool roll or gauze, and taped in position.

48.4 EXCISION OF RHEUMATOID SYNOVIOMA (Figs 48.11 and 48.12)

This is performed using an identical approach to the excision of ganglion.

Figure 48.11 Rheumatoid 'nodule' may be excised as for a ganglion.

Figure 48.12 Rheumatoid 'nodule'.

CHAPTER 49

Caudal epidural and intravenous regional anaesthesia

Chapter 8 covers all of the commonly used methods of anaesthesia suitable for minor surgery and, where possible, these are the techniques which can be recommended. However, there are rare situations where a caudal epidural anaesthetic or intravenous regional anaesthesia (Bier's block) might need to be given. Both carry risks but, provided the doctor is fully aware of these risks and takes appropriate action to minimize them, and has full facilities to deal with any complications, they are useful techniques and are included in this section of advanced minor surgical techniques.

49.1 EPIDURAL ANAESTHESIA

This method of anaesthesia has achieved great popularity, particularly in the obstetric and general surgery fields. Basically, a sterile solution of dilute local anaesthetic is introduced through a lumbar puncture-type needle into the extradural space, in contrast to a spinal anaesthetic where the solution is injected into the cerebrospinal fluid. The technique of high epidural anaesthesia is beyond the scope of this book, but caudal epidural anaesthesia is included as a valuable method of pain relief in patients with acute low back pain accompanied by muscle spasm, such as is found in prolapsed intervertebral disc lesions.

49.1.1 Technique of caudal epidural anaesthesia

The following items are required:

- 50 ml syringe filled with 40 ml 0.9% saline plus 10 ml 0.5% bupivacaine (Marcain)
- 2 ml syringe filled with methylprednisolone 80 mg (Depo-Medrone)

- 2 ml syringe with 1% lignocaine
- 20 swg spinal needle 3½ in. (8.9 cm) long
- Sterile dressing pack.

The patient is placed prone on the operating theatre table or couch and a cushion placed under the pelvis to tilt the sacrum upwards.

Povidone–iodine (Betadine) alcoholic solution is painted over the overlying skin and 2 ml of 1% lignocaine is injected through to the sacral hiatus. The spinal needle is now inserted through the hiatus and just below the cornua. Some difficulty may be encountered in determining the exact angle, but it tends to be parallel to the surface of the fifth sacral segment (Fig. 49.1).

After inserting the spinal needle to 5 cm the stylus is withdrawn and no fluid should be seen. If cerebrospinal fluid is seen, the procedure should be abandoned and repeated on another occasion. If blood is seen, the needle should be moved slightly until bleeding ceases.

The saline/marcain mixture is now injected very slowly, taking 5–10 min.

After 40 ml has been injected, 2 ml of methylprednisolone is injected through the same needle, followed by the remaining 10 ml saline/ Marcain solution. The needle is withdrawn. After the injection the patient is left lying prone for 5–10 min before turning to the supine position. The patient may return home 30 min later.

Provided an absolutely meticulous aseptic technique is employed, this is a valuable method of pain relief which can be used in general practice.

Figure 49.1 (a, b) Models to show caudal epidural injection.

49.2 INTRAVENOUS REGIONAL ANAESTHESIA (BIER'S BLOCK)

The danger of intravenous regional block is that of cuff failure, whereby a large bolus of local anaesthetic is released into the circulation, resulting in major convulsions and even death.

Provided meticulous care is taken, two pneumatic tourniquets are used and good resuscitation facilities are available, this is an extremely useful method of producing total anaesthesia, muscle relaxation and a bloodless operating field in an arm or leg, and enables the general practitioner to increase the scope of minor surgery to include such operations as excision of ganglion, removal of foreign bodies, exploration, reduction of simple fractures, and even release of trigger finger and decompression of the carpal tunnel.

The technique was first described by August Bier in 1908 using procaine as the anaesthetic [51], but it was not until 1963 that the method achieved popularity using lignocaine [52]. As a result of the numerous side-effects of this drug, in 1965 the editorial of the *Journal of the American Medical Association* advised against the use of intravenous regional anaesthesia until safer agents were available.

By 1971 prilocaine had been recommended by Thorn-Alquist [53] and bupivacaine by Ware [54], who further reported favourably using bupivacaine in 1979 [55]. In 1983 serious side-effects were reported from various centres using bupivacaine for intravenous regional anaesthesia, and the drug of choice now appears to be prilocaine (Citanest). A review of the Bier's block technique by Pattison [56] in 1984 concluded that it is a safe, simple, effective and well-tolerated method of regional anaesthesia. He could find no long-term complications attributable to the technique. The method consists of exsanguinating the limb and injecting a large volume of dilute anaesthetic intravenously through an indwelling needle; this passes retrogradely via the veins, venules, capillaries, arterioles and arteries, thence to skin, muscle and the whole limb, producing anaesthesia and muscle relaxation. Up to 1 h operating time is obtained in a bloodless field with total anaesthesia and muscle relaxation.

The following items are required for an intravenous regional block:

- orthopaedic pneumatic tourniquet
- standard sphygmomanometer and cuff
- 3 in. (7.7 cm) Esmarch bandage
- intravenous cannula size 18 swg (0.09 cm metric)
- 40 ml 0.5% prilocaine plain (Citanest).

49.2.1 Technique of Bier's block for the arm

1. An intravenous cannula is inserted in a vein on the opposite limb. This is taped in position: it gives access to the circulation throughout the operation and may be used to administer any premedication drugs intravenously (Fig. 49.2).
2. Cotton-wool padding is applied around the upper arm and an orthopaedic pneumatic tourniquet applied over it.

Figure 49.2 An intravenous premedication injection of midazolam and fentanyl is given.

3. A sphygmomanometer cuff (or second orthopaedic tourniquet) is applied distal to the first tourniquet, covered with a non-stretch bandage and inflated to just below arterial pressure. This distends the veins at the wrist. This second tourniquet acts as a safeguard should the first tourniquet fail (Fig. 49.3).

Figure 49.3 An orthopaedic tourniquet and a sphygmomanometer cuff are applied to the upper arm and bandaged in place.

Figure 49.4 After inflating one cuff to 80 mmHg, an intravenous cannula is inserted in a suitable vein.

Figure 49.5 The cuff is now deflated and the stylus withdrawn, leaving the cannula which is connected to a 1 ml syringe and prilocaine.

Figure 49.6 The arm is elevated and an Esmarch bandage applied. The cuff is inflated to 300 mmHg and the bandage removed.

4. The 18 swg (0.09 cm) intravenous cannula is now inserted in a suitable vein and strapped in position with adhesive tape, and the sphygmomanometer deflated (Fig. 49.4). A 1 ml syringe containing prilocaine is attached to the cannula and strapped in place (Fig. 49.5).

5. The arm is elevated and the limb exsanguinated using the elastic Esmarch bandage, starting at the fingers, carefully over the indwelling cannula and syringe, tightly over the forearm and extending to, and covering, the second tourniquet (Fig. 49.6).

6. The orthopaedic tourniquet is now inflated to above arterial pressure (in practice 250 mmHg) and the Esmarch bandage removed. At this stage, the arm is exsanguinated but there is still a cannula fixed inside a vein.

7. Next, 30 ml of 0.5% prilocaine is now slowly injected through the intravenous cannula, and the second cuff inflated to above arterial pressure. The reason for the interval between inflating the first and second tourniquets is to allow some prilocaine to infiltrate below the second cuff, producing anaesthesia and reducing discomfort to the patient (Fig. 49.7).

8. The cannulae are left in place as a means of access to the circulation should any complications arise.

9. Anaesthesia develops in approximately 4 min.

Figure 49.7 After removal of the Esmarch bandage, 30 ml of 0.5% prilocaine is injected through the cannula, which is left in place for safety.

49.2.2 Additional safeguards for intravenous regional anaesthesia

Most of the complications and mishaps following the use of intravenous regional blocks have been due to failure of the pneumatic tourniquet, from either leaking or faulty equipment. This results in a large bolus of local anaesthetic entering the circulation, with possible collapse, convulsions and even death. It is vital that the tourniquet remains inflated above arterial pressure throughout the whole procedure, and in any case should not be deflated in under 15 min from injection to allow most of the anaesthetic to percolate through the tissues from the veins. It has also been shown [57] that even with adequate cuffs, some of the intravenous injection finds its way into the general circulation, through an active interosseous circulation. Because accidental failure of the cuff has such potentially serious consequences, an assistant should be present throughout the whole procedure, with the sole responsibility of the supervision of the cuff checking the pressure continuously, and reporting any signs of reduced pressure. The use of two separate cuffs reduces still further the chances of accidental failure and is to be strongly recommended. If a standard blood-pressure cuff is used for the second back-up tourniquet, it should be bandaged in place with a 4 in. (10.3 cm) non-stretch cotton bandage which will prevent ballooning and loosening of the cuff during inflation. All rubber parts, connections, taps and pressure gauges should be checked for wear before use and replaced if necessary.

Although most conscious patients can tolerate the discomfort of a fully inflated cuff, nevertheless, it does cause pain to some, particularly after about 10–15 min. To obviate this, a premedication intravenous injection of fentanyl 100 µg and midazolam 4 mg is valuable and enables the cuff to be tolerated.

Full resuscitation facilities should always be immediately available if this method of anaesthesia is used.

Specialist minor surgery

CHAPTER 50

Plastic and reconstructive surgery

The aim of all procedures on the skin is to remove the offending lesion adequately and replace it with a less noticeable scar. Every physician is duty bound to inform the patient that they will be replacing the excised lesion, be it benign or malignant, with a scar of unpredictable nature. In the event of a suspected malignancy there is more justification for the production of a scar; however, these patients need to be as completely informed as the patient undergoing removal of benign lesions for cosmetic purposes. Lesions which are suspected of being malignant need to be completely excised, so the whole lesion may be subjected to histology. If the lesion is large then a punch or small incisional biopsy may be used to confirm the diagnosis. However, it must be borne in mind that this may affect the histological interpretation of the completely excised lesions. In particular, with malignant melanomas it is essential to know the depth of the tumour to establish prognosis and the need for any adjuvant therapy. An incisional punch biopsy may remove the deepest part of the lesion and result in less than optimal treatment.

All types of lesion may be treated by excision, shaving or curettage, and again the predictability of the scar varies with each of these techniques. However, in certain areas it may be wiser to accept the appearance of the benign lesion rather than take the risk of an unpredictable scar. Those areas which are prone to particularly bad scarring are the shoulders and deltoid region and the area overlying the sternum.

50.1 CHOICE OF INCISION

The choice of skin incision will have an effect on the outcome of the scar. The scar should be placed within a natural line, either within a wrinkle or skin crease, or at least parallel to it. In the face and neck the direction of these lines can often be found by asking the patient to frown, close their eyelids tightly or purse their lips. In a child or young adult it may be difficult to establish the direction of the skin line and it is sometimes necessary to excise a lesion around its borders as a circle and then observe the direction of skin pull before completing the ellipse and closing the wound. Scars outside the head and neck tend to take longer to heal and in general remain more conspicuous and have a greater tendency to stretch. In areas of hair-bearing skin it is necessary to make the incision in the direction of the hair follicles thus avoiding a strip of hairless skin around the scar. Elsewhere all incisions should be made in a perpendicular direction which avoids any shelving of the skin edge, allows accurate apposition and improves overall scar healing.

A long, straight scar tends to be more eye-catching as it crosses natural lines. Long scars are also more prone to contracture and can distort surrounding normal tissue. The linear effect of such scars can be disguised by the use of single or multiple Z-plasties which break up the direction of contracture and turn the scar in a parallel direction with normal skin creases (Fig. 50.1).

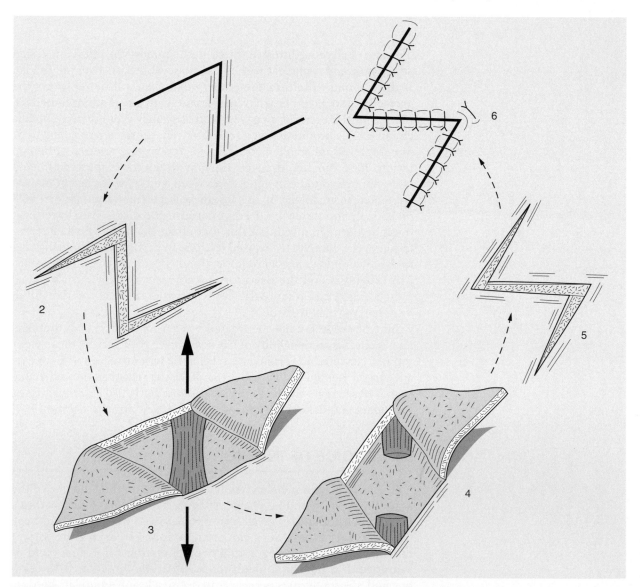

Figure 50.1   Z-plasty – a zig-zag incision with the perpendicular part of the incision over the contracture as shown in picture 1, skin is undermined and released, the contracture is then divided as in picture 4 and the skin flaps are then transposed so that the middle limb of the Z-plasty is now 90° to the original line of contracture as shown in picture 6. Reprinted from *Fundamental Techniques in Plastic Surgery*, I.A. McGregor, by permission of the publisher Churchill Livingstone.

50.2 SUTURING TECHNIQUES

The type of suture required over different areas of the body varies according to the strength of closure required and also the thickness of the skin. Apposition of the skin edges needs to be extremely accurate to optimize the scar. Fine instruments, needles and sutures must be used and atraumatic tissue handling is essential. Skin-hooks are the least damaging instrument, although they can be cumbersome to use. If forceps are used to hold the skin edges then minimal pressure should be applied to avoid crushing and devitalizing the wound margin. Accurate placement of the suture is essential: the needles are curved and should be passed through the skin edge in a circular motion by a rotating movement of the wrist (Fig. 50.2).

It is essential to avoid tension when closing wounds. It may be necessary to enlarge an ellipse to reduce the tension, undermine at the level of the subcutaneous fat or even use appropriate rotational advancement flaps to decrease the tension. The type of suture generally used over different bodies and their size is shown in Table 50.1.

When a circular or oval wound is closed the ensuing tension may cause an elevation or dog-ear at the wound's ends. It is better to extend

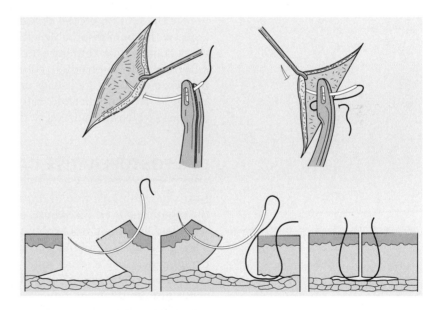

Figure 50.2 Needle passing through wound. Reprinted from *Fundamental Techniques in Plastic Surgery*, I.A. McGregor, by permission of the publisher Churchill Livingstone.

Table 50.1 Size and type of suture required for suturing the skin at different positions in the body

Location	Size of suture	Absorbable/nonabsorbable	Example
Face	5.0 or 6.0	Non-absorbable	Nylon or Prolene
Hand	5.0	Non-absorbable	Nylon or Prolene
Leg and arm	5.0 or 4.0	Non-absorbable	Nylon or Prolene
Trunk	4.0	Absorbable	PDS/Monocryl/Vicryl
Scalp	3.0	Non-absorbable	Prolene

PDS, polydioxanone suture.

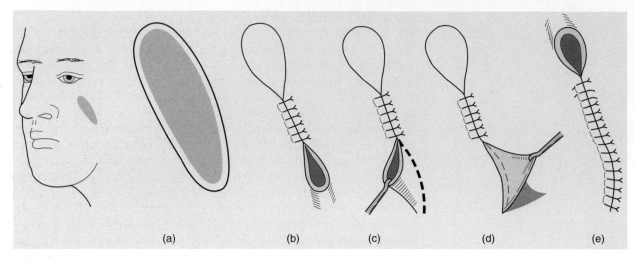

(a)   (b)   (c)   (d)   (e)

Figure 50.3 Dog-ear correction. Reprinted from *Fundamental Techniques in Plastic Surgery*, I.A. McGregor, by permission of the publisher Churchill Livingstone.

the incision to produce a flat, lengthened scar which avoids the more obvious contour defect (Fig. 50.3).

It may be necessary in larger wounds of the trunk or in the limbs to use an absorbable suture in the deep layers to close the wound and to take the tension off the skin closure before closing the superficial layers with a non-absorbable suture. It is also possible in the trunk to use a subcuticular running stitch and it is certainly advisable to use an absorbable interrupted suture below this to take the tension. Absorbable sutures are usually best avoided in the hand or face as they can lead to unpredictable rates of absorption and inflammatory response which may adversely affect the outcome of the scar.

50.3 POSTOPERATIVE CARE

In the face minimal wound dressing is required, particularly around the mouth and eyes. Elsewhere, simple adhesive dressing may be used to protect the wound from rubbing on clothing and absorb any minimal ooze from the wound. As long as the wound remains dry then the dressing may be left intact until the sutures are removed. The timing of suture removal varies for different parts of the body, as different areas heal at different rates according to their blood supply. It is necessary to leave the sutures in long enough for the wound to have gained enough strength to prevent dehiscence. However, if the sutures are left in too long there is increased risk of suture track marks developing and thus resulting in a unpleasant-looking cross-hatched scar. Table 50.2 gives a general indication of times at which sutures should be removed. These may vary according to the tension of the wound and factors which may delay wound healing, such as steroid medication or diabetes.

Subcuticular sutures may be left in for slightly longer as this will avoid the cross-hatching; however, if they are left in for too long it may be difficult to remove them, particularly if they are not of monofilament

Table 50.2 Maximum time for suture removal for different locations

Location	Time of suture removal (days)
Eyelid	3
Face	5
Hand	14
Upperlimb	14
Trunk	14–21
Lowerlimb	14–21

material. It must be remembered that all wounds will gape once a lesion has been excised and the resulting defect may appear much larger than the excised lesion. Undermining has been mentioned as one possible technique for reducing the tension of closure. It may be necessary to use some type of rotation or advancement flap to reduce the tension and some examples are shown in Fig. 50.4.

If it is obvious that the wound will not close without considerable tension then specialist advice may be required. All wounds should then be dressed with a non-adherent dressing and an appropriate referral made, whereupon it may be necessary to skin-graft the defect.

Skin grafts used may be of split thickness or full thickness. Skin-thickness grafts include the epidermis and a variable thickness of dermis, but leave sufficient thickness of skin on the donor site to allow healing by secondary intention. Full-thickness grafts include the full thickness of the dermis and must be taken from an area where there is sufficient skin to allow direct closure. Grafts will take on any bed which has an adequate blood supply and therefore should not be placed directly on to bone, tendon or cartilage. Skin-graft take is detrimentally affected by infection and therefore grafts should only be placed on a surgically clean site. The success of the graft is also affected by sheering forces through the graft during the early phases of healing and it may therefore be necessary to splint any area where a graft is applied.

50.4 SCARRING

Initially all scars tend to be red and swollen. The degree of inflammation is variable, as is the time taken for the scar to settle. The normal healing process takes many months to be completed. Ideally, a smooth, flat, linear, pale scar is achieved. However, such a sequence is not always the case and weakness within the scar may result in stretching and atrophy of the scar, resulting in a widened hollow scar. On some occasions there is an excessive tissue reaction, particularly

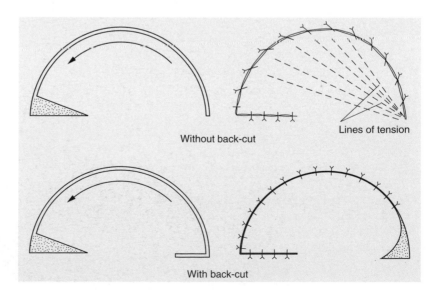

Figure 50.4 Rotation and advancement flaps. Reprinted from *Fundamental Techniques in Plastic Surgery*, I.A. McGregor, by permission of the publisher Churchill Livingstone.

Without back-cut

Lines of tension

With back-cut

within the dermis, and the scar never settles from its red active state and forms into a hypertrophic or keloid scar. A hypertrophic scar is one in which there is excess healing scar tissue that is held within the boundary of the scar itself. A keloid scar shows a similar reaction but tends to be more florid and the scar actually spreads beyond the margins of the original scar. These scars on occasion can be extremely distressing, not only in their appearance, but also as they can be very irritating, painful and itchy. The treatment of these scars involves a lot of patient compliance, understanding and support. Nearly all of these scars should be treated conservatively as further surgery runs an extremely large risk of even more severe recurrence. The mainstays of treatment are pressure and application of steroid, either topically or via intralesional injection. In the most severe circumstances is may be necessary to use a further excision followed by radiotherapy, but this still does not by any means guarantee an improved outlook and may lay the patient open to the risk of developing malignancy in the surrounding skin in the long-term future.

Minor operations in ophthalmology

> Now one eyelid must he held open by the assistant, the other by the surgeon. There-upon the surgeon passes a sharp hook, the point of which has been a little incurved under the edge of the pterygium and fixes the hook in it ...
>
> *Celsus, 30* AD

If one is to tackle minor operations in or around the eye a sound knowledge of the anatomy of ocular structures is essential. Using basic examination equipment including a pen torch, cotton-wool buds and a hand-held direct ophthalmoscope, most ocular structures can be examined. The visual acuity using a Snellen's type chart should be recorded before lid surgery.

Section 51.1 will cover specialized examination techniques including lid eversion, tear film estimation and lacrimal syringe and probing.

Section 51.2 will cover minor surgical procedures including incision and curettage of meibomian cysts, removal of lid lesions, incisional and excisional biopsy, management of entropion and the treatment of corneal exposure.

51.1 EXAMINATION TECHNIQUES

51.1.1 Lid eversion (Fig. 51.1)

Eversion of the upper lid allows inspection of the superior tarso-conjunctival surface and is essential if a subtarsal foreign body is suspected. Prior to the procedure a drop of local anaesthetic (G. Benoxinate 0.4%) is inserted. The patient is seated comfortably and asked to look down to the floor. The operator should sit facing the patient. Whilst pulling on the upper lid lashes a glass rod or cotton-wool bud is used to apply gentle pressure to the skin overlying the upper border of the tarsal plate. The patient is encouraged neither to squeeze their eyelids nor to look upwards. The lid is everted so that the upper edge of the tarsal plate is rolled over the lid margin. This allows examination of the tarsoconjunctival surface of upper lid.

51.1.2 Tear film estimation

Assessment of tear film

- Fluorescein staining: fluorescein dye when placed in the tear film will detect epithelial defects and identify corneal erosions, ulcers

Figure 51.1 How to evert the upper eye-lid. Gentle pressure is applied on the upper border of the tarsal plate whilst at the same time, traction is applied to the eye-lashes.

Gentle pressure on upper border of tarsal plate

Traction on lashes

or foreign bodies. A drop of fluorescein solution made up of 1% fluorescein sodium drops mixed with normal saline can be inserted into the lower fornix. Alternatively, a fluorescein strip can be moistened and placed at a similar location. It is essential that the fluorescein is not used in those patients wearing soft contact lenses, as the dye can become incorporated into the lens material.

■ Rose Bengal staining: degenerative or dead cells stain with Rose Bengal 1%. This facilitates the diagnosis of keratoconjunctivitis sicca and corneal exposure. Rose Bengal is a very irritant solution and topical local anaesthetic should be inserted prior to Rose Bengal.

■ Fluorescein break-up time (FBT): this is a useful method of qualifying the tear film. A drop of dilute fluorescein solution is inserted and the patient instructed to blink once and then keep the eyes open. When the corneal tear film first forms it is an intact layer. The time (in seconds) is recorded until this intact film breaks up with the development of lacunae. Such a pattern normally occurs after at least 10 seconds. A more rapid FBT reflects a reduction in the quality or quantity of the tear film.

Filter paper
hung over
lower lid

Figure 51.2 Schirmer's test for tear-film estimation. A strip of filter paper is hung over the lower lid as shown.

Schirmer's test (Fig 51.2)

To quantify tear production small strips of filter paper, 4×30 mm, are placed over the lower lid margin for a 5 min period. The degree of moistening can be measured and used as a quantitative assessment of tear film production. In general, after 5 min at least 15 mm of the filter paper is moistened. In those with a significantly reduced tear film production less than 5 mm of moistening occurs.

51.1.3 Lacrimal syringing

Epiphora is a relatively common symptom and frequently encountered in the older age group. Watering may result from poor orbicularis tone with reduction of the lacrimal tear pump mechanism. Ectropion, with outward turning of the lower lid, leads to displacement of the inferior puncta which moves away from the tear lake, resulting in epiphora. A blockage of the distal part of the lacrimal drainage system may also present as watering. Careful examination of the patient's lid position and movement may identify the cause for watering. Tear drainage can be assessed by estimation of the speed at which fluorescein is cleared from the tear film.

Further information will be obtained by syringing the lacrimal system. A good light and examination couch are essential. A Nettleship dilator and a lacrimal cannula attached to a 5 ml syringe containing normal saline are required. It is important that the patient is comfortable throughout the procedure and a drop of local anaesthetic (G.Benoxinate 0.4%) should be inserted prior to undertaking syringing. The lower puncta is gently enlarged using the Nettleship dilator. This procedure is more easily performed if the lower lid is drawn slightly laterally and the dilator is lubricated with an

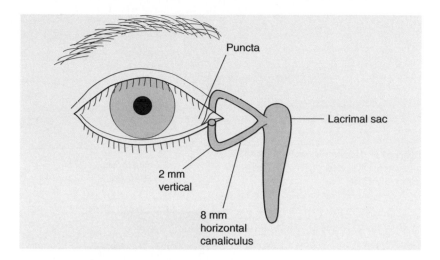

Figure 51.3   The lacrimal drainage system.

ophthalmic ointment. The course of the lower canaliculus should be followed, taking account of the initial 2 mm vertical portion (Fig. 51.3). Despite local anaesthetic drops mild discomfort is often felt as the puncta is stretched. Saline is then injected through the inferior canaliculus. If the system is patent the patient tastes the salt water at the back of the throat as the saline drains through the nasolacrimal duct which opens into the inferior meatus in the nose.

51.2 SURGICAL PROCEDURES

51.2.1 Incision and curettage of meibomian cyst

A meibomian cyst is a cystic swelling occurring within the upper or lower tarsal plates of the lids (Figs 51.4 and 51.5). It represents a retention cyst of the meibomian glands and is generally precipitated by lid margin disease in the form of blepharitis and meibomianitis. Meibomian cysts should initially be treated conservatively with hot compresses and antibiotic ointment. If secondary infection has occurred

Figure 51.4   A typical meibomian cyst (chalazion) in the upper eye-lid.

Figure 51.5   Meibomian cyst shown by everting the eye-lid

Figure 51.6   Incision and curettage of meibomian cyst pointing through the skin – use a *horizontal* incision.

Figure 51.7   Applying topical anaesthetic drops.

Figure 51.8   Injecting local anaesthetic around the cyst.

Figure 51.9   The Chalazion ring clamp.

Figure 51.10   Applying the chalazion clamp to the eye-lid, with the meibomian cyst situated within the ring of the clamp.

a course of systemic antibiotics is necessary. In its chronic form a meibomian cyst appears as a well-localized nodule. The overlying conjunctiva may be engorged but in the centre of the cyst pressure of its contents often cause a central pallid patch on the tarsoconjunctival surface. It is essential to examine the tarsoconjunctival surface before proceeding with incision and curettage, and particularly in atypical or recurring meibomian cysts it is important to consider a meibomian gland carcinoma.

Figure 51.11 Incision and curettage of meibomian cyst through the conjunctival surface using a *vertical* incision.

Figure 51.12 Incising a meibomian cyst using a sharp-pointed scalpel.

Figure 51.13 The chalazion curette.

Figure 51.14 Using the curette to clean out the contents of the meibomian cyst.

Incision and curettage is generally best performed through the tarso-conjunctival surface, although if the lesion has discharged through the skin incision and curettage should be performed through the skin using an incision parallel to the skin margin (Fig. 51.6). Local anaesthesia is generally achieved with a solution of 1% lignocaine containing adrenaline 1:200 000 accompanied by topical anaesthesia using one or two drops of Benoxinate 0.4% (Fig. 51.7). 2 ml of 1% lignocaine with adrenaline are infiltrated into the lid skin around the meibomian cyst using a 25 gauge needle (Fig. 51.8). To reduce the discomfort of local anaesthesia the solution should be warmed to body temperature and, if necessary, a preinjection using a dilute solution of 1% lignocaine with normal saline (1:10) can be employed. After infiltration gentle pressure on the eyelid helps to disperse the local anaesthetic agent. A chalazion clamp (Figs 51.9 and 51.10) is applied over the cyst with its open surface on the tarsoconjunctiva. The lid is then everted and the cyst incised vertically through the tarsoconjunctiva perpendicular to the lid margin, taking care not to involve the lid margin in the incision (Figs 51.11 and 51.12). Once the cyst is opened the contents are evacuated and the walls of the cyst are scraped using a sharp chalazion curette (Figs 51.13 and 51.14). Any abnormal tissue should be sent for histology to exclude malignancy. Antibiotic ointment is then inserted and a pressure dressing using two eye-pads placed for 15 min. The eye is then re-dressed with a lighter pad and antibiotic ointment, generally Oc. Chloramphenicol, is inserted into the eye and continued twice a day for 3 days.

51.2.2 Surgical excision of minor lid lesions

Any surgery to the lid should avoid cutting through the lid margin. Superficial skin lesions frequently occur on the lid margin and can safely be removed by a shave excision technique applying cautery to the base of the lesion. As lid skin is a common site of malignant lesions any suspicious areas which have been excised should be sent for histology. Any malignant lid lesion requires excision with adequate tumour clearance and should not be undertaken as a minor procedure. If the lesion is large an incisional biopsy may be necessary. This is best performed removing an ellipse of the lesion involving a section of normal lid skin along the normal skin line. Care should be taken to avoid distorting the lid skin and in particular attention should be paid to avoiding the development of a lower lid ectropion.

Entropion

Involutional lid changes, including laxity of the medial canthal tendon, age-related enophthalmus and laxity of the tarsal plate made worse by upward migration of the preseptal orbicularis, all lead to the development of an involutional or spastic entropion. The lash margin then lies in contact with the globe and is a source of extreme discomfort and irritation. Corneal abrasion and ulceration may result (Figs 51.15 and 51.16). Lid taping to stabilize the lid margin may be advised, although this is often unsuccessful as a long-term treatment. Definitive entropion correction generally requires specialist skills, but entropion is very well managed in the short term by the insertion of everting sutures. These stabilize the lower lid and restore normal lid position for a significant period, often up to 18 months. This procedure is done following the injection of a

Figure 51.15 Typical entropion.

Figure 51.16 Entropion showing injury to the conjunctiva.

Figure 51.17 Entropion – post-everting sutures.

local anaesthetic (1% lignocaine with adrenaline). Three double-ended 5/0 catgut sutures are inserted (Fig. 51.17). The knots are cut short and left in place. More definitive entropion correction can be planned at a later date.

Management of corneal exposure

The development of a seventh nerve palsy, either as Bell's palsy or as a result of oral pathology damaging the seventh nerve along its course, leads to poor closure with the risk of ocular exposure. Regular lubricant drops and ointment are often sufficient to protect the eye. Taping, particularly at night, may further improve closure. Where evidence of corneal breakdown is occurring, a traction suture (4/0 Nylon) can be inserted into the upper lid to facilitate closure. More permanent procedures such as a tarsorrhaphy or inducing a protective ptosis using botulinum toxin may be necessary if the cornea shows evidence of decompensation.

CHAPTER 52

Dental problems in general practice

The purpose of this chapter is to help those practitioners who are faced with a dental problem and may be in an area where access to a dental surgeon is not easily possible. Because some dental problems may be quite difficult to manage, where possible it is recommended that the patient is referred and treated by a dental specialist.

52.1 INTRODUCTION

The aim of dental treatment is to alleviate pain and discomfort relating to the teeth and mouth problems. Nearly all patients with dental pain are apprehensive, so some of the most important aspects of dental care are to relax the patient, give reassurance and explain to them what is the problem and what can be done to alleviate their symptoms.

52.2 MEDICAL HISTORY

It is vital to check carefully the patient's medical history before embarking on any treatment. To this end, it is essential to ascertain any heart problems which may require antibiotic prophylactic cover. Is there a history of hepatitis B or human immunodeficiency virus (HIV) infection which would alert the operator to the risks of needle-stick injury from sharp instruments or teeth? Are there any blood disorders such as haemophilia or sickle-cell anaemia, or is the patient on aspirin or anticoagulants? It is also important to ascertain any other medication being taken by the patient which might interact with local anaesthetics or drugs to be used. Any history of drug allergies should also be noted, particularly penicillin, as well as any abnormal reactions to previous anaesthetics.

52.3 EXTRAORAL SIGNS

At the first assessment, it is important to check for any extraoral signs, noticing the colour of the skin, any swellings of the face, and any signs of herpes zoster infection, any discharge from the nostril or ear which may be giving referred pain to the mouth or teeth.

52.4 DIFFERENTIAL DIAGNOSIS OF SWELLINGS OF THE FACE

When the operator is confronted with a patient with a swollen face, it is helpful to consider the following possible diagnoses:

- mumps is usually bilateral, affecting the parotid and submandibular glands
- cysts are quite common
- tumours may be suspected from the history, loose teeth and with no pain; in the UK they are still relatively rare
- salivary-gland obstruction, usually from a calculus, is usually unilateral; the swelling appears when food is tasted and gradually subsides
- Oedema may be from infection or be a result of an allergic reaction
- trauma and bruising are usually fairly obvious and will be confirmed from the history
- radiographs can be helpful in establishing a diagnosis in many of the above.

It must be remembered that asymmetry or swelling may also be part of normal anatomy.

52.5 DIFFERENTIAL DIAGNOSIS OF FACIAL PAIN

This can be one of the hardest problems for both physician and dental surgeon, with the patient being referred backwards and forwards between two or more specialists before the final diagnosis is made. It is helpful to consider the following before deciding on the cause of the pain:

- temporomandibular joint dysfunction
- maxillary sinusitis
- earache
- bruxism (tooth-grinding at night)
- atypical facial neuralgia
- trigeminal neuralgia
- primary herpetic infection.

52.6 DENTAL HISTORY AND INTRAORAL EXAMINATION

The patient is asked to describe the problem and to clarify the pain: is it bearable, constant or annoying, are they unable to chew, is it worse with cold, is it made worse by heat, are they kept awake at night, are they in extreme pain or in agony, and is the pain intermittent or continuous?

The patient is also asked whether they are aware of any swelling or unable to open their mouth, and whether they have had any recent dental treatment. Examination inside the mouth may reveal infection, swelling, cellulitis or discharge.

52.7 SYMPTOMS, POSSIBLE DIAGNOSIS AND TREATMENT

- Mild ache, pain with sweet foods, or a hot or cold sensation (try ethyl chloride) of short duration: it may be possible to rescue the tooth with excavation of the caries and applying a dressing of zinc oxide and oil of cloves on the base of the cavity.
- Sharp and more durable pain: may be treated as above but there is a greater risk of exposing the nerve and loss of the tooth.
- Constant pain and awake at night: this is more likely to involve the nerve and will require extraction if no conservation techniques are available.
- Tooth tender when tapped, pain with hot food or drink, tenderness in the buccal sulcus and redness of the tissues an signifies early abscess caused by a dying nerve or infected gum pocket (which may be associated with an impacted or buried tooth): appropriate antibiotics are given and the tooth may require extraction.
- Swelling around the roots in buccal (or rarely lingual) tissues indicates an abscess: antibiotics are given to heal and extraction is carried out when ready.
- Pain which is constant and quite acute can be caused by acute necrotizing ulcerative gingivitis (ANUG); with white–grey sloughing of interdental gingival tissue and a characteristic smell: treatment is with chlorhexidine mouthwash (corsodyl) and metronidazole for 3 days.
- Pain can be caused by a primary herpetic infection, usually in very young children. Intraoral inflammation and transient vesicles are present, and the patient is unable to eat and has an elevated temperature: it may be necessary to give systemic acyclovir.
- Pain after an extraction can be caused by a dry socket (periostitis) or by periodontitis or pulpitis in a neighbouring tooth: a dry socket is treated by dressing with Alvogyl after washing with saline or cleaning with a pledglet of cotton wool.

It is possible to have referred pain from upper teeth to lower teeth and vice versa, but always on the same side (right or left). The pain can refer to the ear, face, head and occasionally arm, but again, always on the same side.

Radiographs, if available, are very useful at this stage

52.8 DENTAL CARIES

A simple, first-aid treatment for dental caries is to excavate with a spoon excavator, and dress with oil of cloves or a temporary dressing, Kalzinol or IRM, filing any rough edges with a nail emery board or rounded diamond nail-file. If an abscess has developed, it will be necessary to treat this with amoxycillin and metronidazole and allow any swelling to subside or drain surgically, and then to return for a possible extraction 10 days later. Extractions are relatively rare these days, but may be the best alternative when facilities do not allow a choice.

52.9 TRAUMA

Trauma to teeth is commonly as a result of sports injuries, falls, road-traffic accidents and fights.

Where the deciduous teeth, especially incisors, are involved usually no treatment is needed and they will return into place naturally. They usually discolour later owing to pulp death and will require treatment later if a permanent tooth. Anterior permanent teeth are usually not a priority and may be treated after a period of healing of associated soft-tissue damage.

Sharp edges can be smoothed with a rounded end nail-file. The exception is if the tooth is very loose and painful, with the risk of inhaling or swallowing it; in this case an extraction is needed unless splinting is an option.

52.10 TREATMENT OF DENTAL ABSCESSES

Any abscesses should be drained intraorally if possible but this can be quite difficult until sufficiently localized and superficial. The patient will obtain great relief after the operation.

52.10.1 Technique

1. A topical anaesthetic spray or gel is applied.
2. A superficial injection of local anaesthetic, 1–2 mm deep, given.
3. The abscess is incised using a Blake size 15 blade.
4. The abscess is gently squeezed until all pus is expressed.

Dental abscesses may be as small as 1 cm across within the mouth (Fig. 52.23) or affect the whole face, which can be swollen and the eye closed with oedema. Pain may not be a feature and antibiotics may not be needed.

52.11 DENTAL EXTRACTIONS

As mentioned earlier, before one embarks on any dental extraction, the patient's medical and dental history is important and should be taken carefully. The practitioner must always be gentle and remove a tooth gradually. It is helpful to have all sets of instruments in trays which can be autoclaved quickly and easily (Figs 52.1–52.5).

52.11.1 Anaesthesia

A knowledge of the anatomy of the skull and the nerve supply to the mouth is essential in understanding the various nerve-block techniques to be described (Figs 52.6 and 52.7).

Figure 52.1 Standard dental examination tray.

Figure 52.2 Tray for local anaesthetics.

Figure 52.3 Extraction tray.

Figure 52.4   Instruments for surgical exposure of roots.

Figure 52.5   Materials for temporary dressings.

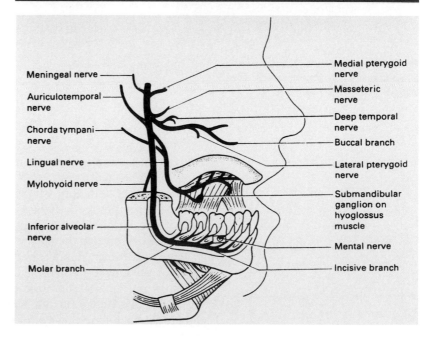

Figure 52.6   Showing the branches of the mandibular nerve. Taken from *Heinemann Dental Handbook*, p. 28.

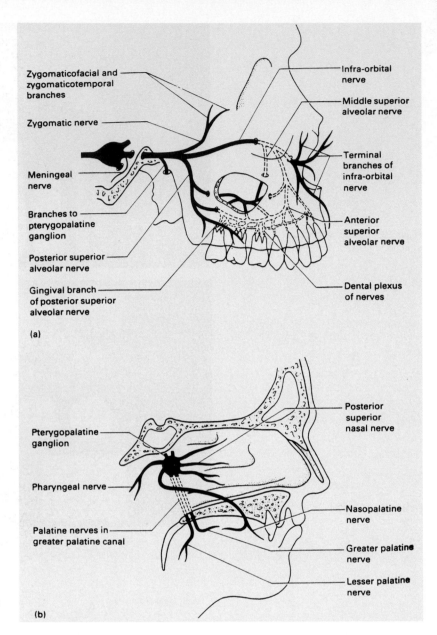

Figure 52.7 (a) The maxillary nerve, (b) Branches of the pterygopalatine nerve. Taken from *Heinemann Dental Handbook* p. 25.

Anaesthesia and infiltration using lignocaine dental cartridges is used for upper teeth and some lower teeth (Figs 52.8–52.10). Both sides are infiltrated, approximately 1 cm deep buccally and 1.5 mm palatally for upper teeth using a 30 swg 'short' needle (0.3×21 mm) with a long bevel. The intraligamental or periodontal membrane is infiltrated by inserting the needle down the side of the root (Fig. 52.11).

The practitioner should always test whether the anaesthetic has taken by pushing a probe or sharp instrument gradually and forcibly down the periodontal membrane before extraction.

Local anaesthetics do not work well in the presence of pus or inflammation, and in these situations larger volumes may be needed,

Figure 52.8 Upper pre-molar/canine injection site.

Figure 52.9 Injection site for upper molar tooth.

or treatment delayed until the infection has subsided. The one exception to this is where the teeth are very loose and the injection can be given down the periodontal membrane.

52.11.2 Choice of anaesthetic

Inferior dental block

A standard dental syringe and local anaesthetic cartridge are used, with either a short (30 swg) or long (27 swg) needle and a short bevel. The nerve block can usually be accomplished using the shorter needle and is more comfortable (Figs 52.16 and 52.24). This block is used for the permanent lower molars and second premolars, as well as canines and incisors. (Note that the lower, central incisors require additional anaesthetic from the opposite side, i.e. a mental nerve block as well.)

Figure 52.10 Injection site for upper incisor tooth.

Figure 52.11 Periodontal injection of local anaesthetic.

An inferior dental block should not be given on both sides simultaneously owing to difficulty with swallowing and tongue reflexes.

The technique for inferior dental block is as follows:

1. The patient is asked to open their mouth as wide as possible.
2. The ridge behind the last molar palpated.
3. The thumb is placed in the retromolar fossa.
4. The needle is inserted near the tip of the thumb on a line just above the occlusal plane of the teeth, just lingually.
5. The needle is inserted 5 mm and injection made very slowly and continuously.
6. The operator turns it horizontally, at a 40° angle across the dorsum of the tongue, and advances until bone contact is made.
7. The needle is withdrawn slightly and the remainder of the cartridge injected very slowly.
8. A buccal injection is needed for extractions of lower molars (Figs 52.15 and 52.24).

Mental nerve block

This is used for the lower first premolars and anterior teeth (Fig. 52.14). Injection should not be into the mental nerve itself, and the needle should always be withdrawn slightly before injecting. This block needs to be accompanied by a lingual infiltration.

Nasopalatine nerve block

This is given by the incisive papilla just behind the central incisors. It is quite painful and only a very small amount of anaesthetic is needed (Fig. 52.12).

Greater (posterior) palatine nerve block (see Fig. 52.13)

Periodontal (intraligamental) injection. This is useful for loose teeth, or to back up a difficult case which is resistant to local anaesthesia (Fig. 52.11).

Figure 52.12 Palatal injection for incisors (Incisal papilla).

Figure 52.13 Palatal foramen injection site for upper molars.

Figure 52.14 Mental nerve injection for 1st premolar and canine and incisors.

Figure 52.15 Buccal infiltration injection for lower molars.

Figure 52.16 Inferior dental nerve block for all teeth up to the midline.

Figure 52.17 Use of Couplands elevator on a lower molar tooth.

52.11.3 Position of operator and patient

Good lighting is essential. The patient should be sitting upright with the operator's arm level with the patient's mouth. The operator should stand in front of the patient for upper right or left and lower left extractions, but behind the patient for extractions on the lower right. The practitioner should be prepared to lie the patient down quickly if they feel faint or if they actually faint.

52.11.4 Technique for extractions

1. The Coupland's or periosteal elevator is pushed into the gingivae to free the attachment of the tooth to the alveolar bone (Fig. 52.17).
2. The instrument is pushed to separate and lever off the alveolar bone support.
3. It is elevated to loosen against secure neighbouring teeth (Fig. 52.26).
4. Forceps are chosen (preferred by the author for most extractions) for deciduous upper or lower molars (Figs 52.18–52.22).

Figure 52.18 Use of forceps on a lower incisor.

Figure 52.19 Use of upper forceps on upper molar.

Figure 52.20 Use of elevator on upper molar.

Figure 52.21 Use of forceps on lower molar.

Figure 52.22 Use of upper forceps on upper pre-molar.

5. The instrument is pushed down past alveolar support.
6. It is moved from side to side.
7. Movement is in a small circle, with gradually increasing movement.
8. The operator feels for the direction of give and the path of direction of the root pattern.
9. The tooth usually gives buccally, and is gradually levered out and pulled (Fig. 52.27).
10. The cheek, lips and opposing teeth are protected with a pack.
11. The use of force on the crown of the tooth to lever or pull must be avoided as it will break.
12. For single-rooted teeth, the forceps are pushed up into the gum and rotated gently clockwise then anticlockwise, gradually increasing the movement.
13. Once the periodontal fibres give, the forceps are swung lingual to buccal.

Figure 52.23 Lower molar buccal abscess.

Figure 52.24   Lower molar inferior dental nerve block.

Figure 52.25   Lower molar buccal local anaesthetic.

Figure 52.26   Lower molar elevator.

Figure 52.27 Lower molar extraction.

14. For two-rooted teeth or premolars, movement from the buccal to lingual direction in small increments, and gradually increasing the force as necessary.
15. The operator must pull carefully to avoid breaking the apices of the roots.

Where a tooth fractures, any part of the root may be left, particularly in an emergency situation, unless it easy to elevate. Fortunately, they are not usually a cause of pain.

52.12 COMPLICATIONS OF EXTRACTIONS

■ The patient faints or hyperventilates, or there may be other unrelated medical emergencies.
■ Postoperative pain may be variable in degree and timing owing to the trauma of extraction or a dry socket. In most cases simple analgesics and anti-inflammatory drugs are all that are needed.
■ Bleeding, which may require suturing.
■ Soft-tissue swelling, which may require antibiotics.

52.13 SOME DOS AND DON'TS

The practitioner should:

■ ask a local dentist for some practice sessions
■ understand the anatomy of the jaws, nerves, blood supply and the teeth
■ avoid injections in the presence of an abscess (local anaesthetic will not work)
■ avoid solid difficult molar teeth until practised
■ not rely on the crown for force, but place pressure on roots
■ avoid using molar forceps. The smallest, most delicate instruments adequate for the job (root forceps) should be used, as the crown of the tooth can sheer off with too much force
■ with difficult extractions avoid persisting for a long time. It will be easier to repeat the procedure in 3–4 days' time owing to the natural inflammation and loosening of the periodontal tissues

- avoid very carious teeth until experienced, especially if caries is below the gum/bone level (divide roots and elevate if molar)
- avoid extractions if visibility is poor
- avoid extracting traumatized teeth, i.e. incisors, deciduous or permanent, at the time of trauma as they rarely cause pain, and may be reassessed 1 week later
- avoid tearing the attached gingivae: they should be separated from the tooth first to avoid causing unnecessary persistent bleeding
- avoid high-pressure intraligamentary periodontal syringe or intrabony injections for extractions
- treat every patient as if they were hepatitis B or HIV positive.

52.14 BLEEDING AND SUTURING

It is occasionally necessary to suture a bleeding tooth socket. Packing for 15 min should be tried first, and if this does not control bleeding, a suture should be inserted. Suturing should also be used if the medical history suggests a bleeding tendency, and also if the patient is on aspirin or is very apprehensive. Interrupted black silk is the preferred suture material: it is soft and ties easily, and is easily seen when the sutures are removed 4–7 days later.

52.15 PROPHYLACTIC COVER AGAINST BACTERIAL ENDOCARDITIS

Antibiotic cover should be used where the patient has a history of cardiac defects, rheumatic fever, St Vitus's dance (chorea), where there is an arterial prosthesis or where there are significant cardiac murmurs.

The recommended drug regime is as follows:

- amoxycillin 3 g sachet is given 1 h before the operation (half-dose if aged under 5 years); only two doses per month and none for 3–4 months
- if the patient is allergic to amoxycillin, or has had a recent dose, clindamycin 600 mg may be used (half-dose under 5)
- chlorhexidine mouthwash is used 5 min before the procedure and kept in the mouth for 2–3 min undiluted.

52.16 ANTIBIOTIC REGIME FOR INFECTIONS

Antibiotics are not routinely needed; a hot salt-water mouthwash is often sufficient with or without a chlorhexadine mouthwash. Where antibiotics are deemed necessary, the following may be used:

- amoxycillin 250 mg qds for 5 days
- metronidazole 200 mg tds for 5 days
- amoxycillin 3 g sachet stat, with a second dose at a 6–8 h interval
- phenoxymethyl penicillin 250 mg qds for 5 days.

In severe cases a combination of the above may be used, e.g. starting with a 3 g sachet of amoxycillin and continuing with an alternative. Where the patient is sensitive to penicillin or any of the above, erythromycin or tetracycline may be used.

52.17 RECOMMENDED INSTRUMENTS

Each practitioner has their own favourite instruments, but the following have been found to be of most use for dental surgery:

- oil of cloves
- dental mouth mirror
- right-angled probe
- Briault probe
- basic periodontal examination probe (BPE)
- hygienist sickle scalers no. 6 and 7
- college tweezers
- flat plastic mixing spatula
- mixing pad
- topical anaesthetic gel
- cotton bud to apply topical gel
- normal local anaesthetic syringe with cartridges and needles
- upper premolar forceps, deciduous 108 and 76 (adult size)
- lower premolar forceps, deciduous 102 and 74 (adult size)
- Coupland's elevators, various sizes
- Cryer's elevators, left and right
- Swann Morton scalpel handle no. B3 and blades no.15
- perioesteal elevator
- Austin flap retractor
- mosquito needle holders
- suture scissors
- black silk sutures and needle
- cotton-wool rolls
- cotton-wool pledglets
- Septodont 'Pharmaethyl', ethyl chloride spray
- Septodont 'Cimpat'
- Septodont 'Alvogyl'
- De Trey 'Kalzinol'
- De Trey 'IRM'

Suppliers include Henry Schein Procare, Claudius Ash and Wright-Cottrel.

Appendix 52.1

Sample questionnaire to be completed by patients giving a medical history:

	No	Yes – details please
■ Are you receiving/attending treatment from a doctor, hospital, clinic or specialist?		
■ Are you taking any medicines, tablets, creams, ointments, injections, from your doctor?		
■ Are you taking or have you taken steroids in the last two years?		
■ Are you allergic to any medicines, foods or materials?		
■ Do you carry a warning card?		
■ Have you had any blood tests, inoculations, etc.?		
■ Have you had a bad reaction to general or local anaesthetic?		
■ Do you have arthritis?		
■ Do you bruise easily of following a tooth extraction, surgery or injury have you or your family bled so as to cause you to be worried?		
■ Have you been hospitalized? If YES what for and when?		
■ Do you suffer from bronchitis, asthma or other chest conditions?		
■ Have you ever had your blood refused by the blood transfusion service?		
■ Have you ever been told you have a heart murmur, heart problem, heart attack, angina, blood pressure?		
■ Do you have fainting attacks, giddiness, blackouts or epilepsy?		
■ Do you have diabetes or does anyone in your family?		
■ Do you ever get ulcers or cold sore?		
■ Have you had rheumatic fever or chorea (St Vitus's dance)?		
■ Do you have a pacemaker, or have you had any form or heart surgery?		
■ Do you suffer from hay fever, eczema or any other allergy?		
■ Have you had a joint replacement?		
■ Are there any other aspects concerning your health that you think the dentist should know about? If so please use this space.		
■ Has there been any change in your health since you last attended?		

Completed by Patient/Guardian*

Signed: . . . .   Date: . . . .

Administration

Providing information to the patient

Patients who are about to have an operation, whether major or minor, are anxious, and it is a common experience that, despite discussing the details of their forthcoming operation, most of the information is either not heard or soon forgotten. This also applies after the operation is completed, when the doctor and nurse have spent a considerable amount of time and think that they have covered all the relevant points.

When an operation has been performed under an intravenous premedication injection of a benzodiazepine such as midazolam or diazepam, it is almost universal that the patient will remember nothing of what was said.

This can have profound psychological and even medicolegal implications, but can be prevented in almost all situations by the judicious use of preprinted information leaflets which may be given to the patient both before and immediately after their operation. There can then be absolutely no doubt about what was intended, what to expect, when to seek further help, when to return for dressings or suture removal, and what sort of result can be anticipated.

If contact numbers are also included the patient will feel able to seek help both at an early stage, and also appropriately should there be any queries.

The following information sheets are some of those used by the author. Each doctor can design his or her own sheets for their own particular situation, which can be kept in a loose-leaf folder for immediate use.

Some information sheets are included as examples.

The Surgery

1. Carpal tunnel – preoperative information

1 The median nerve passes through a tight space at the wrist called the **carpal tunnel** – occasionally it becomes compressed in this tunnel causing pins and needles in the fingers, and pain which can extend up the forearm.

2 Some settle with splinting, others with tablets, and others following a steroid injection into the tunnel itself. However, when symptoms persist despite these medical measures, it is necessary to decompress the nerve surgically.

3 This will be done under a local anaesthetic supplemented by a premedication injection of a mild sedative and analgesic, and the operation will take about 30 minutes in all.

4 **YOU SHOULD NOT DRIVE A CAR FOR AT LEAST 24 HOURS**

5 Please make arrangements to be driven home 2 hours after the time of your operation.

6 Your hand will be bandaged and in a sling. The bandage needs to be left in place and not disturbed for 14 days when the stitch will be removed. The sling may be removed after 24 hours if comfortable.

7 It is advisable not to work for 2 weeks until after the stitch is removed.

8 If you have any questions, please do not hesitate to contact the surgery.

The Surgery

1A. Carpal tunnel operation – postoperative instructions

1 The median nerve passes through a narrow tunnel at the wrist, and your symptoms of pain and pins and needles have been due to pressure on this nerve.

2 The operation consisted of splitting the thick tissue which lies in front of the nerve, thus releasing the nerve and removing the pressure.

3 It may take several months before the symptoms disappear, depending on how long the nerve has been trapped; in some instances the pain and pins and needles disappear immediately, but the majority improve gradually. Where muscle wasting has occurred around the base of the thumb and little finger, release of the nerve will not improve this, but will at least prevent it becoming any worse.

4 Keep the arm in a sling for two days, and do not disturb the bandage for fourteen days.

5 There is only one single nylon suture holding the wound together; please make an appointment to have this stitch removed on

_____ at _____

6 Please make an appointment in six weeks' time to check that the scar is healing satisfactorily, and that the symptoms are improving.

7 If you have any queries, please do not hesitate to telephone the surgery.

The Surgery
2. Ingrowing toe-nails – postoperative instructions (phenol)

1   A small strip of nail, including the nail-bed has been removed, and the base treated with pure phenol to prevent this strip from regrowing again.

2   When you arrive home, please rest on a setee with the feet elevated on a cushion for the remainder of the day – this reduces the discomfort and the tendency to bleeding.

3   Any simple analgesic tablet such as paracetamol may be taken for any postoperative discomfort.

4   Please make an appointment to see our nurse on

_____ at _____

and a second appointment to see our nurse on

_____ at _____

5   If you have any queries, please do not hesitate to telephone the surgery.

The Surgery
2A. Ingrowing toe-nails – postoperative instructions (wedge)

1   A small strip of nail on the infected side has been removed, including the nail-bed, to prevent this narrow strip from regrowing.

2   Normally, there is just one stitch which needs to be removed on the 7th postoperative day.

3   When you arrive home, please rest on a settee with the feet elevated on a cushion for the remainder of the day – this reduces discomfort, minimizes bleeding, and helps healing.

4   Any simple analgesic tablet such as paracetamol may be taken for any post-operative discomfort.

5   Please make an appointment to see our practice nurse on

_____ at _____

and a second appointment to have the stitch removed on

_____ at _____

6   If you have any queries, please do not hesitate to telephone the surgery.

The Surgery
2B. Ingrowing toe-nails – postoperative instructions (R.W.)

1   A small strip of nail on the infected side has been removed, together with any messy 'granulations'.

2   Using a radio-surgical unit, the nail-bed beneath this small strip of nail has been destroyed by passing a very high-frequency electric current through it.

3   This means that the remaining nail will eventually be very slightly narrower, reducing the chances of an ingrowing nail happening again.

4   When you arrive home, please rest on a setee with the feet elevated on a cushion for the remainder of the day – this reduces any discomfort, minimizes bleeding, and helps healing.

5   Any simple analgesic tablet such as paracetamol may be taken for any postoperative discomfort.

6   Please make an appointment to see our practice nurse on

_____ at _____

7   If you have any queries, please do not hesitate to telephone the surgery.

The Surgery
3. Injection treatment for varicose veins

Injection treatment for varicose veins consists of injecting an irritant fluid into the vein and applying a firm dressing over the injection site. The object of the treatment is to create a controlled inflammation inside the vein, and then by compressing the inflamed surfaces together, hope that they will adhere to each other, thus obliterating the lumen of the vein.

The following instructions should be followed:

1   The bandages should be left on (day and night) for **3 weeks**. Some discomfort should be expected during the first few days, in a small number of patients, it can be very painful, in which case you should take any simple analgesic tablet such as paracetamol, aspirin, codeine or neurofen at regular intervals until the pain subsides.

2   If the outer layers of the bandages work loose or begin to dig into the skin, it is helpful to carefully remove the outer bandage whilst lying down, and then to reapply it firmly from the toes up to the knees, making sure not to disturb the pressure-pads overlying the injection sites in the veins.

3   **Walk at least 3 miles every day**

4   If you wish to have a bath or shower, the bandaged leg may be kept dry by putting it inside a large waterproof polythene bag (e.g. bin-liner) with two elastic bands around the top.

5   After 3 weeks, please make an appointment to see your doctor or the nurse to have the bandages removed.

6   If you have any queries, please do not hesitate to contact the surgery.

The Surgery
3A. Stab-avulsion varicose veins – information sheet

Varicose veins may be treated by elastic support stockings, injections, stripping, or most recently by stab-avulsions.

In stab-avulsion treatment, small 3 mm incisions are made in the skin overlying the vein, which is then gently pulled out. Multiple incisions are made, depending on the extent and severity of the veins. Normally no stitches are needed, and the incisions are closed with just Steri-strips with a small gauze dressing covering them. Elastic bandages are then applied over the dressings and remain in place for 2 weeks.

1   You may have a light meal before coming to the surgery if you wish.

2   If your leg is hairy, **please shave it** before you come – this will help with the application of the Steri-strips, and make it easier for you to remove them!

3   Ladies should wear a loose-fitting skirt.

4   Men should wear a pair of shorts under their trousers.

5   Please bring loose-fitting shoes or slippers to wear home as your foot will have several layers of bandages.

PLEASE ARRANGE TRANSPORT HOME 2 HOURS AFTER THE TIME OF YOUR OPERATION

Under **NO** circumstances must you drive yourself home, or drive a car for at least 24 hours.

When you arrive home, **go immediately to bed** and remain there for at least 12 hours. Gentle walking is encouraged.

You will need to take one week off work, possibly two, depending on how comfortable the leg is, and what your job entails.

If your doctor has given you a prescription for special bandages or elastic stockings, collect them from the chemist and bring them with you on the day of the operation.

You will be given a postoperative instruction sheet on the day of the operation.

If you have any questions, please do not hesitate to telephone the surgery.

The Surgery

3B. Stab-avulsion varicose veins – postoperative instructions

1   In this form of treatment, a small incision has been made in the skin adjacent to the varicose vein and a small segment of vein removed. Multiple incisions are made, depending on the extent and severity of the veins. Normally no stitches are used, and the incisions closed with just Steri-strips, covered by a small dressing, elastic bandages and Tubi-grip.

2   To prevent any bleeding on the way home, an additional strong elastic bandage has been applied over all the above bandages, and this may be removed after you are in bed at home.

3   When you arrive home, **go immediately to bed and remain there for 12 hours**. This is essential, and is to allow the small blood vessels under the skin to seal off and let the bandages apply an even pressure over the leg.

4   Bleeding can occasionally occur under the bandages and some soak through. Should this occur, remain in bed, lie flat, and raise the foot; as the blood is coming from a vein and not an artery, raising the leg will stop the bleeding. If, however, you are concerned, please contact this surgery and speak to one of the doctors.

5   **Keep the bandages on for 10 days**.

6   If they feel uncomfortable or are working loose, it is permissible to reapply them yourself – do this lying down rather than standing, and endeavour to keep an even pressure from the toes to the top of the dressing.

7   Gentle walking each day is helpful.

8   On the 10th day, take off the Tubi-grip and elastic bandage and have a bath. This will soak off the Steri-strips and dressings.

9   Bruising and discoloration is common at this stage and is harmless; it is due to blood collecting under the skin, and disappears over the next few weeks.

10   Reapply the Tubi-grip for another 4 days.

11   Make an appointment to see one of our practice nurses **2 weeks** after the date of your operation to check that everything is healing satisfactorily.

12   **TWO MONTHS** after your operation, would you make an appointment to see your doctor for a final check.

13   If you have any queries, please do not hesitate to contact the surgery.

The Surgery
3C. Varicose veins – information leaflet

1 Varicose veins below the knee can be treated by injections (sclerotherapy).

2 This involves a series of injections into the segments of veins and the application of a pressure-bandage for 3 weeks.

3 The solution used for the injections is an irritant and the object is to produce a controlled area of phlebitis within the vein, and by applying pressure with the bandage, it is hoped to occlude the vein.

4 During the three weeks following injections, it is essential that you walk at least three miles every day – this is extremely important to avoid the risk of developing a deep-vein thrombosis.

5 The treatment itself will take about 15–20 minutes, and you will have an elastic bandage applied over the leg, covered with a Tubi-grip bandage and possibly a third bandage as well!

6 This means you should bring a very loose-fitting shoe with you in order to be able to walk afterwards.

7 The bandage will need to be in place for three weeks and must be kept dry – this means covering the bandaged leg with a plastic bag (bin-liners are ideal) with rubber bands round the top, if you wish to have a quick bath or shower.

8 On the day of the injections, we will give you another information leaflet explaining how to look after the leg and bandages.

9 If you have any questions, please do not hesitate to ask one of the doctors or nurses.

The Surgery
4. Injection treatment for ganglion

A ganglion is a cyst filled with clear jelly; it is often situated near a joint, and may cause pain and slowly increase in size. Some eventually rupture spontaneously and disappear, but this may not happen for up to three years.

1 Injection treatment consists of drawing off the jelly from the ganglion, and then injecting an irritant fluid into the empty cyst.

2 This causes an inflammation within the ganglion. A pressure bandage is then applied with the object of compressing the inflamed surfaces and thus obliterating the cyst.

3 **Please keep the bandage in place for 2 weeks**

4 If it works loose, you may reapply it firmly, but do not disturb the pressure-pad overlying the ganglion.

5 At the end of 2 weeks, you may remove the pad and bandage, and normally no further follow-up visits are needed.

6 This treatment carries an 80% cure rate and has the advantage that there is no scar. If however, you are in the 20% which recur, the same treatment can be offered again.

7 If you have any queries, please do not hesitate to contact the surgery.

The Surgery
4A. Information sheet – ganglion

1   A ganglion is a cyst filled with clear jelly.

2   They usually occur near an underlying joint, particularly at the wrist and fingers, and can cause pain or discomfort.

3   It is possible they arise from a leak of lubricating jelly in the joint through the tissues, to the skin, where they appear as a smooth, tender swelling.

4   Many ganglia, if left alone, will eventually disappear on their own, but this may take many years.

5   An old-fashioned treatment used to be to hit it with the 'Family Bible' in the hope of bursting it and releasing the jelly under the skin. Unfortunately, this treatment was never very successful, and there was a high recurrence rate!

6   Small ganglia on the fingers can be pricked with a sterile needle, and the jelly squeezed out. If a firm tape is then applied around two-thirds of the finger for 6 weeks, this carries an 80% cure rate, and can always be repeated if the first attempt fails.

7   Larger ganglia around the wrist can be cut out, but even this carries a 20% recurrence rate, so is not always the preferred treatment unless everyone is desperate!

8   At this surgery, we offer a treatment called **aspiration and sclerose** which involves putting a small amount of local anaesthetic in the skin, inserting a needle into the ganglion, and sucking out the jelly. We then inject a small quantity of sclerosant, which makes the inside of the cyst sticky, and then apply a firm compression bandage for the next 2 weeks.

9   The object of this bandage is to press the front and back walls of the cyst together in the hope that they will stick together and seal off the little hole through which the jelly has leaked.

10 This treatment also carries an 80% cure rate, but has the advantage that it does not leave a scar, and should the ganglion recur, we can always repeat the treatment.

The Surgery

5. Instructions following treatment with liquid nitrogen

1   Liquid nitrogen destroys tissues by freezing to minus 196 degrees Celsius. This results in ice forming inside the cells, and as this thaws, it causes cell death. It also releases the wart virus into the surrounding tissue, which in turn stimulates the body's immune system to produce antibodies against the wart virus. This explains why other warts on the body often disappear after treating the main warts.

2   Immediately following treatment, apart from a slight discomfort, it will look as if nothing has happened to the skin.

3   Gradually, over the next few days, swelling, reddening and sometimes, blistering will occur.

4   Following this stage, healing occurs, which is usually remarkably pain-free, and leaves only a very slight scar, or none at all.

5   In dark skins, there is usually an area of depigmentation following cryotherapy, this normally recovers over the following year.

6   Reaction to liquid nitrogen is very variable; in some patients quite alarming-looking blisters can occur together with swelling of the surrounding tissues. Despite this, satifactory healing occurs.

7   Keep the treated area dry for 6 days if at all possible – it does not need any dressing unless blistering occurs, in which case, just a simple non-stick dressing may be applied. If a blister occurs, it is quite in order to prick it with a sterile needle to drain any fluid, and then apply a clean dry dressing.

8   More than one treatment may be required.

9   If you have any queries, please do not hesitate to contact the surgery.

The Surgery

6. Electrocautery – postoperative instructions

1 Many warts, moles, naevi and keratoses can be removed with a scalpel or curette, and the base cauterized with the electrocautery. This stops any bleeding.

2 Alternatively, the mole may be removed entirely with the electro-cautery or a high-frequency electrosurgical unit. This cuts through the tissues and seals any bleeding points simultaneously, thus avoiding the need for any stitches, and in many cases gives a neater scar.

3 After cautery, healing occurs over the next few weeks.

4 It is helpful to keep the area dry for 2 or 3 days.

5 When you remove any dressing, you may find a reddened, weeping area, which forms a dry crust. This will then separate leaving a bright pink area, and may even form another crust.

6 Try not to pick off any scabs or crusts, but allow to come away naturally.

7 The bright pink area will slowly fade to match the surrounding skin over a period of 18 months to 2 years.

8 Where possible, every specimen is sent for routine examination under a microscope to establish an exact diagnosis. We normally receive the results back from the laboratory after 10 days. You can assume that if you have not heard from us, the lesion was harmless, but we are happy to give you the result personally if you contact the surgery.

9 If you have any queries, please do not hesitate to contact the surgery.

The Surgery

7. Meibomian cysts – postoperative instructions

1 A meibomian cyst occurs inside the eyelid, and is caused by a blockage of one of the little lubricating glands.

2 Treatment consists of incising the cyst under a local anaesthetic.

3 This is done from inside the lid, so there will not be any visible scar.

4 After the operation, eye-ointment is applied, and a pad and bandage put on; this is to protect the eye against dust, etc. on the way home as the eye will still be anaesthetized.

5 The pad and bandage may be removed after four hours.

6 Do not be alarmed when you remove the pad – there will be a mixture of ointment, secretions and blood which can look alarming!

7 Gently clean the eyelids with warm water and a face-flannel.

8 Thereafter, apply the chloramphenicol eye-drops three times a day for one week.

9 It is not normally necessary to see you again, but if you have any queries, please do not hesitate to contact the surgery.

The Surgery
8. Tongue-tie – preoperative and postoperative instructions

1   The fibrous band holding down the tongue can usually be divided under a local anaesthetic.

2   One hour before your operation, apply the local anaesthetic solution on a dental cotton-wool roll to the area below the tongue. It is helpful to renew the anaesthetic solution three or four times until that part of the mouth feels completely 'numb'.

3   Do not have hot drinks from now on, until normal sensation returns, as there would be a risk of burning the inside of the mouth. Likewise, avoid biting on the inside of the cheek with the teeth.

4   Following the operation, rinse the mouth out with warm water or mouth-rinse three or four times a day until healing has taken place.

5   Bleeding is unusual – however, should it occur, it may easily be controlled by applying a clean dressing or handkerchief and pressing firmly for at least **10 minutes by the clock**.

6   Normally, no follow-up is necessary. If you do have any queries, please do not hesitate to contact the surgery.

The Surgery
9. Hormone implants

1 Most of the symptoms occurring at the menopause are due to a deficiency of oestrogens.

2 Hormone-replacement therapy consists of giving oestrogens to the patient, and in the majority of women, all the symptoms are relieved. As well as relieving symptoms, it has been shown to offer protection against osteoporosis (thinning of the bones), heart-disease and stroke, and can even lower the levels of cholesterol.

3 Oestrogens may be given as tablets, adhesive patches, creams or implants.

4 A hormone implant consists of a small tablet of pure oestradiol (the naturally occurring hormone in the body) which is inserted just under the skin. This is done under a local anaesthetic and the skin closed either with a single stitch or by skin-closure adhesive Steri-strips.

5 The implant slowly dissolves, releasing the oestradiol over a period of six months.

6 If you have had a hysterectomy, hormone replacement is very simple as you will only need oestrogens. If, however, you still have a uterus, you will need additional progesterone, and this can be given intermittently each month to bring on a period, or continuously when it may be possible to avoid having a period.

7 Some patients feel their implant has 'worn off' in less than 6 months and feel they would like another at shorter intervals. This is generally not advisable nor necessary as blood tests show the level of circulating oestradiol is still adequate, and another implant would raise the levels too much. Thus, unless your doctor has recommended otherwise, we suggest **one implant every 6 months** will give the best results.

8 **After 5 months please would you make an appointment to see our Practice Nurse.** This will enable us to offer a simple check-up, answer any questions about HRT and at this visit we can give you a prescription for the next implant.

9 At this visit, you can also make an appointment for your next implant.

The Surgery
10. Patient information leaflet – basal cell carcinoma

1   A basal cell carcinoma (also known as a rodent ulcer or BCC) is a type of skin tumour which is increasing in frequency in this country.

2   It is thought to arise from previous repeated exposures to severe ultraviolet light causing sunburn, up to 40 years previously.

3   They are **not** malignant cancers, i.e. they do **not** spread to other parts of the body producing secondary tumours, but slowly grow, and if not treated, become larger and larger, slowly invading deeper tissues beneath the surface.

4   Small basal cell cancers can be treated in a variety of ways – some are excised surgically and the wound stitched, others are treated with radiotherapy, some with liquid nitrogen cryotherapy, and others by removing with a steel spoon and cauterizing the base several times with a diathermy or electrocautery.

5   Whichever method is chosen, it is **essential** to have meticulous follow-up for several years – your doctor will let you know how this should be done in your case.

6   As a general guide, however, if there are no signs of any lumps reappearing in the scar of the original tumour, all is well. If you think there may be a recurrence, **please contact your doctor for advice**.

The Surgery
11. Care of wounds which have been sutured

1 When suturing a wound, the object is to obtain the neatest scar possible.

2 This is achieved at the time of the operation by inserting many fine sutures, rather than a few, widely spaced, thick sutures.

3 It is also helped by designing the scar such that the minimum tension occurs on the skin edges.

4 As well as sutures, we sometimes use sterile self-adhesive strips (Steri-strips) to support the edges of the wound while it is healing.

5 Where the wound is deep, we also insert absorbable sutures under the skin to give additional support during healing.

6 The timing of the removal of sutures is critical – if they are left in too long, 'cross-hatching' can occur leaving permanent scars, whereas if they are removed too soon, the edges of the wound can gape open.

7 Where there is little tension on the skin, e.g. the face, the sutures may be removed after only a few days, but where there is considerable tension, e.g. over the knee, shoulder or back, we need to leave them in for a much longer time.

8 You can help to achieve the neatest scar yourself by following the following simple rules: (a) Where the wound is open to the air (e.g. on the face and scalp) keep it **dry** for at least 48 hours. (b) Where the wound is covered, keep it **dry** and do not disturb the dressing – this will prevent any infection.

9 **Please make an appointment with our nurse to have the stitches removed on.**

_____ at _____

10 If the wound looks reddened or discharging, or you are at all concerned, please do not hesitate to contact the surgery.

11 We may apply Steri-strips to the wound after the stitches have been removed – this is to give external support; it helps to leave these in place for as long as possible.

12 In certain sites such as the arm and shoulder, it is helpful to apply Steri-strip support for several weeks after the stitches have been removed.

The Surgery

12. Removal of skin lesions by radiosurgery

1   Radiosurgery is a new method of treating many skin lesions using high-frequency radiowaves (4 million Hertz) which cuts through the skin and also seals off any small bleeding vessels.

2   This tends to give superior cosmetic results to conventional surgical excision or electrocautery.

3   At the end of the treatment, a small plaster is usually applied – please keep this in place **for 2 days**.

4   After this time, the plaster may be removed and the area cleaned gently with warm, soapy water.

5   Healing can take from one to four weeks, depending on the size of the original lesion; during this time, it helps to keep the wound clean and moist, by regularly washing with warm, soapy water – about six times a day, using soft cotton wool. Do not rub the area too vigorously or it may bleed. If bleeding does occur, it may be stopped by covering with a small dressing and pressing firmly with the finger for 10 minutes.

6   Normally no other treatment is necessary, but if the area becomes very messy or inflamed or develops a reddened surrounding area which seems to be spreading, **please contact the surgery for advice**.

7   Initially the wound will be moist, with a slight discharge. This will gradually dry, and may form a thin scab on the surface. Try not to pick this off but leave to separate naturally.

8   At this stage, the wound will appear bright red and dry.

9   Over the next few weeks, the reddened area will gradually fade, and eventually, after about 18 months, should match the surrounding skin.

10   The majority of all lesions are sent to the hospital for routine examination under a microscope, and we normally receive the full histological report after 10 days.

11   If you have any concerns, please do not hesitate to contact the surgery.

The Surgery

13. Advice about 'Moles' and 'Naevi'

1   Moles (naevi) occur on everyone.

2   The majority are harmless and remain harmless, but in recent years there has been a marked increase in three types of mole:
(a) basal cell carcinoma
(b) squamous cell carcinoma
(c) malignant melanoma.

3   It is now realized that exposure to sunlight increases the chances of developing melanoma and skin cancers. There may be a delay of ten to forty years between exposure and the development of a skin tumour.

4   Basal cell cancers (rodent ulcers) and squamous cell cancers are thought to arise in people who have repeated exposure to strong sunlight (e.g. farm workers) They start as a small raised, circular lesion, slightly translucent with very small blood vessels crossing the surface, they are commonly seen on the face. Basal cell carcinomas are not malignant (i.e. don't spread to distant parts of the body), but just tend to get bigger and invade local tissues. Treatment is removal surgically.

5   Malignant melanoma is the most serious of the skin tumours. It is thought to arise following one episode of severe blistering sunburn many years previously. It can spread to glands and other parts of the body, so early diagnosis and treatment is essential. Treatment is by wide surgical excision.

6   The most important advice is to seek medical help for any mole which **has recently changed,** i.e. changed colour, changed size, or has started to bleed or itch.

7   Some facts about melanoma:
(a) They are commonly more than 1 cm in diameter
(b) They are irregular in outline
(c) They are usually multicoloured, black, brown, pink and red
(d) The mole has recently changed size or colour
(e) It may itch
(f) They are common in fair-skinned people
(g) They are very rare before puberty
(h) They may be raised above the surface of the skin
(i) They are more common in people who already have more than 50 pre-existing moles.

8   **IF IN DOUBT SEEK MEDICAL ADVICE**

9   **Prevention:**
(a) Although everyone likes a suntan and enjoys the warmth of sunbathing, overexposure to sunlight is definitely bad for you.
(b) Therefore, avoid exposure to sun.
(c) Avoid getting accidentally sunburned.
(d) Protect children from sunlight.
(e) Use high-factor sun barrier cream (factor 15 or above)
(f) Don't use sunbeds
(g) Cover any dark moles before exposure to sunlight with total sunblock cream or clothing.

13. *(Continued.)*

OTHER HARMLESS SKIN LESIONS

Benign intradermal naevus – a raised, circular mole

Melanocytic naevus – a coloured mole

Juvenile melanoma – very dark, usually in children – harmless

Solar keratosis – flaky, warty lesion

Seborrhoeic wart – coloured, warty lesion, usually on trunk

Hand warts and verrucae – harmless but a nuisance – caused by a virus

Blue naevus – black/blue small circular raised spot

Keratoacanthoma – rapidly growing warty lesion with rough centre

Molluscum contagiosum – small, pearly spots with dimple in centre – can spread

Histiocytoma (dermatofibroma) – Hard nodule in the skin – pale – harmless.

TERMINOLOGY

Solar – related to exposure to sunlight

Actinic – also related to sunlight

Melanocytic – coloured

Benign – harmless

Intradermal – in the skin

Naevus – another name for a mole.

The Surgery
14. Information sheet – warts

1. Warts are caused by a virus, and are therefore spread by contact.

2. Verrucae are warts on the sole of the foot.

3. If left alone, the majority of warts and verrucae will eventually disappear. This is because the body has built up a high enough level of immunity to the wart virus, and at this stage the wart is destroyed.

4. When warts disappear spontaneously, they do not leave a scar.

5. Treatments are many and varied! As with most conditions in medicine, where there are many different treatments available, it usually means none of them is particularly effective!

6. Simple remedies can be purchased from the chemists and consist of paints, ointments and plasters. It is important to follow the instructions.

7. Where there are large numbers of warts or verrucae, no treatment seems to be very good, and it probably means waiting patiently until they disappear on their own.

8. Large, single, stubborn warts can be treated either with liquid nitrogen or surgically. Liquid nitrogen destroys the wart by freezing to $-196°C$ and is very effective in many cases.

9. If this fails, we can remove the wart surgically, or with a radiowave surgical instrument.

10. **It is important to realize that no treatment can offer a 100% guarantee of cure**. Even with very thorough treatment, they can return, so you should be aware of this possibility.

The Surgery
15. Tennis elbow

1   Tennis elbow is diagnosed by a very painful spot over the outer bony part of the elbow.

2   It is thought to be due to tearing of a few tendon fibres where they are attached to the bone at the elbow – usually as a result of repeated muscle strain (such as playing tennis).

3   If left to nature, all tennis elbows eventually recover, but it may take several years.

4   Various treatments have been suggested, but none is very successful.

5   Injection with steroid and local anaesthetic gives about the best results when other treatments have failed.

6   The injection itself can be quite painful, and during the next two or three days, the pain may be very severe and require strong pain-killers.

7   After a few days, if the injection has been successful, the original pain disappears.

8   Unfortunately, if you are still overusing the arm, a tennis elbow can recur.

9   Following an injection, it is helpful to rest the elbow for two days, avoiding any heavy lifting and repetetive movements.

10   Up to three injections can be given, but each becomes less effective, and if symptoms persist after three injections, it is better to live with it, knowing that it will eventually clear on its own.

11   In very rare cases, an operation can be offered if symptoms are extremely severe, but even this cannot guarantee a cure!

The Surgery

16. The treatment of piles (haemorrhoids)

1   Piles are merely veins inside the anus.

2   They can bleed or even prolapse.

3   Bleeding, when it occurs, is usually painless and bright red.

4   Treatment is important to abolish any bleeding, otherwise more serious conditions such as tumours and ulcers may be missed.

5   Simple piles can be treated with creams and suppositories.

6   Where these measures fail, injections and/or banding may be offered.

7   Where injections are done, a small volume of oily phenol is injected above the pile, and this causes it to shrink over the next 6 weeks.

8   Where 'banding' is done, a small neoprene band is applied to the loose lining above the pile, and this pulls the pile away from the anus, preventing it prolapsing. The band eventually drops off.

9   Both injections and banding are remarkably pain free. A slight discomfort may be experienced during the procedure, but this soon passes off.

10 Improvement occurs gradually over the following 6 weeks.

11 To help recovery, please note the following instructions:
(a) Avoid becoming constipated.
(b) Drink plenty of water (more than six glasses daily)
(c) Do not sit for a long time on the toilet (i.e. do not take a library book in the 'loo'). Wait until you feel you need to have your bowels open, and then go quickly. Sitting and straining makes piles worse.

(d) Eat plenty of fruit and vegetables in your diet.

12 You may notice bleeding during the first 6 weeks following injections or banding – this is quite normal.

13 **Bleeding which occurs after 6 weeks should be reported.**

14 If you have any concerns, please do not hesitate to contact the surgery.

CHAPTER 54

Medicolegal aspects of minor surgery*

Many doctors contemplating minor surgery are worried about possible medicolegal implications, and even litigation. Fortunately, up to the present time, minor surgery in general practice has not been a 'high-risk' area as far as medicolegal problems are concerned; at the time of writing minor surgery accounts for 2.5% of medical negligence claims settled by the Medical Defence Union (MDU) on behalf of general practitioner (GP) members in the UK. This chapter covers those aspects which will enable the doctor to offer a high standard of care, so that his or her technique will not be open to criticism, and to reduce the risk of harm to his or her patients.

54.1 SURGICAL SKILL

All doctors must evaluate their surgical proficiency before offering a minor surgery service to patients; to this end it is good practice to approach a local consultant surgical colleague to discuss any problems, and to ask for guidance and support in the future. This is usually more than willingly given.

As experience grows, doctors may wish to extend their range of surgical skills; it is important always to ensure that they have received adequate instruction and supervised practice before embarking on any new minor operation.

54.2 PREOPERATIVE ASSESSMENT OF THE PATIENT

Careful preoperative assessment of the lesion and a patient's suitability for minor surgery is fundamental to safety. Where the doctor suspects a malignant melanoma, or basal cell or squamous cell carcinoma, the patient should be referred urgently to a specialist colleague for assessment.

Certain patients such as very young children, elderly, frail patients, and the psychiatrically disturbed may find difficulty in coping with a

*Based on the booklet 'Problems in general practice – minor surgery' by Patrick Dando, Stephen Green and Julie Price of the Medical Defence Union Ltd.

procedure done under local anaesthesia, or may find difficulties with mobility during the postoperative period. It would, therefore, be wise to refer such patients.

Knowledge about the patient's past medical history and current medication is extremely important. Such conditions as diabetes, peripheral vascular disease, skin sepsis and previous keloid scar formation would be possible contraindications to operation, as would treatment with anticoagulants and long-term steroids. Patients taking any medication which affects coagulation and haemostasis such as warfarin, aspirin, non-steroidal anti-inflammatory drugs and the oral contraceptive pill should be given careful assessment. In certain circumstances, stopping the medication one week prior to surgery may be advisable.

Certain lesions have predictable difficulties: sebaceous cysts on the back of the neck can be quite difficult to remove or extremely vascular, and frequently difficult to anaesthetize adequately. Similarly, lipomata, particularly in the midline on the back, or large lipomata over the shoulder may be found to extend deeper than originally anticipated and are better referred.

Recurrent lesions may also be better referred, as fibrous scarring may make accurate dissection difficult. Keloid scars should never be revised as a larger keloid scar will certainly recur. The skin over the anterior tibial surface heals poorly, so care needs to be taken in removing any lesion in this site.

54.3 CONSENT

For most minor surgical procedures in general practice, oral consent is adequate. If the doctor feels that a written consent form is necessary, this should be signed by both the patient and the doctor only after the whole procedure has been carefully explained to, and understood by the patient. Written consent should be obtained for vasectomy (Chapter 39). The fact that consent has been obtained should be recorded in the patient's notes, together with any warning about visible scars or risk of keloid formation. It is also important to explain to the patient what alternative treatments are available, what to expect at operation, that there will inevitably be a scar (it is surprising how many patients assume that they can have an operation without a scar) and how much time off work may be needed, and to ensure they have adequate transport home. Keloid scarring is more likely on the anterior chest wall, deltoid, shoulder and back of neck, particularly in patients of Afro-Caribbean origin.

54.4 HISTOLOGY

Because surprises can always occur, it is good practice to send every specimen for histological examination. This is not only establishes an accurate diagnosis, but also improves the doctor's diagnostic acumen. Where a laboratory finds that it cannot deal with all specimens, one of two alternative courses of action is possible.

1. Selected specimens should be fixed, mounted in paraffin wax, but filed away, only to be sectioned and examined if a subsequent query arises.
2. The consultant histopathologist should provide written criteria to define those lesions which do not need to be sent for routine examination.

The usual fixative is 10% formaldehyde in normal saline; this is toxic and should be kept away from young children. The specimen should be carefully labelled with the patient's name and address and the nature of the specimen.

It is not sufficient just to send every specimen for routine histological examination; it is essential that a foolproof system is evolved whereby every histology report is personally seen by the doctor. To this end, a 'histology book' can be recommended (Chapter 19), whereby the patient's name and address, specimen, clinical diagnosis and histological diagnosis are recorded. By putting a tick opposite each entry when the report is received and noted, any missing reports can easily be identified.

54.5 DANGER AREAS

Before making an incision, a thorough knowledge of the underlying anatomy is essential, particularly the surface markings of nerves, arteries and tendons.

The axilla, femoral triangle, neck and wrist are complicated areas anatomically, and great caution needs to be exercised. If it pulsates, it must not be touched. Incisions in the line of skin creases will give the neatest scars (Chapter 10).

Superficial nerves may be damaged in the following three areas:

1. the posterior triangle of the neck (spinal accessory nerve)
2. the lateral side of the popliteal fossa (common peroneal nerve)
3. the side of the jaw (mandibular branch of the facial nerve).

Operations on the face, particularly for cosmetic reasons, should be given careful consideration, and if necessary referred to a plastic surgeon. Skin closure can be difficult on the tip of the nose and pinna of the ear; similarly, the doctor should beware of excising lesions near the eyes, particularly near the nasolachrymal ducts.

Before suturing lacerations following trauma, the GP must ensure that there are no foreign bodies still present, and that no neurovascular or tendon or joint damage has occurred. If necessary a radiological examination may be arranged, and the patient's tetanus immunization status should be checked.

54.6 INFECTION

It is essential that all surgical instruments are properly sterilized [5, 58]; this requires the use of an autoclave or hot-air oven, or central sterile supplies department (CSSD) facilities (Chapter 6). Given this, infection rates for GP minor surgery are very low.

For both patients' and doctors' safety, gloves should be worn. No doctor should operate if he or she has any infection, particularly one involving the hands.

All healthcare workers, including GPs and their assistants offering minor surgery, who perform 'exposure-prone procedures' should be immunized against hepatitis B if non-immune, and their response to the vaccine should be checked. Detailed guidance is contained in HSG (93)40. This defines 'exposure-prone procedures' as those where there is a risk that injury to a healthcare worker will result in his or her blood contaminating a patient's open tissues. Those who are e-antigen positive must not carry out such procedures.

It is worth considering giving prophylactic antibiotics to those patients with a history of rheumatic fever, a pacemaker, artificial heart valves or any artificial joint.

If electrocautery or diathermy is to be used, spirit-based antiseptics be avoided, as they may ignite. Joint injections and aspirations must be done under completely aseptic conditions.

54.7 ANAESTHETICS

As a general guide, local anaesthetics are remarkably safe, but the doctor should be aware of the maximum dose for each preparation used (see Chapter 8). Lignocaine should be used cautiously in patients with cardiac and hepatic disease. Lignocaine with added adrenaline should not be used on any digit, the tip of the nose, ear, penis or scrotum.

Nerve blocks in experienced hands provide safe and efficient means of anaesthesia, but if the doctor is considering using an intravenous regional block (Bier's block), scrupulous attention to detail must be observed, an assistant should **always** be present to monitor the tourniquet, a double sphygmomanometer cuff employed and full resuscitation facilities available (Chapters 8 and 49). Similar safeguards also apply where intravenous diazepam or midazolam is used, and the doctor should be aware that benzodiazepines may cause not only amnesia, but also hallucinations.

54.8 PRODUCT LIABILITY

Under the Consumer Protection Act 1987, it is now necessary for a doctor to record the batch numbers and source of supply of all drugs, anaesthetics and suture materials used for minor surgery. All equipment used should be properly maintained and records kept that this has been done. Such records need to be kept for 11 years.

54.9 MISHAPS

In the unlikely event of a mishap, it is sensible to inform the patient immediately of the facts, with the simple courtesy of a sincere apology, and to ensure that arrangements can be set in hand to rectify the problem quickly. Such action should be recorded in the patient's notes, and advice sought from the doctor's medical defence organization.

54.10 RISK MANAGEMENT ANALYSIS

An analysis of 26 claims settled by the MDU on behalf of its members over 5 years showed that 65% patients were female and 58% patients were aged between 20 and 45 years.

The types of minor surgery involved were as follows:

vasectomy	4%
cryosurgery	8%
chemicals	15%
sclerotherapy	4%
aspiration	4%
ligation	4%
electro-cautery	4%
circumcision	4%
intra-articular injection	23%
excision/biopsy	26%

Five of the above procedures accounted for 80% of the settled claims, namely:

- excision/biopsy
- intra-articular/periarticular injections
- application of chemicals
- cryosurgery
- vasectomy.

Forty-six per cent of claims involved issues related to lack of consent or lack of information and the most common complaints were of pain and scarring.

Adverse outcomes included the following:

postoperative pain	33%
scarring	26%
burns	11%
wound infection	7%
nerve damage	7%
necrosis	4%
septic arthritis	4%
discoloured skin	2%
haematoma	2%
bleeding	2%
ischaemia	2%

54.11 MINIMIZING THE RISK OF A CLAIM

54.11.1 Excisions

- Surgery of the face, particularly in young adults, should ideally be referred to a specialist.
- One should beware of operating on the shoulder, chest and deltoid as these areas are prone to keloid scar formation.
- Excision of a hypertrophic scar is better referred to a specialist.

- Practice nurses should always seek the opinion of the GP if a wound is not healing satisfactorily.
- It is advisable to have an agreed protocol covering postoperative care and when to remove sutures.
- Removal of sutures and the state of the wound should be recorded.
- Patients should be given an information leaflet covering follow-up arrangements and what to do if there are any complications.

54.11.2 Intra-articular and periarticular injections

- Full aseptic precautions are essential.
- One should avoid injecting infected areas.
- Urgent referral is needed if it is suspected that a joint is infected.
- Particular care is needed to avoid damage to the local neural or vascular structures.

54.11.3 Chemicals

- Phenol must always be kept separate from lignocaine and cleaning agents.
- The bottle must only be opened when required.
- Phenol must be kept in a locked cupboard.
- Protective jelly should be used to surround the skin before applying silver nitrate.

54.11.4 Cryosurgery

- Cryosurgery may cause blistering and scarring.
- The recommended freeze–thaw cycle is 10–15 seconds repeated at 3-weekly intervals.
- Patients should be warned of possible scarring and this fact recorded in the notes.
- Doctors should be adequately trained before using a cryospray or cryoprobe.

54.11.5 Electro-cautery

- Spirit-based skin cleaners should be avoided when undertaking electrocautery.
- Care should be taken that the cautery does not touch dressings, swabs, etc.

Fortunately, with appropriate selection and care, such problems are exceedingly rare and should not deter a doctor from offering a minor surgery service to his or her patients.

The general practitioner and the National Health Service

I hope the House will not hesitate to tell the British Medical Association that we look forward to this Act starting on 5th July 1948 and that we expect the Medical Profession to take their proper part in it because we are satisfied that there is nothing in it that any doctor should be otherwise than proud to acknowledge.

Aneurin Bevan, 1897–1960

55.1 REMUNERATION

The remuneration of a general practitioner working within the National Health Service (NHS) is derived from the number of patients registered on his or her 'list', together with additional item-of-service payments and allowances as follows [59]:

- basic practice allowance (para. 12)
- practice in designated area (para. 14)
- seniority payments (para. 16)
- employment of an assistant (para. 18)
- associate allowance (para. 19)
- deprivation payments (para. 20)
- standard capitation fees (para. 21)
- child health surveillance fees (para. 22)
- registration fees (para. 23)
- night visit fees (para. 24)
- target payment childhood immunizations (para. 25)
- target payment for preschool boosters (para. 26)
- vaccinations and immunizations (para. 27)
- schedule of procedures eligible for a fee (para. 27)
- target payments for cervical cytology (para. 28)
- contraceptive services (para. 29)
- health promotion and chronic disease management (para. 30)
- maternity medical services (para. 31)
- temporary residents (para. 32)
- fees for emergency treatment (para. 33)
- fees for services of an anaesthetist (para. 34)

- fee for arrest of dental haemorrhage (para. 35)
- fee for immediately necessary treatment (para. 36)
- postgraduate education allowance (para. 37)
- GP registrar scheme (para. 38)
- doctors' retainer scheme (para. 39)
- fee for teaching undergraduate medical students (para. 40)
- fee for minor surgery (para. 42)
- rural practice payments (para. 43)
- supply of drugs and appliances (para. 44)
- inducement payments (para. 45)
- payments for temporary cover (para. 46)
- locum cover for education courses (para. 47)
- additional payments during sickness (para. 48)
- additional payments during confinement (para. 49)
- prolonged study leave (para. 50)
- payments under rents and rates (para. 51)
- payments for practice staff (para. 52)
- improvement grants (para. 56)
- London initiative zone workforce flexibilities (para. 57)
- GP computer reimbursement scheme (para. 58)
- cover for GMPs relieved of out-of-hours duties (para. 82)
- drugs
- DMO reports
- others.

Before considering these paragraphs, it is important to clarify when a doctor may charge a fee. Under their terms of service, general practitioners (GPs) are expressly forbidden from asking for, or receiving, payment for, or token in lieu of, the provision of any medical service for any patient registered with them under the NHS [59]. The only exceptions which are allowed are for certain documents, private certificates and vaccination certificates. A GP is allowed to accept private fee-paying patients, provided they are not already registered with the GP or his or her partners under the NHS, and charges may be made to such patients for all medical services rendered.

In the past it was suggested that a GP could request the removal of a NHS patient from his or her list for 3 months and treat the patient privately, in which case the charging of a fee is allowable. Although this is perfectly legal, most doctors would not be happy to do it and it cannot be recommended.

An item-of-service fee is payable for a minor surgical operation performed on a patient receiving emergency medical treatment who is not registered with that GP, or with any of his or her partners. In this case, form FP32 is completed, provided the emergency was not caused by the use of a motor vehicle on the road. What constitutes a minor surgical operation is not defined in this section of the regulations.

Likewise, a separate item-of-service fee is payable for the administration of a general anaesthetic, provided a second qualified doctor (not a trainee GP) is in attendance and personally administers the anaesthetic. This is claimed on form FP31. Thus, although the number of general anaesthetics given in general practice outside hospital is decreasing, there is a recognition by the Department of Health that the administration of a general anaesthetic qualifies for an additional payment. No such item-of-service payment exists for the administration of any local anaesthetic, be it infiltration, nerve block or epidural. It is possible, however, to obtain indirect reimbursement by careful use of the 'Red Book' utilizing paragraph 44.13 for all injections, anaesthetics, suture materials, intrauterine contraceptive devices and skin closure strips, as follows.

1. The doctor personally purchases all injections, anaesthetics, sutures, coils and skin closure strips.
2. For each patient where any of the above are used, and which the doctor or their nurse personally administers, the doctor writes the items on a standard FP10 prescription form.
3. The patient pays no prescription charge, irrespective of age or exemption category.
4. Once per month, all prescriptions are sent to the Central Prescription Pricing Bureau together with a claim form FP34, duly signed.
5. The doctor is subsequently refunded as follows: (a) the basic price of the item used; (b) an 'on-cost' allowance; (c) a 'container' allowance; and (d) a dispensing fee.

This results in a very small profit on each item prescribed. As an example, for the excision of a sebaceous cyst, the practitioner could submit prescriptions for three items used, namely local anaesthetic, suture materials and Steri-strips.

In addition to utilizing paragraph 44.13, savings may be achieved by writing a prescription for certain drugs, dressings and appliances used for any surgical procedure, giving it to the patient, who then brings it back for use by the doctor on that particular patient. However, it must not be overlooked that the general medical practitioner already receives a few pence each year included in the patient's capitation fee to take account of the occasional bandage and dressing.

Items which may be obtained on prescription include the following:

- all bandages, whatever type and size
- Elastoplast bandages
- eye-pad and bandage
- triangular bandages
- cotton wool, lint, gamgee and gauze
- catheters and drainage bags
- self adhesive tapes
- povidone–iodine alcoholic solution
- any drugs, ointments, creams and drops
- injections and insufflations used.

55.2 1990 CONTRACT

Under the Government Contract introduced in 1990, minor surgery was recognized for the first time and a limited payment scheme introduced (SFA 42.1–42.6). In order for a GP to be able to claim the fees for minor surgical procedures he or she must apply to be included in the Family Health Services Authority's 'Minor Surgery List'. This usually entails an inspection of the premises and equipment, together with record-keeping, sterilization, histology and resuscitation facilities, and suitable instruments and rooms. The GP may also have to demonstrate competence in the various procedures on the list.

55.3 MINOR SURGERY PROCEDURES

■ Injections:
intra-articular
periarticular
varicose veins
haemorrhoid
■ aspiration:
joints
cysts
bursae
hydrocele
incisions
abscesses
cysts
thrombosed piles
■ excisions:
sebaceous cysts
lipoma
■ skin lesions for histology:
intradermal naevi, papilloma, dermatofibroma and similar conditions
removal of toe-nails (partial and complete)
curette, cautery and cryocautery
warts and verrucae
other skin lesions (e.g. molluscum contagiosum)
■ other:
removal of foreign bodies
nasal cautery.

A fee will be payable where a GP has performed 15 operations included in the above list in any quarter. Where more than 15 minor operations have been performed, no additional fee is payable.

A GP in a group practice may delegate his or her minor surgery to a partner provided he or she is also on the 'Minor Surgery List'. Thus, a practice of four doctors, where one partner chooses to do all the minor surgery, can claim a fee for 60 minor operations in any one quarter.

55.4 OFFERING A MINOR SURGERY SERVICE TO COLLEAGUES

By approaching the Local Health Authority and/or Primary Care Group for the locality it is possible for GPs to become 'providers' and to negotiate a contract to undertake a set number of minor operations per year for neighbouring colleagues.

55.5 OBTAINING HELP FROM HEALTH AUTHORITIES

The majority of health authorities will welcome GPs undertaking their own minor surgery, and if approached, will generally be very willing to offer help. Advice about the choice and variety of surgical instruments can always be obtained by approaching the district supplies officer, operating theatre sisters or the central sterile supplies department (CSSD) manager. The hospital will usually have favourable arrangements for bulk-buying surgical instruments and will often be able to include the GP in their scheme.

Similarly, the hospital supplies officer may know of obsolete items such as operating theatre tables, lights, trolleys and other such equipment which may be purchased by the GP for a nominal sum.

If the practitioner intends to use CSSD instrument packs, it is worth discussing with the hospital the possibility of using their autoclaves, particularly if the hospital is near the GP's surgery. Some Health Districts make a small service charge for CSSD facilities, while others waive this charge in recognition of the considerable financial savings resulting from the GP undertaking minor surgery. Either way, pre-packed pre-sterilized instrument sets are invaluable and greatly increase the scope and safety of what can be done. Where the doctor is well known to the hospital, certain less-used instrument packs such as abdominal paracentesis, lumbar puncture or chest aspiration sets may be loaned to save the practitioner having to purchase instruments.

55.6 COLLABORATION WITH CONSULTANT COLLEAGUES

It is always a good policy to obtain the support of local consultant surgeons should advice or help be required. In general, this is willingly given and improves relationships. Assuming that GPs only tackle what they feel they can safely complete, the need for help seldom arises, but it is reassuring to know that it is there if required.

55.7 THE PRIVATE PATIENT

GPs are entitled to treat private patients as well as to accept NHS patients. Where a doctor has an exclusively private practice and no NHS patients, arrangements are straightforward: the doctor charges for all medical services rendered, and included in these may be fees for minor surgical operations. There is no set scale of fees and this is left entirely to the discretion of the doctor. Where a GP has a predominantly NHS list of patients, he or she is still entitled to accept fee-paying patients, but the overall earnings from private practice should not exceed 10% of the total practice income, otherwise the GP will be liable to forfeit certain allowances.

If a patient is treated privately, he or she cannot be registered as a NHS patient with that doctor or any of his or her partners, neither can the patient be given a NHS prescription and the doctor cannot utilize paragraph 44.13 of the Statement of Fees and Allowances. Thus, the fee for the operation must include the cost of all drugs, anaesthetics, suture materials, service charges and dressings used.

Surgical instrument and equipment suppliers

UK

ACER Medical Technology Ltd, 3, Hillgrove Business Park, Nazeing Road, Nazeing, Essex EN9 2HB. Tel: 01992 982085. Fax: 01992 893 721 (ROWMED Cryoprobe)

Astra Pharmaccuticals Ltd, Home Park Estate, Kings Langley, Herts WD4 8DH. Tel: 01923 266191 (local anaesthetics)

Brymill Cryogenic Systems (UK) Ltd, 204 Blakes Avenue, Witney, Oxfordshire OX8 6UD. Tel: 0800 838 274 (cryosurgical equipment)

Caterham Surgical Supplies Ltd, 89a Gloucester Road, Croydon, Surrey CR0 2DN. Tel: 020 8683 1103. Fax: 020 8683 1105 (varicose vein forceps)

Chilworth Medicals, 19 Beach Road, Burton Bradstock, Dorset DT6 4RF. Tel/Fax: 01308 898 150 (infrared coagulator)

Cryomedical Instruments Ltd, Cryo-tec House, Goods Road, Belper, Derbyshire DE56 1UU. Tel: 01623 424200

Doctors' Shop, Miller Freeman House, 30 Calderwood Street, London SE18 6QH. Tel: 020 8309 7000 (general equipment)

Doherty Medical Hospital Equipment, 278 Alma Road, Enfield, Middlesex EN3 7BH. Tel: 020 8804 1244

Eschmann Equipment Ltd, Peter Road, Lancing, West Sussex BN15 8TJ. Tel: 01903 761122. Fax: 01903 766793 (theatre equipment)

Ethicon Sutures Ltd, P.O. Box 408, Bankhead Avenue, Edinburgh EH11 4HE. Tel: 0131 453 5555. Telex: 727222 (wound closure products, skin adhesives)

Philip Harris Medical Ltd, Hazelwell Lane, Stirchley, Birmingham B30 2PS. Tel: 0121 433 3030. Fax: 0121 433 4400

Henleys Medical Supplies Ltd, Brownfields, Welwyn Garden City, Herts AL7 1AN. Tel: 01707 333164. Fax: 01707 334795. Telex: 28942

Kimberley Clark Ltd, 1 Tower View, Kings Hill, West Malling, Kent ME19 4HA. Tel: 01732 594000. Fax: 01732 594001 (paper towels and dispensers)

Laerdal Medical Ltd, Laerdal House, Goodmead Road, Orpington, Kent BR6 0HX. Tel: 01689 876634 (resuscitation equipment)

Ledu Lamps Ltd, 12 Barmeston Road, London SE6 3BF. Tel: 020 8265 1681 (lights)

Limbs & Things Ltd, Radnor Business Centre, Radnor Road, Horfield, Bristol BS7 8QS. Tel: 01179 446 466. Fax: 01179 446 222

3-M United Kingdom, 3-M House, P.O. Box 1 Market Place, Bracknell, Berks RG12 1JU. Tel: 01344 858000 (Steri-strips and skin staplers)

Medinox International Ltd, Crown House, Hornbeam Square North, Harrogate, North Yorkshire HG2 8TD. Tel: 01423 873232 (Fern cryosurgical instruments)

Nova Instruments Ltd, Mill House, 127 Newgatestreet Road, Goffs Oak, Herts EN7 5RX. Tel: 01707 875600 (chiropody instruments)

Prospect Medical Ltd, Unit 5, Sherburn Enterprise Centre, Aviation Road, Sherburn in Elmet, Leeds LS25 6NB. Tel: 01977 680033. Fax: 01977 680044. E-mail: sterilisers@prospect73.freeserve.co.uk (radiosurgery, general instruments and equipment)

Rimmer Bros Ltd, 18/19 Aylesbury Street, Clerkenwell, London EC1R 0DD. Tel: 020 7251 6494 (electric cauteries)

Rocket of London, Imperial Way, Watford, Herts WD2 4XX. Tel: 01923 239791. Telex: 922531 (surgical instruments)

Henry Schein Procare, 23–25 Merrick Road, Southall, Middlesex UB2 4AU. Tel: 08700 102043. Fax: 020 8235 5010. Website: www.henryschein.co.uk (dental instruments and equipment)

Schuco International London Ltd, Lyndhurst Avenue, London N12 0NE. Tel: 020 8368 1642. Telex: 893312 (Hyfrecator)

Stiefel Laboratories (UK) Ltd, Holtspur Lane, Wooburn Green, High Wycombe, Bucks HP10 0AU. Tel: 01628 524966. Fax: 01628 810021. Telex: 849312 (biopsy instruments, curettes)

S.T.D. Products Ltd, Field Yard, Plough Lane, Hereford HR4 0EL. Tel: 01432 353 684. Telex: 35421 (sclerosants for varicose veins)

Warecrest Ltd, Unit D4, Cowdray Centre, Cowdray Avenue, Colchester, Essex CO1 1BW. Tel: 01206 761404 (C282 rechargeable cautery)

Welch Allyn UK Ltd, Cublington Road, Aston Abbotts, Bucks HP22 4ND. Tel: 01296 682140. Fax: 01296 682 104 (lighting, instruments, monitors)

NORTH AMERICA AND CANADA

Aaron Medical Industries, P.O. Box 261196, Tampa, FL 33685, USA (disposable electrocauteries)

American Hospital Services, 7080 River Road, Suite 131, Richmond, BC V0X 1X5, Canada

Amsco Canada, 77 Hale Road, Brampton, Ontario L0W 3J9, Canada

Bard Canada Inc., 2345 Stanfield Road, Mississauga, Ontario L4Y 3Y3, Canada

Birtcher Corporation, 4051 N. Arden Drive, El Monte, CA 91734, USA. Tel: (213) 575 8144. TWX9105873445 (Hyfrecator)

Brymill Corporation, P.O. Box 2392, Veron, CT 06066, USA. Tel: (203) 875 2460. Fax: (203) 872 2371 (cryosurgical equipment)

Clement Clarke Inc., 6947 Americana Parkway, Reynoldsburg, Columbus, OH 43068, USA

Cyanamid Canada Inc., Davis and Geck, 2255 Shepherd Avenue, Willowdale, Ontario M2J 4Y5, Canada

Downs Surgical Inc., 2500 Park Central Boulevard, Decatur, GA 30035, USA

Downs Surgical Canada, 5715 McAdam Road, Mississauga, Ontario L4Z 1PG, Canada

Electro-Med, 3278 Oak Street, Victoria, BC V0X IP7, Canada

Ellman International Inc., 1135 Railroad Avenue, Hewlett, NY 11557, USA. Tel: (516) 569-1482. Fax: (516) 569-0201 (radiosurgical instruments)

Ethicon Inc., Route No. 22, Somerville, NJ 08876, USA. Tel: 201 524 0400. Telex: 833487

Fern Medical, Suite 1500, 50 Milk Street, Boston, MA 02109, USA. Tel: 617 338 6563. Fax: 617 451 2589 (cryotherapy equipment)

Frigitronics of Connecticut Inc., 770 River Road, Shelton, CT 06484, USA.
Tel: 203/929-6321

Owen/Galderma, 6201 South Freeway, P.O. Box 6600, Fort Worth, TX 76115, USA

Johnson & Johnson Inc., 2155 Pie IX Boulevard, Montreal, Quebec HIV 2E4, Canada

Keeler Instruments Ltd. 456 Parkway, Lawrence Park Industrial District, Broombal, PA 19008, USA Tel: 215 353 4350. Telex 831370.

Kimberley Clark Co., 1400 Holcomb Bridge Road, Roswell, GA 30076, USA

Laerdal Medical Corporation, 1 Labriola Court, Armonk, NY 10504, USA

Ledu Corporation, 25 Lindeman Drive, P.O. Box 358, Trumbull CT 06611, USA. Tel: 203 3715500 (lamps)

3M, 3M Centre, St Paul, MN 55101, USA

Omnis Surgical Inc., 1425 Lake Cook Road, Deerfield, IL 60015, USA. Tel: 312 480 5600

Physio Control International, 11811 Willows Road, Redmond, WA 98052-1013, USA. Tel: (206) 881-4000. Telex: 320166 PHYSIO RDMD (cardiac monitors and defibrillators)

Roboz Surgical Instruments, 810 18th St. N.W., Washington DC 20006, USA

Scican, 260 Yorkland Boulevard, Toronto, Ontario M2J IR7, Canada. Tel: 416 491 5000. Fax: 416 491 5040 (cryotherapy equipment)

Chas F. Thackray (USA) Inc., 175-X Nev. Boston Street, Woburn, MA 01801, USA. Tel: (617) 935-6831

Wallach Surgical Devices Inc., 291 Pepe's Farm Road, Milford, CT 06460, USA. Tel: (203) 783-1818. Fax: (203) 783-1825 (cryosurgical equipment)

APPENDIX B

Corresponding trade names for drugs named in the book

Drug	UK	Canada	USA
Lignocaine	Xylocaine	Xylocaine	Octocaine
Prilocaine	Citanest	Unavailable	Xylonest
Bupivacaine	Marcain	Marcaine	Marcain
Chlorhexidine	Hibitane	Hibitane	Hibiclens
Povidone–iodine	Betadine	Betadine	Isodine
Diazepam	Valium	Valium	Valium
Sodiumtetradecyl	STD	Trombovar	Sotradecol
Glutaraldehyde	Cidex	Cidex	
Atropine	Atropine	Atropine	Atropine
Ethyl chloride	Ethyl chloride	Ethylchloride	Ethyl chloride
Pethidine	Pethidine	Demerol	Demerol
Entonox	Entonox	Entonox	
Methylprednisolone	Depo-Medrone	Depo-Medrol	
Triamcinolone	Lederspan	Aristocort	
Chloramphenicol	Chloromycetin	Chloromycetin	Chloromycetin
Adrenaline	Adrenaline	Epinephrine	Epineprine

References

1. Brown JS (1979) Minor operations in general practice. *Br Med J* **i**, 1609–1610.
2. Robertson B (1982) Minor surgery in general practice saves resources. *BMA News Review*, November, p. iv.
3. St John Ambulance; St Andrew's Ambulance Association; The British Red Cross Society. *First Aid Manual*, 7th edn (1997).
4. DHSS (1986) Booklet 3, AIDS – *Guidance for Surgeons, Anaesthetists, Dentists and their Teams Dealing with Patients Infected with HTLV*, p. 111. DHSS, London.
5. Department of Health (1988) *An Evaluation of Portable Steam Sterilisers for Unwrapped Instruments and Utensils.* Ref. HE1 No. 185.
6. Langer K (1861) Ueber die Spaltbarkeit der Cutis. S-B *Akad Wiss Wien Math-Nat* K1 **43**, 23.
7. Froman S (1939) *The Surgery of Injury and Plastic Repair.* Williams and Wilkins, Baltimore, MD, p. 50.
8. Berson M (1948) *Atlas of Plastic Surgery.* Grune and Stratton, New York, p. 3.
9. Barsky A (1950) *Principles and Practice of Plastic Surgery.* Williams and Wilkins, Baltimore, MD, p. 38.
10. Smith F (1950) *Plastic and Reconstructive Surgery – A Manual of Management.* WB Saunders, London, p. **213**.
11. Kraissl C (1951) The selection of appropriate lines for elective surgical incisions. *Plast Reconstr Surg* **8**, 1.
12. Eberhart NM (1911) *A Working Manual of High Frequency Currents.* New Medicine Publishing, Chicago, IL.
13. Morton ER (1910) The use of solid carbon dioxide. *Lancet* **ii**, 1268–1270.
14. White AC (1899) Liquid air in medicine and surgery. *Med Rec* 2899, **56**, 109.
15. Lloyd Williams K, Holden HB (1975) Cryosurgery in general and ENT surgery. *Br J Hosp Med* **14**, 25.
16. Chamberlain, G (1975) Cryosurgery in gynaecology. *Br J Hosp Med* **14**, 26–37.
17. Hopkins P (1982) *Proceedings of the Fifth Meeting of the American College of Cryosurgery,* New Orleans, USA, p. 12.
18. Hopkins P (1983) Cryosurgery by the general practitioner. *Practitioner* **227**, 1861–1873.
19. Colver GB, Dawber RPR (1989) Cryosurgery – the principles and simple practice. *Clin Exp Dermatol* **14**, 1–6.
20. Holt PJA (1988) Cryotherapy for skin cancer. *Br J Dermatol* **119**, 231–240.
21. Yates VM, Scott MM, Carter ED (1988) Rupture of tendons after cryotherapy for hand wart. *Br Med J* **297**, 1106.
22. Ruscoe MNJ (1990) Audit in general practice. *Br Med J* **300**, 50.
23. Metcalfe DHH (1989) Audit in general practice. *Br Med J* **299**, 1293–1294.
24. Dammers, Veering & Vermeulen (1999) Injection with methylprednisolone proximal to the carpal tunnel: randomised double blind trial. *Br Med J* **319**, 884–886.
25. Frost FA, Jessen B, Siggard Anderson (1980) A controlled, double blind comparison of mepivacaine injection versus saline injection for myofascial pain. *Lancet* **i**, 499–500.

26. Nash JR. (1979) Sclerotherapy for hydrocele and epididymal cysts. *Br J Surg* **66**, 289.

27. Haye KR, Maiti H (1985) Self treatment of condylomata acuminate using 0.5% podophyllin resin. *Practitioner* **229**, 37–39.

28. Dagnall JC (1981) The history, development and current status of nail matrix phenolisation. *Chiropodist* 315.

29. Boll OF (1945) Surgical correction of ingrowing toe-nails. *J Natl Assoc Chiropod* **35**(4), 8.

30. Suppan RJ, Ritchilin JD (1962) A non-debilitating procedure for ingrown toe-nail. *J Am Pediatr Assoc* **52**, 900.

31. Barrish SJ (1969) The phenol–alcohol technique. *Curr Podiatr* **18**(7), 18.

32. Sykes PA, Kerr R (1988) Treatment of ingrowing toe-nails by surgeons and chiropodists. *Br Med J* **297**, 335–336.

33. Ellis H (1984) Sigmoidoscopy. *Update* **1**, 981–984.

34. Ellis H (1984) Rectal bleeding and the general practitioner. *Cancer Care* **1**(4) 4.

35. Brown JS (1983) Sigmoidoscopy in general practice. *R Coll Gen Pract* **33**, 822.

36. Goligher JC (1967) *Surgery of the Argus, Rectum, and Colon.* Baillière Tindall and Cassell, London, p. 120.

37. Gabriel WB (1956) Minor ano-rectal operations. In *Pye's Surgical Handicraft.* John Wright, Bristol, p. 426.

38. Lewis MI (1972) Cryosurgical haemorrhoidectomy. *Dis Colon Rectum* 128.

39. Alexander-Williams J (1982) The management of piles. *Br Med J* **285**, 1137–1139.

40. Barron J (1963) Office ligation of internal haemorrhoids. *Am J Surg* **105**, 563–570.

41. Steinberg DM, Liegois H, Alexander-Williams J (1975) Long term review of the results of rubber band ligation of haemorrhoids. *Br J Surg* **62**, 144–146.

42. Panda AP *et al.* (1975) Treatment of haemorrhoids by rubber band ligation. *Digestion* **12**, 85.

43. Lord PH (1975) Conservative management of haemorrhoids 2 – dilation treatment. *Clin Gastroenterol* **4**, 601.

44. Fegan WG (1983) Continuous compression technique of injecting varicose veins. *Lancet* **ii**, 109.

45. Fegan WG (1967) *Varicose Veins, Compression Sclerotherapy.* Heinemann, London.

46. Feathers RS (1981) Varicose veins in women. *Matern. Child Health* **6**, 318–324.

47. Studd J (1986) A practical guide to HRT. *MIMS Mag.* **1**, 21–22.

48. Yeates WK (1984) Vasectomy. *Update* **28**, 1229–1234.

49. McEvedy BV (1962) Simple ganglia. *Br J Surg* **49** (218), 584–594.

50. Brett MS (1977) Operations for ganglion. In *Operative Surgery – The Hand* (Eds Rob and Smith). Butterworth, London, p. 369.

51. Bier A (1908) Ueber einen neuer weg Localanaesthesie an den Gliedmassen zu erzeugen. *Arch Klin Chir* **86**, 1007.

52. Holmes C McK (1963) Intravenous regional analgesia; a useful method of producing analgesia of the limbs. *Lancet* **i**, 245–247.

53. Thorn-Alquist AM (1971) Intravenous regional anaesthesia; a seven year survey. *Acta Anaesthesiol Scand* (Suppl.), 40.

54. Ware RJ (1975) *Anaesthesia* **30**, 817.

55. Ware RJ (1979) Intravenous regional anaesthesia using bupivacaine. *Paraesthesia* **34**, 231–235.

56. Pattison CW (1984) A review of the Bier's block technique. *Practitioner* **228**, 235–237.

57. Mason MA (1983) Regional anaesthesia with bopivacaine. *Lancet* **ii**, 1085.

58. British Medical Association. *A Code of Practice for Sterilisation of Instruments and Control of Cross-Infection.* BMA London.

59. *The National Health Service (General Medical and Pharmaceutical Services)* (1982) Regulations SI 1982 No. 1283, Sch. I, Pt I, para. 32–34.

Selected further reading

RADIOSURGERY

Bisaccia E, Scarborough D (1995) Blepharoplasty with radiosurgical instrumentation. *Cosmetic Dermatol* **8**, 1207–1208.

Cresswell CC (1992) Introduction to electro-surgery. *Br Podiatr Med* **47**, 11–14.

Garden JM, O'Banion MK, Shelnitz LS, *et al.* (1988) Papillomavirus in the vapor of carbon dioxide laser-treated verrucae. *JAMA* **259**, 1199–1202.

Henry F (1989) Interet du bistouri haute frequence en chirurgie plastique. *Extrait Ann Cir Plast Esthet* **34**, 65.

Hettinger D (1995) Excision of planter fibroma via radiowave technique. A review of the literature and a case report. Personal communication.

Hettinger D, Valinsky M, Nuccio G, Lim R (1991) Nail matrixectomies using radio-wave technique. *J Am Podiatr Med Assoc* **81**, 317–321.

Hurwitz JJ, Johnson D, Howard D, Molgat YM (1993) High frequency radiowave electrosection of full-thickness eyelid tissues. *Can J Ophthalmol* **28**, 62–64.

Kendall MW (1988) Radiosurgery: an advanced technique for performing nail matrixectomies. *Podiatr Manage* **7**, 53.

McGlamry ED (1987) *Comprehensive Textbook of Foot Surgery,* Vol. II. Williams and Wilkins, Baltimore, MD.

Pollack SV (1991) *Electrosurgery of the Skin.* Churchill Livingstone, New York.

Pearce JA (1986) *Electrosurgery.* John Wiley and Sons, New York.

Pfenninger JL, DeWitt DE (1994) Radiofrequency surgery. In *Procedures for Primary Care Physicians.* Mosby, pp. 91–101.

Saidi MH, Setzlter FD, Sadler RK, *et al.* (1994) Comparison of office loop electrosurgical conization and cold knife conization. *J Am Assoc Gynaecol Laparosc* **1**, 135–139.

Sebben J (1988) Electrosurgery: high frequency modulation. *J Dermatol Surg Oncol* **14**, 367–371.

Sebben J (1988) Electrosurgery principles: cutting current and cutaneous surgery – Part 1. *J Dermatol Surg Oncol* **14**, 29–32.

Sebben JE (1989) *Cutaneous Electrosurgery.* Year Book Medical Publishers, Chicago, IL.

Sherman AJ (1992) *Oral Electrosurgery, An Illustrated Clinical Guide.* Martin Dunitz, London.

Turjansky E, Stolar E (1994) *Lesiones de Piel y Mucosas Tecnicas Terapeuticas.* EDAMA, Argentina.

Turner RJ, Cohen RA, Voet RL, *et al.* (1992) Analysis of tissue margins of cone biopsy specimens obtained with 'cold knife', and Nd:YAG lasers and a radiofrequency surgical unit. *J Reprod Med* **37**, 607–610.

Valinsky M (1990) Treatment of verrucae via radio-wave surgery. *J Am Podiatr Med Assoc* **80**, 482–488.

Waldman SR (1993) Management of superficial skin lesions in a cosmetic surgery practice. *Plastic and Reconstructive Surgery of the Head and Neck. Proceedings of the 5th International Symposium,* Chap. 120.

Waldman SR (1994) Transconjunctival blepharoplasty minimising the risks of lower lid blepharoplasty. *Facial Plastic Surg* **10**, 27–41.

White WF (1986) Radiosurgery – an advancement over the scalpel in many procedures. *Podiatr Prod Rep* **3**, 16.

Wyre HW (1977) Extirpation of warts by a loop electrode and cutting current. *J Dermatol Surg* **3**, 520–522.

DENTISTRY

Heinemann Dental Handbook. Heinemann Medical Books, Oxford (1990).

Oxford Handbook of Clinical Dentistry. Oxford University Press, Oxford (1991).

Essentials of Dental Surgery and Pathology, 5th edn. Churchill Livingstone, Edinburgh (1991).

Clinical Dentistry in Health and Disease, Vol. 2, *The Mouth and Perioral Tissues*. Heinemann Medical Books (1989).

Index

Page numbers appearing in **bold** refer to figures and page numbers appearing in *italic* refer to tables

1990 Contract recognizing minor surgery 451–2

Abdominal
  ascites 183–4
  paracentesis 184–8
    instruments required **12–13**, 17, 184
    technique 184–8
Abscess
  incision of 193–4
  perineal 46
  web-space **194**
  See also Bartholin's abscesses
Accessory
  auricle 342, **344**
  digits 117
Achilles tendon, steroid injection 182
Acromioclavicular joint 169
Acrylic resin aerosol dressings 102
Actinic keratosis **352**
  radiosurgery **328**
Acute psychiatric crisis 356
Adhesive putty, cryotherapy 136–7
Adrenaline, local anaesthetic with 60, 65
AIDS 47–8
Allergic reaction 355
Anaesthesia 44
  Bier's block 36, 61, 385
  caudal epidural 383–8
  general 68
  infiltration *see* Local anaesthesia
  medicolegal aspects 446
  topical or surface 57–8
  see also Local anaesthesia and bloodless field; Nerve blocks
Analgesia 66–7
  see also Entonox
Anaphylactic reaction 355
Anatomical
  danger areas 445
  snuff-box, radial nerve block **64**
Ankle joint, aspiration and steroid 181–2
  injection **182**

Antibacterial dressings 102
Antiseptic solutions 50
  inflammable, hazards 120
Anus
  manual dilatation 274
  and rectum, anatomy **262**
Appointment book 151, **153**
Arteries, iatrogenic damage 156
Aspiration
  abdominal ascites 12–13, 17, 184–8
  Bartholin's abscess 287, **288**
  breast
    cyst 190–1
    lump 189
  cysts and bursae 190–2
  pleural effusions 188, **189**
  and sclerosant injection, ganglia 308–9
Assessment, preoperative 55–6
Assisting in minor surgery 43–5
Atrophy of tissues, tennis elbow steroid injection 166
Audit 158–9
Auricle, accessory **343**, **344**
Auriscope speculum, cryotherapy **136**
Autoclaves **34**, **52**
  guidelines for selecting 52–3

Bacterial endocarditis 417
Baker's cyst 181
Ball-ended coagulation electrode, radiosurgery **317**
Bartholin's cysts and abscesses 194, 287, **288**
Basal cell carcinoma 196, **197**, 211, **212**
  electrocautery 117
  histological appearance **146**
  information leaflet 435
Battery packs, rechargeable 21
Bicipital tendonitis 169–70
Bier's block 61, 385–8
  orthopaedic pneumatic tourniquet **36**
  safeguards 388
  technique for arm 385, **386**, **387**, **388**

Biopsy
  cryobiopsy **138**, **139**
  excisional **256**
  incisional 254, **255**
  lymph gland 303–4
    needle 189, **190**, 257
    punch 251, **252**, **253**, **254**
    shave 250, **251**
  sigmoidoscopy 264
    forceps 264, **265**
  techniques 249–57
  temporal artery 350–1
Bipolar
  diathermy machine 121
  forceps **122**
    radiosurgery **303**
Birtcher hyfrecator **31**, 121
Blanket stitch, sutures 84
Blood vessel, visible 70
Bloodless field and local anaesthesia, *see* Local anaesthesia and bloodless field
Boiling 50–1
  electric boiling water disinfector **51**
Bowen's disease 212–13
  leg **212**
Braided silk 84
Bravery certificates 156, **157**
Breast
  aspiration
    cysts 190–1
    lump, needle 189
  training aid model **73**
Brush cytology 284
Burners, electrocautery 28–31, **112**, **113**, **114**
  cold-point **115**
Bursae, aspiration 190–2

C28 cordless rechargeable electro-cautery 26, **30**, **112**, **113**
Candida infections 46
Capillary bleeding 70
Carbolic acid *see* Phenol
Carbon dioxide, cryotherapy 128
Carcinoma *in situ* 212–13

Cardiac
    arrest 356–9
        box **358**
    defibrillators *see* Defibrillators
    monitor 33
    pacemakers *see* Pacemakers
Carpal tunnel
    decompression 363–8
        anaesthetic and bloodless field
        364–5
        technique 365, **366**, **367**
    diagnosis 170–1
    information leaflets 424
    injection 170–3
        needle entry **172**, **173**
        technique 171–3
Carpometacarpel joint 175–6
Carpet-layer's knee 181
Catgut 84
    suture, transfixing ganglion 307
Caudal epidural anaesthesia 383–8
    injection models **384**
Cauterization *see* Chemical cauteri-
    zation; Cryotherapy; Diathermy;
    Electrocautery, Cautery
    burners *see* Burners, electrocautery
    comparison, treatment methods *38*
    and curette 203, **222**, **223**, 224
    light transformer 112
Cellular naevus **197**
Cerebrovascular attack 355–6
Cervical
    cytology 283
    dysplasia, radiosurgery 336
    erosions
        cryosurgery 284–5
        diathermy 285
        electrocautery 117, 285
        silver nitrate cauterization 108,
        284
        smear 283
            instruments required **283**
Chalazion *see* Meibomian cysts
Chemical cauterization 107–10
Chemicals, care of 448
Chevalier Jackson biopsy forceps **265**
Chondrodermatitis helicis chronicus
    352
Circumcision 345-6
    dissection **345**
    'three-in-one' fraenal stitch **346**
Claim, reducing risks of 447–8
Clergyman's knee 181
Clinical waste disposal 23, 36
Clips
    skin closure 86–7
    removal 106

Coagulation, diathermy 123
Coalminer's knee 181
Coated polyglactin 910: 85
Collaboration with consultant col-
    leagues 453
Complications 156
Concealed haemorrhage 355
Condylomata
    acuminata 225
    electrocautery 117
Congenital accessory digits 342, **343**
    electrocautery 117
    ligation 332
Conjunctiva
    chronic conjunctivitis, chemical
        cauterization 109
    surface anaesthesia 57–8
Consent 444
Consent form
    vasectomy 297
    medicolegal aspects 444
Consultant colleagues, collaboration
    with 453
Contamination, accidental 49
Continuous sutures 84
Convulsion, following vasovagal
    attack 354
Cornea, surface anaesthesia 58
Corneal exposure 403
Costochondritis 183
Cotton
    conforming bandages 102
    surgical tubular stockinette **103–4**
Cotton-wool applicator, liquid nitrogen
    132, 135, **136**
Counselling
    IUCD insertion 288
    preoperative, vasectomy 296
Cross infection 8
Cryo jet **131**
Cryobiopsy **138**, **139**
Cryoprobes **35**, 129, **130**, **131**
    technique 134
    for use with
        liquid nitrogen **134**, 135
        nitrous oxide **128**, **129**
Cryospray, liquid nitrogen **132**, 133
Cryosurgical equipment 128–37
    C5-76 liquid nitrogen cryotherapy
        unit **132**
Cryotherapy 448
    cervical erosions 284–5
    comparison, treatment methods *38*
    contraindications and dangers 137–8
    ganglion, finger **140**
    genital warts 286
    indications for 127–8

information leaflets 141, 431
ingrowing toe-nails 241
internal haemorrhoids 270, **271**
Little's area, epistaxis 259
mechanism of 126–7
with radiosurgery 314
skin lesions, treatment 127, *140*
solar keratosis **129**
success rates *140*
warts and verrucae **130**, **133**,
    138–9, 224–6
Central sterile supplies department,
    sterilization by 11, 17, 24, 34, 50,
    53
Cupboards, operating theatre 22
Curette and cautery 203, 222–4
Cutaneous horn **216**
Cylindroma 204
Cysts
    aspiration 190–2
    Baker's 181
    breast, aspiration 190–1
    ear-lobe **231**, 341
        chemical cauterization 109–10
    epidermal 195, **231**
        appearance and histology **143**
        removal from finger **229**
    epididymal 110
    meibomian *see* Meibomian cysts
    popliteal 181
    sebaceous *see* Sebaceous cysts
    thyroid, aspiration 191
Cytological examination of fluids 257

Defibrillation 356
Defibrillators 21, 32–3, **356**, **357**
Dental
    abscess **414**
        caries 406
        history 404, 405, 419
        trauma 407
    anaesthesia 407, **408**, 410–13, **415**
        injection sites **411**, **412**, **413**
    antibiotic regimes 417–18
    extractions 407, **408**
        bleeding and suturing 417
        complications 416
        instruments **408**, **409**, 418
        techniques **413–16**
    sinus 197
    syringe **16**, 36
DeQuervain's disease, steroid
    injection 175
Dermatofibroma 204
    appearance and histology **148**
Dermatological minor surgery 195–8
    see also Skin

Desiccation, diathermy **122**
Dexon 85
Diabetic syringes and needles,
    infiltration
    anaesthesia **59**
Diathermy
    apparatus **31**
    cervical erosions 125
    Little's area, epistaxis 259
    skin preparation 55
    unipolar 121–5
    see also Hyfrecaror
Digits
    congenital accessory 342, **343**
        electrocautery 117
Digital nerve blocks 65
Disinfectant dispensers 35
Disposable
    cauteries 119–20
    electrocautery **113**
    proctoscopes 261
    sigmoidoscopes 264
    sterile skin biopsy punch **252**
Dissection 79
Documentation 43
Dog-ear, avoidance and removal **79**,
    80, 393, **394**
Domestic pressure cookers, improvised
    sterilization 54
Drains 87
Dressings
    reasons for using 101–2
    types of 102–4
Drugs and trade names *457*
Dry heat sterilization 34, 52

Ear
    ear lobe cysts 341
        chemical cauterization 109
    foreign body removal 340–1
    keratoacanthoma, curette and
        cautery 205, **206**
    sebaceous cyst removal **231**
Elasticated
    bandages 103
    net stockinette 103
    tubular stockinette **103**
Elbow
    golfer's elbow 167
    intra-articular injections 167–8
    tennis elbow 164–7
Electrical safety 21
    radiosurgery 320, 321
Electrocautery 39, 111–20, 448
    appearance, base of lesion removed
        with **114**
    equipment **28–31**, **112–15**

instrument comparison 119–20
instruments required 113
information leaflets 155
power sources **111–13**
skin preparation 55
uses 116–19
    cervical erosions 117
    Little's area, epistaxis 117
    skin tags **114**, 116
    spider naevi **115**, 118
    squamous papilloma **116**
    subungual haematoma 117
    warts and verrucas 118
Electrodes, radiosurgery
    ball-ended coagulation **317**
    ingrowing toe-nails **332**
    nail matrixectomy **333**
    nail spicule electrode **334**
    needle electrode **316**
    tungsten-wire loop **317**
Ellman
    Dento-Surg 90 Watt radiosurgical
        unit 315
    Surgitron FFPF radiosurgical unit
        32, **304**
Embolism, pulmonary 355
Emla cream, topical anaesthesia 58
Endocervical polypi, removal of 294
Endometrial cell samplers 283
Entonox 35, **67**
    giving set **67**
    removal, splinters 339
Entropion 402–3
    electrocautery 117
    surgical treatment 402
Epidermal cysts 192
    appearance and histology **143**
    removal from finger 229
    see also Sebaceous cysts
Epididymal cysts, aspiration and
    injection 110, 192
Epidural anaesthesia *see* Caudal
    epidural anaesthesia
Epilation **335**
Epileptic convulsion 354
Epiphora 398
Episiotomy, repair 286, **287**
    surgical anatomy **286**
Epistaxis 258–60
    acute bleed 260
    chemical cauterization 108
    electrocautery 117, 259
Equipment purchase 453
    supply sources 16, 454–6
Eruptive angioma *see* Granuloma
    pyogenicum
Esmarch bandage **66**

Ethilon 84
Ethyl chloride spray, anaesthesia 57
Excision 79, **80**
    ganglia 307–8, 378–82
    gland 304
    lipoma 232–3
    precautionary notes 447–8
    rheumatoid synovioma **368–9**
    skin lesions, general technique
        100, 200–2
    warts 224
    wedge, ingrowing toe-nails
        241–2
    Zadik operation **245**
Eye
    conjunctiva
        chronic conjunctivitis 109
        and cornea, surface anaesthesia
            57
        examination techniques 397–8
    eye-lid
        eversion **397**
        lesions 402–3
        multiple skin tags **217**
        papilloma **217**
    foreign body removal 239
    surgery, skin preparation 55

Facial swelling or pain 404–5, 406
Family bible, ganglion treatment
    method 306
Fern cryoprobe **131**
Fibrolipoma **218**
Filiform warts on neck **217**
Finger
    mucous cyst 309, **310**
    removal, epidermal cyst **229**
First-aid box 37
Fish-hooks, removal **346**
Fistulae, chemical cauterization of
    chronic 108
Flaps, rotation and advancement **395**
Foot, steroid injection 181–3
Forceps, bipolar **123**, **315**
Foreign body removal
    ear 341
    eye 341
    fish-hooks **346**
    local anaesthesia and bloodless
        field 345
    subungual splinter removal 339
Formalin, aqueous 221
Freezing, anaesthesia 57
Freeze–thaw cycle, cryotherapy 126,
    128, 131, 132, **133**
Fulguration 31, **122**
Fungal infection, nails 248

Gabriel's haemorrhoid syringe 13, **15**
Ganglia 197, 305–10
  aspiration and sclerosant injection
    308–9
  excision 307–8, 378–82
  information leaflet **154**
  over interphalangeal joint,
    cryotherapy **140**
  mucous cyst on finger **309–10**
  steroid injection 178
  treatment 306–8
    indications for 306
  typical **305**
  on wrist **307**
Gases, boiling points *126*
General practitioner and National
  Health Service 449–53
Gillies combined needle holder and
  scissors 11
Glenohumeral joint 169
Glue *see* Tissue: adhesive
Glutaraldehyde 34, 50, 221
Golfer's elbow, steroid injection 167
Granulations
  chemical cauterization 107, 108, 109
  vaginal vault following
    hysterectomy 285
Granuloma pyogenicum 196, 206, **207**
  chemical cauterization 108
  electrocautery 117
Gynaecology, minor surgery 283–94
Haemangioma
  appearance and histology **148**
  diathermy 124
  lip 118, **341**, **342**
Haemoarthritis, knee 180
Haemorrhage 156
  concealed 355
Haemorrhoids
  chemical cauterization 110
  first-degree 269
  information leaflet 442
  instruments required 13, **14**, **15**
  internal, treatment 270–3
  prolepsy 269
  second-degree 269
  third-degree 269
  thrombosed external **267–8**
  visualization *see* Proctoscope: use of
Haemostasis 70
  electrocautery 116
Hand
  sensory innervation **62**
  steroid injection
    carpal tunnel 170–3
    DeQuervain's disease 175
    first carpometacarpal joint 175–6

interphalangeal joints 177
  metacarpophalangeal joints 176
  radiocarpal joint 175
  trigger finger 173–4
Hayes Martin skin punch biopy
  instrument **214**
Head-mounted spotlights 27, **28**
Health authorities, obtaining help
  from 453
Hepatitis viruses 47
High-frequency currents, diathermy
  123–4
Hip joint, steroid injection around 178
Histoacryl blue tissue adhesive **92**, 93
Histiocytoma 196, 198, 204
  appearance and histology **148**
Histology 142–9
  book 43, **149**, **445**
  cryobiopsy **138**, **139**
  medicolegal aspects 444–5
  needle biopsy 189, **190**, 257
  specimens
    appearance comparison, radio-
      surgical and scalpel cut **319**
    radiosurgery 319
  see also Lymph gland biopsy
HIV infection 47–8
  control guidelines 48–9
Hormone implants, HRT 290–4
  information leaflet **386**
  technique **291–4**
Hot water disinfectors 34
Hot-air
  hand driers 36
  ovens **51**
    improvised sterilization 54
Housemaid's knee 181
Hydrocele, aspiration and injection
  110, 191–2
  technique 191
Hyfrecator **31**, 39
  Birtcher, **31**, **121**
  comparison, treatment methods *38*
Hypertrophic lesions 196–7

Illumination
  operating theatre 22, **26–8**
  proctoscope 13, **15**
Incisions 765, 391–2
  abscesses 193–4
  sebaceous cyst removal **228**
  skin lesions 200–2
  with tenotomy knife, ganglia 306, **307**

Infection control
  book 49
  guidelines 46–9

medicolegal aspects of 445–6
Infiltration anaesthesia *see* Local
  anaesthesia
Inflammable antiseptics, hazards 120
Information leaflets 43, 150–1
  advice, moles and naevi 438–9
  basal cell carcinoma 435
  care of sutured wounds 436
  carpal tunnel 424
  cryotherapy 141, 431
    liquid nitrogen cryotherapy 431
  electrocautery 432
  ganglia 430
    injecting 429
  haemorrhoids 442
  hormone implants 434
  ingrowing toe-nails 425–6
  meibomian cysts 432
  radiosurgery 243, 437
  tennis elbow 441
  tongue-tie **433**
  varicose veins 426, 429
    stab avulsion 427–8
  warts 440
Infrared coagulator 271, **272**
Ingrowing toe-nail 234–45, 332–4
  cryotherapy 241
  infected **235**
  information leaflets **154**
  instruments required 15, **16**, 236
  medical treatments 235–6
  nail matrix phenolization 109,
    236–41
  nail-bed ablation 243–5
  postoperative instructions **154**
  radiosurgery 243
  silver nitrate 108
  training aids **73**
  typical 235
  wedge excision 241, **242**
Injections and aspirations
  154–82
Instaclave **52**
Instruments
  choice of 10–15
  commonly used **12**
  and equipment
    care 20, 50–4
    preparation 44
    suppliers 16–17, 454–6
  packs 17–20
    basic **10**, **18**
    minor operations **19**, **20**
    suture 17, **18**
  required for abdominal
    paracentesis 11, **12**, 17
    abscesses, incision 193–4

Bier's block 385
carpal tunnel decompression 364
ganglia, aspiration and sclerosant
    injection 308
ganglia, excision 379
hormone implants **291**
hydrocele, aspiration and injection
    191
ingrowing toe-nails 19
    nail matrix phenolization 236
internal haemorrhoids, injection of
    sclerosing fluid 270
IUCD insertion 288
lipoma, excision 232
lymph gland biopsy 303–4
meibomian cyst removal **13**, 17, **18**
pleural effusion aspiration 188
sebaceous cysts, removal 227
sigmoidoscopy 263–4
skin lesions, routine minor surgery
    199
skin tags and papillomata 215
suturing 17, **18**
thrombosed external haemorrhoids
    267
trigger finger, release 369
varicose veins
    sclerotherapy 278
    stab avulsion 372–7
vasectomy 295, 297
warts, excision 224
warts and verrucac, curette and
    cautery 222–3
    ties 87–8
Internal haemorrhoids, treatment
    269–74
    cryotherapy 270, **271**
    infrared photocoagulation 271,
        272–3
    injection, sclerosing fluid 270, **271**
    manual dilatation, anus 274
    neoprene band ligation 273, **274**
    types of 269
Interphalangeal joints, steroid injec-
    tion 177
Interrupted sutures 83
    mattress 83
    plain 83
Intra-articular steroid injections 167
    common sites **179**
    knee **180**
Intradermal
    continuous suture *see* Subcuticular
        suture
    lesions, electrocautery 118
    naevi 196, 198, 203
        appearance and histology **145**

curette and cautery 203
    radiosurgery **325–30**, 331–2
Intraocular pressure, measurement
    see
    Glaucoma
Intravenous regional anaesthesia *see*
    Bier's block
Intrauterine contraceptive device
    (IUCD)
    insertion 288–90
        diagram **289**
        technique 288–90
    removal of lost 290

Juvenile melanoma 209

Kaposi's sarcoma 48
Keloid scars 213, 444
    appearance and histology **147**
Keratoacanthoma 196, 198, 205–6
    appearance and histology **146**
    curette and cautery **206**
    electrocautery 118
    typical and atypical **206**
Knee
    aspiration and steroid injection
        179–81
    osteoarthritis 180
Knots, suturing **88–9**

Lacerations deeper than expected 99
    over anterior surface, tibia **100**
    scalp, method of closing **82**, **93**
    suturing 95–100
        technique 96–7
    tissue adhesive 92, **93**
Lacrimal duct, syringing 398, **399**
Langer lines, incisions 76, **77**
Larynx, surface anaesthesia 58
Lateral epicondylitis *see* Tennis
    elbow
Ligation
    congenital accessory digit **343**
    neoprene band, internal haemor-
        rhoids 273, **274**
Lighting *see* Illumination
Lip
    haemangioma 118, **341–2**
    squamous cell carcinoma, appear-
        ance and histology **147**
Lipoma 197
    antecubital fossa **232**
        removal **233**
    excision 232–3
Liquid nitrogen 35, 126–7, 131
    Cryo-jet **131**
    CS-76 cryotherapy unit **132**

handling 137–8
information leaflets 141, 151
methods of using **132–4**
probes for use with **134–5**
warts and verrucae 224–5
Little Sister autoclaves 3: **52**
    Mk II **34**
Little's area, cauterizing 117, 259
Lloyd-Davies sigmoidoscope 13, **14**,
    250, **251**
Local anaesthesia 13, 44
    abdominal paracentesis 184
    ankle joint injection **182**
    hydrocele, aspiration and injection
        191–2
    infiltrating
        base of lesion **203**
        skin **201**
    instruments required 14, 15
    intradermal naevus removal **203**
    and median nerve 172
    meibomian cysts removal 240
    nail matrix phenolization **237**
    pleural effusions, aspiration 188
    radiosurgery 312
    skin lesions, excision 201
    suturing 96, 97
    technique in general practice 68
Local anaesthesia and bloodless field
    65–6
    carpal tunnel decompression
        364–5
    foreign body removal 334
    ganglia, excision 379–80
    nail matrix phenolization 237
    trigger finger, release of 370
Local anaesthetics 58–9
    choice of 60
    maximum dose 60–1
    mechanisms of action 60
    toxicity 61
Lower limb
    anatomy 275–6
    Langer lines 77
Lymph gland biopsy 303–4
    selection of patients 303
    technique **304**

McDonald's double-ended dissector
    11
McGiveny neoprene band ligator **274**
McIndoe scissors 11, 79
Mains-operated cauteries 119
Malignant
    lesions 197
    see also Basal cell carcinoma;
        Squamous cell carcinoma

melanoma 209–10
appearance and histology **147**
on leg **210**
lentigo **210**
nodular 210
prognosis 211
recurrence and metastatic
spread **210**
superficial nodular amelanotic
211
superficial spreading **210**
Mandibular nerve **409**
Marsupialization, Bertholin's abesess
287, **288**
Mattress suture 83, 90
Maxillary nerve **410**
Medial epicondylitis *see* Golfer's
elbow
Median nerve block **64**, 65
carpal tunnel
decompression in 363–8
injection 170–3
local anaesthesia 172
Medicolegal aspects 443–8
Meibomian cysts 397–403
appearance **399**
instruments required 12, **13**, 17,
400–1
postoperative instructions 155
removal **400–1**
training aid **72**
Melanoma
juvenile 209
malignant **147**, 209, **210**, 211
Meralgia paraesthetica, steroid
injection 179
Mersilk 84
Metacarpophalangeal joints, steroid
injection 176–7
sites for **176**
Metatarsophalangeal joint, steroid
injection 182–3
Minor operating list **151**
Minor surgery
advantages and disadvantages 7, *8*
5-year analysis *152*
instruments **10**, 11–21
procedures 452
scope and limitations 6–7
services to colleagues 452
Mistakes 446
Moles, patient information
leaflet **389**
Molluscum contagiosum 196, 209
appearance and histology **144**
chemical cauterization 109
electrocautery 118

single lesion **209**
topical anaesthesia 58
Monochloroacetic acid 110, **220**
warts and verrucae 219–26
Monofilament
polyamide 6 and 66: 84
polypropylene 84–5
Music during minor surgery 40
Myocardial infarction 354–5

Naevi
blue *see* dermal melanocytoma,
benign **148**
cellular **197**
dermal melanocytoma benign **148**
evolution **143**, 148
intradermal 196, 198, 203
curette and cautery **203**
radiosurgery 325–30, **331–2**, **337**
melanocytic, benign **144**, 148–9
patient advice about **389**
pigmented **79–80**, **207**
port-wine 186
spider 207, **208**, 349–50
electrocautery **115**, 118
unipolar diathermy 124
strawberry 196, 198, **200**
Nail chisel 15, **16**
matrix phenolization 236–40
matrixectomy electrode **333**
spicule electrode **334**
Nail-bed ablation 243–5
phenol appearance following **247**
recurrent nail spicule **334**
Zadik operation 245
Nails
fungal infections 46
normal 195–6
see also Ingrowing toe-nail
Nasal *see* Nose
National Health Service and the general practitioner 449–53
Naunton Morgan
proctoscope 13, **15**, 249
rectal speculum 262
Needle
biopsy 189, **190**
breast cysts **189**
holder 11
puncture, topical anaesthesia 58
sizes 36
Needlestick injury 49
Neoplastic lesions *see* Malignant
Neoprene ligation, internal haemorrhoids 273, 274
Nerve blocks 61–5
Nerves, iatrogenic damage 156

Netelast 103
Nipples, supernumerary 344
Nitrous oxide 128
cryoprobe **129**, **130**, 131
Wallach LLSOX cryosurgical
instrument **128**
Nobecutane 102
Nodular malignant melanoma 188
Non-adherent dressings 102
Non-disposable proctoscopes 261–2
North American and Canadian
instrument and equipment
suppliers 455–6
Nose
cellular naevus 197
foreign body removal 340–1
nasal
cavity, surface anaesthesia 58
polypi 342
Novafil 85
Nurse–patient relationship 43
Oestradiol implants 290–4
Olecranon bursitis 167
One-hand tie, sutures 87–8
Onychogryphosis 246, **247**
appearance **246**
nail removal **246**
phenol ablation **247**
Operating theatre 4, **5**, 22–40
alternative layout 37
fixtures and fittings 22–3
lighting **26–8**
positioning patient 43–4
stool 25
table **25**
Operations list, organizing 146
Ophthalmology
cautery designed for **112**
minor operations 397–403
Orthopaedic pneumatic tourniquet
36, **66**
Osteoarthritis, knee 180

Pacemakers
post-mortem removal 344
radiosurgery 320
typical site **344**
Paper towels and sheets **23–4**
Papilloma 196, 215–18
diathermy 125
scalp, electrocautery **116**
Paronychia
chemical cauterization of chronic
109
thumb **194**
Paterson biopsy forceps **265**
Pathogens, common 46

Patient
informing the 151–3, 424
reassurance 43
see also Information leaflets
Perianal haematoma *see* Thrombosed
external haemorrhoids
Perineal abscess 46
tinorescein semicircles, correct
positions 245
Pharynx
surface anaesthesia 58
Phenol
chemical cauterization 109–10
hydrocele, aspiration and injection
110, 180, 181
information leaflet, ingrowing
toe-nails 425–6
internal haemorrhoids, injection 110
nail matrix phenolization 109,
236–41
nail-bed ablation 243–5
recurrent nail spicule 334
Photocoagulation
internal haemorrhoids 271, **272–3**
Little's area, epistaxis 259
Pigmented naevi **79–80, 203**
radiosurgery **328**
suture after removal **209**
Pig's trotters, training aid **71**
Pilar cysts *see* Sebaceous cysts
Pillar offauces, squamous
papillomation posterior **216**
Pilosebaceous unit, normal skin 195
Pinch-grafts 342
varicose ulcers 346, **347–9**
Planned sessions 42
Plantar fasciitis, steroid injection
182
Plastic
instruments, care of 20
surgery 391–6
Pleural effusion
aspiration 188
needle insertion **189**
Podophyllin 220
Polybutester 85
Polyglycolic acid synthetic absorbable
sutures 85
Polypoid malignant melanoma,
appearance and histology **140**
Popliteal cyst 181
Posterior tibial nerve block **59**, 62
Postoperative
complications 156
information leaflets, *see*
Information leaflets
recovery and after-care 43

Practice
nurse 41–5
organization 8–9
Premedication 66
Preoperative
assessment of patient 55–6, 443–4
preparation 55–6
Prepatellar bursitis 181
Prescription, items available on 398
Prestige autoclave **54**
Private patients 453
Probes *see* Cryoprobes
Proctoscopes 13, **15**, 261–2
disposable 261
Naunton Morgan 13, **262**
non-disposable 261–2
St Mark's hospital pattern **15**
use of 261
Product liability and record keeping
446
Profound vasovagal attack, leading to
convulsion 354
Prolapsing haemorrhoids 256
Prolene 84
Proximate stapler
remover **106**
use **86**
Psychiatric crisis, acute 356
Psychological therapy, warts 219
Pulmonary embolism 355
Punch biopsy instruments **252**

Radial nerve block 63, **64**
Radiocarpal joint
site of 175
steroid injection 175
Radiosurgery 32, 311–52
anaesthesia 324
applications **324**, 325
avoiding complications 321
calculation, heat generated 314–15
comparison, treatment methods
38, 39
with cryosurgery 330–1
diagrammatic illustration **312**
electrical frequencies **312**
safety 320, 321
equipment **315–18**
care of 321, **322**, 323
finger switch and bipolar forceps **315**
general guidelines 323
historical background 311–12
information leaflet **388**
learning technique 318–19
miscellaneous uses 337
needle electrode **316**
units **315–16**

obtaining samples for histology
319, 321
postoperative care 332
preparation of patient 323
quick reference chart 322
warnings 320–1
waveforms and modes of action
313, **314,**
Radiosurgical treatment
actinic keratosis **328**
cervical dysplasia 337
coagulation 259
Epilation **335**
ingrowing toe-nails 243, 332, **333–4**
intradermal naevi **325-30**, 331–2, **337**
recurrent nail spicules 334
rhinophyma **336**
seborrhoeic keratosis 336
telangiectasia and thread veins
334–5
vasectomy 337
warts 226
xanthelasmata 336
Rechargeable
battery packs 21
cautery 29, **114,** 119
Reconstructive surgery 391–6
Records 43, 45, 150–1
product liability 446
vasectomy 290
Rectal
bleeding 261
examination, sigmoidoscopy 263
Rectum
and anus, anatomy **262**
view through sigmoidoscope 252
Remuneration 449–51
Resuscitation 353–9
box **33**
equipment 353–4
facilities 32, **33**
kit 353–4
protocol **359**
Retractors, self-retaining 11
Rheumatoid synovioma, excision **382**
Rhinophyma, radiosurgery 325
Ring block 60
nail matrix phenolization 227, 228
Risk management analysis 447
Rodent ulcer *see* Basal cell carcinoma

St George's haemorrhoid-grasping
forceps **274**
St Mark's hospital pattern
proctoscope **15**
Salicylic acid, warts and verrucae 220–1
Salivary duct, removal of stone 341

Scalp
    basal cell carcinoma **212**
    laceration **82**, 346
    papilloma, electrocautery **116**
    typical sebaceous cyst, removal
        228, 229–30
Scalpel
    cut histological specimen **319**
    treatment methods comparison *38*
Scars 395–6
    dog-ear, avoidance and removal **79,
        80**, 393, **394**
    keloid 203
    minimizing **70**, 76–8, 391–2
    skin creases **199, 202**
    skin stapling, result **106**
Schiötz tonometer 243, 244
    technique 244
Schirmer's test **398**
Scrubbing up 44–5
Selerotherapy, varicose veins 278
    complications 267–8
    information leaflet **381**
Sebaccous cysts 196, 227–31
    appearance and histology 143
    histology 230
    instruments 11, 227
    removal 228–30
        alternative method 230
        training aid **73**
    skin preparation 56
    unusual shaped, on neck **231**
Seborrhoeic
    keratosis, radiosurgery 320, 325
    warts 204, **205**
        appearance and histology **145**
        radiosurgery **329**
Self-retaining retractors 11
Semimembranosus bursitis 181
Sharp-spoon curette
    cryobiopsy **138, 139**
    Volkmann **12, 114**
Sharps disposal **23**, 36
Shoulder, painful 168
    injection sites **169**
    technique 168–9
Sigmoidoscope 13, **14**
    Lloyd-Davies 13, **14, 264**
Sigmoidoscopy 263–6
    indications for 263–4
    preparation of patient 265
    technique 266
Silver nitrate cauterization 107–9
    cervical erosions 284
    epistaxis 258
    ingrowing toe-nails 108
Simple interrupted sutures 89

Sinus
    chronic, chemical cauterization 108
    dental 197
Skin
    biopsy **214**, 223
        using scalpel **214**
    clips **86–7**
        removal 106
    closure 81–94
        choice of
    excision, lesions 202
        inversion of edges, avoidance **201**
        strips **81**, 86
    grafting 342, 395–6
    hooks, use of **88**
    incision
        choice of technique **78, 391–2**
    lesions 196–8, 199–214
        chemical cauterization of
            superficial 110
        common, histological
            appearances 142–9
        not requiring treatment 198
        suitable for treatment 196–7
        to avoid 197–8
        treatment by cryotherapy 127
    model, training aids **72–5**
    normal 195–6
        histology **143**
    preparation, preoperative 55–6
    simulators, training aids 71–5
    tags 196, 215–18
        axilla **196, 215**
        electrocautery **114**, 116
        eye-lid, multiple **217**
        picking up and dissecting **217**
    see also Dermatological minor
        surgery
Soft corn treatment 248
Soft tissue steroid injection 163, 183
    common sites **169**
Solar keratosis **204**
    cryotherapy **129**
    diathermy 124
    electrocautery 118
    multiple on hand **204**
Squamous
    cell carcinoma 197
        electrocautery 118
        histological appearance **147**
    cell epithelioma 212
        papilloma
    electrocautery **216**
        typical **215**
Stab avulsion, varicose veins 281, **282,**
    372–7
    information leaflet 427

Stainless steel, care 20–1
Staphylococci 46
Statistical analysis 150–7
Stenosing tenosynovitis *see*
    DeQuervain's disease
Steri-strips **81**
Sterile drapes **7**
    strips 81–2
    supplies 42
Sterilization 5
    and disinfection of instruments 50–4
    improvised methods 53–4
    plastic instruments 20–1
Sterilizers 34
    guidelines for 52–3
    see also Autoclaves
Sternomanubrial joint steroid
    injection 183
Steroid
    cream
        cryotherapy 131, 133
        keloid scarring 213
    injection 164, 165
        common sites **179**
        contraindications 164
        indications for use 164
        soft tissue 183
Stitchcraft 87–92
Stitches *see* Suturing
Stock control 42
Strawberry naevi 196, 198, **200**
Streptococci 46
Subeuticular suture **83**, 84
    removal 105–6
Subtrochanteric bursitis 178
Subungual exostosis 247, **248**
Subungual haematoma 338, **339**
    appearance **338–9**
    electrocautery 117, **339**
    splinter removal 339
Suction equipment **34**
Supernumerary nipples 344
Surface anaesthesia 57–8
Surgical
    skills 443
    techniques 71–5
Suture
    material 84–6
    needle **393**
    removal 394–5
        technique 105–6
        time *395*
    size and type 89, **102–5**, *393*
Suturing **64,** 65
    basic pack 17, **96**
    care of wounds information leaflet
        436

deep tissues 90
   lacerations 95–100
   instruments required 96
   technique 96–7, **98–100**
skin lesions
   excision 200–2
   techniques 393–4
   types of 82–4, **393**
   wound, simple method **82**
   see also Scars, minimizing
Syringes 36

Tachyphylaxis, hormone implants
   292
Tarsal cysts *see* Meibomian cysts
Tattoos, removal 209
Teaching aids *see* Training aids
Tear film estimation 397–8
Telangiectasia and thread veins,
   radiosurgery 334, **335**
Temporal artery
   anatomy **350**
   biopsy 350–1
Tempero-mandibular joint injection
   183
Tendo achilles tendinitis 183
Tendon sheaths, hand
   arrangement of 177
   injection of 177–8
   see also Trigger finger
Tendons, iatrogenic damage 156
Tennis elbow
   alternative treatments 167
   information leaflet **441**
   steroid injection 164–7
      and local anaesthetic 165
      palpation for tender spot **165**
      technique 165–6
Themoelectric coolers 137
Thenar muscle syasting, carpal
   tunnel syndrome **161, 350**
Thread veins and telangiectasia,
   radiosurgery 334, **335**
Thwaites nail clippers 15, **16**
Thyroid cysts, aspiration 191
Tietze's syndrome 183
Time management 42
Tissue
   adhesive 92, **93, 94**, 97
   healing 71
   temperature and survival *127*
Toes, minor operations 334–8
   toe-nails
      fungal infection 248
      see also Ingrowing toe-nail
Tongue
   granuloma pyogenicum 206, **207**

lacerations **100**
   squamous papilloma **216**
Tongue-tie
   division of 351, **352**
   information leaflet 433
Topical anaesthesia 57–8
   creams 58
Tourniquets **36**
Training aids 71–5
   pig's trotters 71
   radiosurgery 318
Treatment room *see* Operating theatre
Tricholemmal cysts *see* Sebaceous
   cysts
Trigger finger release 369–71
   anaesthetic and bloodless field 370
   steroid injection 173–4
   technique 371
Trocar and canula, abdominal
   paracentesis 12, **13**
Tru-cut biopsy needle 189, **190**
Tubegauze 103
Tubigrip 103
Tungsten wire loop electrode,
   radiosurgery **305**
Turban tumour 204

UK instrument and equipment
   suppliers 16, 454–5
Ulnar nerve 167
   block 62, **63**
Ultrasonic cleaning bath **42**
Unipolar diathermy 31, 121–5
   see also Hyfrecator
Upper limb, Lauger lines 77
Urethra, surface anaesthesia 58
Urethral caruncle 287–8

Vaginal vault granulations 285
   chemical cauterization 108
Varicose ulcers, pinch grafts **346–9**
Varicose veins 275–82
   bandages 103
   model, training aid **74**
   patient information sheet 155,
      426–9
   sclerotherapy 278–81
      information leaflets **429**
   selection, patients for treatment
      277–8
   short saphenous, appearance **277**
   stab avulsion 281, **282**, 372–7
      before and after **376**
      information leaflet 427
      marking veins 373
      technique 373–6
   types **276–7**

Vascular skin lesions 196
Vasectomy 295–302
   consent form **296**
   postoperative care 302
   preoperative counselling 295
      records required 295
   technique **297–302, 337**
Vasovagal attacks 354
Verrucae
   cryotherapy 127, **129**, 224–6
   curette and cautery 222, **223**, 224
   diathermy 124
   electrocautery 118
   histological appearance **144**
   multiple **221**
   treatment 219–26
Vertical mattress suture **90**, 91
Vicryl 85
Vital signs, monitoring 39–40
Volkmann sharp-spoon curette 11,
   114, 203

Wallach LLSOX **128**
Warts 196, **200**, 219–26
   cryotherapy 127–8, **133, 139**, 224,
      225–6
   curette and cantery **222**, 224
   diathermy **122**, 124
   electrocautery 118
   excision 224
   filiform, on neck **217**
   genital 221, 286
   histological appearance **144**
   information leaflet 440
   monochloroacetic acid 110, **220**
   radiosurgical treatment 226
seborrhoeic **145**, 204, **205**
   test for cure **221**
   treatment 219–26
   viral DNA 316
Wedge excision, ingrowing toe nails
   241–3
   information leaflet 425
Wrinkle lines, incisions 76, **77**
Wrist, anatomy **171**

Xanthelasmata **340**
   appearance **340**
   chemical cauterization 110
   diathermy 124
   radiosurgery 336
Xanthoma
   chemical cauterization 110
   electrocautery 119

Zadik operation **245**
Z-plasty *392*